Practising Social Inclusion

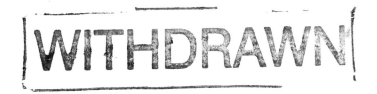

This book explores what is known about what works and why in promoting or practising social inclusion in the variety of fields that deal with human health and wellbeing. It is concerned with research into and/or reflection on the practice of a wide variety of health and social welfare (human services, social care) professionals, as well as community workers, activists, policy makers and researchers.

Our earlier book, *Theorising Social Exclusion*, focused particularly on the role of social and cultural factors in the creation and recreation of categories of exclusion and inclusion. It addressed how individuals and groups come to be seen, or experience themselves, as included and/or excluded. This subsequent book, *Practising Social Inclusion*, moves beyond identifying mechanisms and processes of exclusion to providing answers to the important question of how to actually work towards inclusion, drawing on the research and/or reflective practice that the authors have engaged in. The book is global in its scope, with chapters relating to socially inclusive health and social welfare practice internationally.

The book contributes to the growing debates on social inclusion, which hitherto have often been confined in terms of discipline (e.g. public health, social work), field of practice (e.g. education, disability or youth) or geography (from a single country or continent). Furthermore, the book explores the full range of practice dimensions, including policy, service design, service delivery, community life and research.

This research-based book is relevant to a wide range of different readerships globally. The book addresses issues of concern for those engaged in debates about the provision of health, social welfare and other public services. It will be of interest to academics, policy makers and practitioners in a wide range of fields, including health sciences, public health, health promotion, occupational therapy, disability studies, social work, social policy, social sciences and education.

The editors are all based in the School of Health and Social Development, Deakin University, and are members of the Centre for Health through Action on Social Exclusion (CHASE)

D1381479

Ann Taket holds the Chair in Health and Social Exclusion and is Director of CHASE

Beth R. Crisp is a Professor in Social Work

Melissa Graham is Senior Lecturer in Health Research and Epidemiology

Lisa Hanna is a Senior Lecturer in Public Health

Sophie Goldingay is a Senior Lecturer in Social Work

Linda Wilson is a Lecturer in Disability Studies

Practising Social Inclusion

Edited by
Ann Taket, Beth R. Crisp,
Melissa Graham, Lisa Hanna,
Sophie Goldingay, Linda Wilson

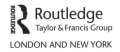

Routledge
Taylor & Francis Group

LONDON AND NEW YORK

First published 2014
by Routledge
2 Park Square, Milton Park, Abingdon, Oxon, OX14 4RN

Simultaneously published in the USA and Canada
by Routledge
711 Third Avenue, New York, NY 10017

Routledge is an imprint of the Taylor & Francis Group, an informa business

British Library Cataloguing in Publication Data
A catalogue record for this book is available from the British Library

Library of Congress Cataloging in Publication Data
  Practising social inclusion / edited by Ann Taket,
  Beth R. Crisp, Melissa Graham, Lisa Hanna,
  Sophie Goldingay, Linda Wilson.
  pages cm
  1. Social integration. 2. Social service. 3. Social policy.
  I. Taket, A. R. (Ann R.)
  HM683.P73 2013
  302.4—dc23
  2012050415

ISBN: 978–0–415–53106–1 (hbk)
ISBN: 978–0–415–53107–8 (pbk)
ISBN: 978–0–203–76679–8 (ebk)

Typeset in Bembo
by Swales & Willis Ltd, Exeter, Devon
Printed by Bell & Bain Ltd, Glasgow

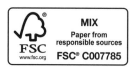

Contents

List of illustrations

Figures

Tables

Contributors

Ndidiamaka Amutah is an Assistant Professor in the Department of Health and Nutrition Sciences at Montclair State University, Upper Montclair, New Jersey, USA.

Sarah Barter-Godfrey is a Lecturer in the School of Health and Human Science, the University of Essex, UK.

Robert Campain is a Research Fellow at Scope, Victoria, Australia.

Beth R. Crisp is a Professor in the School of Health and Social Development, Deakin University, Australia.

Suzanne M. Dolwick Grieb is a Research Fellow in the Johns Hopkins School of Medicine, Baltimore, Maryland, USA.

Faysal El-Kak is a Senior Lecturer in the Department of Health Promotion and Community Health, Faculty of Health Sciences, American University of Beirut, Lebanon.

Michael El-Khoury is a Lecturer in the Department of Health Promotion and Community Health, Faculty of Health Sciences, American University of Beirut, Lebanon.

Peter Fahey is a teacher at St. James Parish School, Sebastopol, Ballarat, Australia.

Peta Farquhar is Research and Community Engagement Officer, Hume City Council, Victoria, Australia.

Nena Foster is a Senior Lecturer in the School of Health, Sport and Bioscience, University of East London, UK.

Jon Fox is a Lecturer at the School of Social Sciences and Psychology at Victoria University, Australia.

Mary Frawley is a teacher at St. James Parish School, Sebastopol, Ballarat, Australia.

Emily Freeman is a doctoral candidate at the London School of Economics, UK.

Mark Furlong is a Senior Lecturer in Social Work in the School of Health and Social Development, Deakin University, Australia.

Jessica Gill is a doctoral candidate in the School of Public Health, La Trobe University, Australia.

Melissa Graham is a Senior Lecturer in Health Research and Epidemiology in the School of Health and Social Development, Deakin University, Australia.

Sophie Goldingay is a Senior Lecturer in Social Work in the School of Health and Social Development, Deakin University, Australia.

Kimberli Hammonds is the Program Manager, DRU Mondawin Healthy Families, Baltimore, USA.

Lisa Hanna is a Senior Lecturer in the School of Health and Social Development, Deakin University, Australia.

Elizabeth Hoban is a medical anthropologist and Senior Lecturer in Public Health, School of Health and Social Development, Deakin University, Australia.

Tamar Kabakian-Khasholian is an Associate Professor in the Department of Health Promotion and Community Health, Faculty of Health Sciences, American University of Beirut, Lebanon.

Natasha Layton is a doctoral candidate in the School of Health and Social Development, Deakin University and a practicing occupational therapist in Victoria, Australia.

Emily Learmonth is the Workplace Learning Project Officer at South East Local Learning and Employment Network, Victoria, Australia.

Rachel Lennon is a doctoral candidate in the School of Public Health, La Trobe University, Australia.

Pranee Liamputtong is a medical anthropologist and holds a Personal Chair in Public Health, School of Public Health, La Trobe University, Australia.

Brian Lynch is the Principal of St. James Parish School, Sebastopol, Ballarat, Australia.

Jihad Makhoul is an Associate Professor in the Department of Health Promotion and Community Health at the American University of Beirut, Lebanon.

Jan Moore is a Lecturer in Public Health and Health Promotion in the School of Health and Social Development, Deakin University, Australia.

Sarah Pollock is the Manager Strategic Projects, Research Development and Advocacy at Mind Australia, and a doctoral candidate in the School of Health and Social Development, Deakin University, Australia.

Scott D. Rhodes is a Professor in the Division of Public Health Sciences at Wake Forest School of Medicine, Winston-Salem, North Carolina, USA.

Michael W. Ross is a Professor of Public Health in the Center for Health Promotion and Prevention Research, The University of Texas, USA.

Julia Shelley is an Associate Professor in Social Epidemiology in the School of Health and Social Development, Deakin University, Australia.

Horace Smith is CEO/President, Group Ministries Baltimore, USA.

Karen Stagnitti has a Personal Chair in Occupational Therapy in the School of Health and Social Development, Deakin University, Australia.

Jason Stowers is a health educator at the Triad Health Project, Greensboro, North Carolina, USA.

Ann Taket holds the Chair in Health and Social Exclusion, in the School of Health and Social Development, Deakin University, Australia.

Erin Wilson is a Senior Lecturer in People, Society and Disability in the School of Health and Social Development, Deakin University, Australia.

Acronyms

ABI	Acquired brain injury
ABS	Australian Bureau of Statistics
ADB	Asian Development Bank
AEDI	Australian Early Development Index
AIHW	Australian Institute of Health and Welfare
AIPC	Australian Institute of Primary Care
ASD	Autistic spectrum disorder
AT	Assistive technology
ATSI	Aboriginal and Torres Strait Islander
BMI	Body mass index
CBPR	Community-based participatory research
CBT	Cognitive–behavioural therapy
CDC	US Centers for Disease Control and Prevention
COAG	Council of Australian Governments
CRPD	Convention on the Rights of Persons with Disabilities
CSCI	Commission for Social Care Inspection (UK)
CSO	Community services organisation
CyBER/M4M	Cyber-Based Education and Referral/Men for Men
DHS	Department of Human Services (Victoria, Australia)
DOHA	Department of Health and Ageing (Australia), in 1988 was Department of Health and Aged Care
EU	European Union
FASD	Foetal alcohol spectrum disorder
FBO	Faith-based organisations
GP	General practitioner, family doctor
GMB	GROUP Ministries Baltimore
GPC	General Pharmaceutical Council (UK)
HIV/AIDS	Human immunodeficiency virus/acquired immunodeficiency syndrome
HOPE	HIV Outreach, Prevention, and Education curriculum
IASSW	International Association of Schools of Social Work
ICF	International Classification of Functioning
ICT	Information and communication technology

IFSW	International Federation of Social Work
ISO	International Organization for Standardization
ISOPIC	Initiative on Standards of Practice in Childbirth
ISP	Individual Support Package
IT	Information technology
JHMI	Johns Hopkins Medical Institutions (USA)
JHSPH	Johns Hopkins Bloomberg School of Public Heath (USA)
LGBT	Lesbian, gay, bisexual and transgender
MSM	Men who have sex with men
NHMRC	National Health and Medical Research Council (Australia)
NHS	National Health Service (UK)
NSW DoH	New South Wales Department of Health (Australia)
NT DoHCS	Northern Territory Department of Health and Community Services (Australia)
NUJ	National Union of Journalists (UK)
OECD	Organisation for Economic Co-operation and Development
PAR	Participatory action research
PFPI	Patient Focus and Public Involvement (Scotland, UK)
PIS	Participant information sheet
PPI	Patient and public involvement
PTSD	Post-traumatic stress disorder
QH	Queensland Health (Australia)
RCT	Randomised controlled trial
REC	Research ethics committee
RK	Resilient Kids, a community-based programme
SAHMSA	Substance Abuse and Mental Health Services Administration (USA)
SDQ	Strengths and Difficulties Questionnaire
STIs	Sexually transmissible infections
TLC	The Life Changing Group
UDHR	Universal Declaration of Human Rights
UK	United Kingdom
UN	United Nations
UNAIDS	Joint United Nations Programme on HIV/AIDS
UNDP	United Nations Development Programme
UNESCO	United Nations Educational, Scientific and Cultural Organization
USA	United States of America
USSR	Union of Soviet Socialist Republics
VAEP	Victorian Aids and Equipment Program (Australia)
WACHS	Wesley Aged Care Housing Service
WHO	World Health Organization

Part I
Introduction

1 Scoping social inclusion practice

Ann Taket, Beth R. Crisp, Melissa Graham,
Lisa Hanna and Sophie Goldingay

Introduction

The overall aim of this book is to explore what is known about promoting or practising social inclusion in the variety of fields that deal with human health and wellbeing. Our emphasis is on the examination of what works and why. So, the book is concerned with research into and/or reflection on a wide variety of professional and community practice.

Our earlier book, *Theorising Social Exclusion* (*TSE*, Taket et al. 2009a) focused particularly upon the role of social and cultural factors in the creation and recreation of categories of exclusion and inclusion, and this is retained here as a strong focus. *TSE* examined how individuals and groups come to be seen as, or experience themselves as, included and/or excluded. The book illustrated how exploring the processes that lie behind exclusion and connectedness helps us understand how these arise, and are played out in everyday life. While the examples presented in *TSE* provided theoretical insights into how practitioners and policy makers may shape their practice to improve wellbeing and reduce social inequity, this book, *Practising Social Inclusion*, provides concrete examples of socially inclusive policies and practices and reflections on their outcomes.

TSE noted that many different understandings about social exclusion are present in the academic literature and within policy discourses. A range of definitions of social exclusion exist, produced in diverse circumstances, each definition to some extent meeting different needs. *TSE*'s purpose was not to craft a detailed genealogy of the term, but rather to illustrate its variety and the necessity of paying close attention to the particular definition(s) that come into play in different policy and practice situations. For the purposes of the present book, our understanding of social exclusion is best expressed in the following, which is created from a merging of two different sources:

> Social exclusion is a complex and multi-dimensional process driven by unequal power relationships interacting across four main dimensions – economic, political, social and cultural – and at different levels including individual, household, group, community, country and global levels. It involves the lack or denial of resources, rights, goods and services, and the

inability to participate in the normal relationships and activities, available to the majority of people in society, whether in economic, social, cultural, or political arenas. It affects both the quality of life of individuals and the equity and cohesion of society as a whole.

Created from Levitas et al. (2007: 9) and Popay et al. (2008: 2)

The intersectional framework we set out in *TSE* had a number of distinctive features in its approach to social exclusion. By extension, these features also underpin the approach to socially inclusive practice we present in this book. First, social inclusion is dynamic, multiple and contingent. Individuals, groups, and communities will usually experience differing degrees of inclusion and connectedness in different domains of life, and these change through time as both external and internal factors change. This complexity demands a nuanced and sophisticated approach to tackling exclusion in both policy and practice. All too often, however, responses are situated within the silo of a particular sector and are based on a binary distinction between excluded and included. In responding to this complexity, we emphasised the importance of a focus on the privileged, as a distinct group within the broader category of the included, and on intersectoral or multisectoral approaches to addressing exclusion. Second is the importance of language in the creation and recreation of exclusion, inclusion and connectedness. We make sense of the world, our understandings of it, and our place in it, through language; our use of language creates, contests and recreates power, authority, and legitimation (Rorty 1989). The discursive construction of social experience sets limits and constraints on the positions of exclusion, inclusion and connectedness that individuals and groups can take up. However individuals and groups are active, resistant agents in these processes and can shape the realm of discursive possibilities. In terms of successful inclusive practice, language is therefore also important.

Connected to this is the importance of a shift in view about identity, as constituted rather than determined (Gordon 1980, Butler 1990). Our analysis of inclusion/exclusion is based on a position of theoretical pluralism, discussed elsewhere as pragmatic pluralism (Rorty 1989; Taket and White 2000) or adaptive pluralism (Chambers 2010). Such a theoretical stance is necessary to do justice to the complexity of the forces and relationships that shape individuals' and groups' experiences of exclusion/inclusion and being excluded/included.

TSE proposed that social exclusion and connection can be considered in three broad spheres of action: individual agency, community and society. This approach has similarities to that of Gallie (2004), who presents his ideas on social isolation by describing three major spheres of sociability: the primary (micro) sphere involving connection to immediate family and household residents; the secondary (meso) sphere regarding interactions with people outside of the household; and the tertiary (macro) sphere involving participation in external structures and the broader environment. There are also resonances with three levels (biographical, life-world and structural) used in Steinert and Pilgram (2007), as well as with the relational framework described in Abrams and Christian (2007), whose analysis distinguishes four different elements: the actors in an exclusion relationship (sources and targets of exclusion); the relationship context (across a series of levels from intrapersonal through to societal and trans-national); the modes/forms of exclusion (ideological/moral, representational, categorical, physical, communicative); and the dynamics of the exclusion relationship (the why and when exclusion happens).

TSE's analysis of how exclusion arises and is perpetuated points to the need for change in both policy and practice. There is a need to move away from 'victim-blaming' approaches that construct exclusion as a deficiency or shortfall in the excluded, rather than arising as a consequence of the complex interactions between a wide range of factors, including the actions of the privileged. The growth of critical and anti-oppressive approaches to practice in social work, as well as the growth of empowerment and strengths-based approaches in health promotion, public health and other public sector services is a partial response to this, but needs to become more widespread in implementation. This will not be an easy task to achieve, as it demands, in many instances, a change in service ethos at all levels of practice.

Social inclusion, according to the theoretical framework utilised in this book, occurs when the participation or involvement achieved in any particular case can be demonstrated to be real rather than tokenistic or manipulative; in other words, reaches the top three rungs of Arnstein's ladder of citizen participation (Arnstein 1969) as shown in Figure 1.1, i.e. citizen control, delegated power and partnership. Achievement of such levels of participation has far-reaching consequences for those involved: 'Autonomy – how much control you have over your life – and the opportunities you have for full social engagement and participation are crucial for health, well-being and longevity' (Marmot 2004: 2).

The individual's experience of inclusion as being associated with feelings of connectedness and belonging, as well as right or entitlement, then is of vital importance. Social inclusion can also thus be seen as the fulfilment of civil,

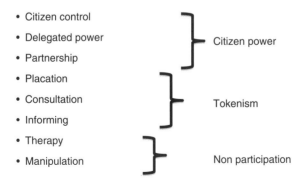

Figure 1.1 Arnstein's ladder of citizen participation

Source: adapted from Arnstein (1969)

political, economic, social and cultural rights (Room 1999; Renner et al. 2007). Rights to participation in political, social and cultural life in society are set out in the Universal Declaration of Human Rights and in the various human rights instruments within the United Nations (UN) system. Rights-based approaches have been developed and used successfully to implement rights to participation (Taket 2012) as has community-based participatory research (considered further in the later section on research).

Klasen (n.d.) suggests a rights-based approach to challenging social exclusion has four advantages, similar to the advantages of Sen's capabilities-based approach (Sen 2000): emphasising firstly that the inability to participate in, and be respected by, mainstream society is a violation of a basic right that should be open to all residents; we note the difference implied if the term 'citizens' were to be substituted for 'residents'. Rights-language considerably strengthens the case for society to ensure that it enables participation and integration of all its members, while also highlighting the role of political, economic and social factors in creating (and maintaining) exclusion in contrast to phrasings that position social exclusion as a 'social' or 'welfare' issue. Secondly, a rights-based approach calls for equal freedoms for all, and thus makes an important distinction between individual choice not to participate in mainstream society, and inability to do so. Thirdly, the diverse abilities of people to make use of opportunities are recognised. Achieving equal capabilities (or the ability to exercise civil and social citizenship rights) may require extra efforts by society to provide equal capabilities to all people. Fourthly, a rights-based approach focuses on ends and not on means. In the remainder of this chapter, and throughout the different parts of the book, different examples of such rights-based approaches to social inclusion are highlighted.

When considering the practice of social inclusion, some aspects of Foucault's theorisation of power are relevant. A critical scrutiny of the construction of the subject/identity and the operation of power is important, as the point of its operation is also the point at which resistance is/can be sited (or sighted). Three of Foucault's methodological precautions in looking at power are of particular pertinence: to examine domination and the material operators of power; to study 'power at the point where its intention . . . is completely invested in its real and effective practices' (Foucault 1976: 97); and to analyse power as something that circulates.

The past thirty years have seen a variety of different initiatives throughout the health and social welfare sectors focusing on user/customer/consumer involvement/engagement/participation. These have arisen in a number of different, albeit overlapping, ways, drawing on different traditions and combinations of circumstance. In some instances they have arisen as a result of intense advocacy by social movements formed by service users and/or their families and carers, for example in the fields of mental health, aged care, disability and women's health (Curtis and Taket 1996; Postle et al. 2005), although it should be noted that some identify the importance of policy failures in creating a climate in which attentiveness to consumer perspectives increased (Tomes 2006).

The HIV/AIDS pandemic saw the rise of a social movement around HIV/AIDS activism, and the use of rights-based approaches, something that was also developing in response to the challenge of poverty and achieving appropriate inclusive development (Taket 2012). Other traditions arose, labelled 'action research' and 'participatory research', and then later a whole tradition labelled 'community-based participatory research', and these are discussed in a later section of this chapter.

In this chapter we now provide an overview of current social inclusion practice in five different sections, focusing in turn on policy, service design, service delivery, community life, and finally research. These sections examine practice around the globe as well as introduce the specific exemplars that form the basis of the chapters in Parts 2 to 6 of this book.

Our consideration of socially inclusive practice in this book has an international focus; contributing chapters represent a range of countries in addition to Australia. In addition, this introductory chapter locates our discussion firmly within a global context by including literature and examples from around the world. Although published formal academic research is dominated by that from high-income countries, there are many excellent exemplars of inclusionary practice from low- and middle-income countries, and indeed important roots of different traditions in such practice lie in precisely these countries.

It is important to recognise that, in a single book, we cannot be comprehensive in our coverage of everything, which is why this chapter is titled 'Scoping Social Inclusion Practice'. We also recognise that inclusionary practice and the literature that captures it is growing rapidly, and that research and practice continue to better inform our understandings of how to practice social inclusion. What we have tried to do, therefore, is explore the range and diversity of inclusionary practice that exists.

Practising inclusion in policy

Over the past decade there has been an increasing focus internationally on social exclusion as an indicator of poor health and wellbeing outcomes. Recently, there has been a clear directive to governments, from the WHO Commission on Social Determinants of Health, that social inclusion is their responsibility and needs to be addressed at the policy level (Popay et al. 2008). In this section we explore this issue in three different ways. First, we look at policies that are specifically about social inclusion. Secondly, we consider how policies can be socially inclusive; in other words, how they can serve to promote social inclusion in the domains in which they are concerned. Finally, we look at the question of inclusion in policy making processes.

Policies on social inclusion

Social inclusion policy has historically focused on reducing poverty with a more recent shift to combating exclusion and increasing inclusion in social domains as well (Atkinson et al. 2005). Where governments have developed and implemented specific policies on social inclusion, these have sought to address past exclusion and its consequences and to promote future inclusion.

Policies on social inclusion developed by the European Union (EU) have served as models on which many countries have based their own policies. In 2005, common EU objectives for social inclusion were agreed, but member states can focus on the policy priorities most relevant to their national context (Commission of the European Communities 2005). Some critics, for example Daly (2007), have argued that this represents a lessening of the priority given to challenging social exclusion.

Table 1.1 provides an overview of the areas covered in the EU social inclusion policy in comparison to selected country-level policies. It should be noted that the list of areas covered in European social inclusion policies continues to develop; this ongoing commitment is demonstrated in the Europe 2020 Strategy, which includes specific attention to social policy aimed at improving social inclusion (Social Protection Committee 2011).

Outside of Europe there has also been a growing focus on social inclusion policy. However, as evident in Table 1.1, despite the United States, Mexico and China having adopted social inclusion policies, they lag behind Europe in terms of scope and coverage. In these countries social inclusion policies are predominantly focused on anti-poverty approaches, lacking the coverage of the broader social determinants of poverty. For example, Silver and Miller (2003) argue that the United States' thinking in regards to social policy is dominated by the 'poverty-line', individualism, discrete programmes, single-focused policies, disjointed approaches and a narrowing of the scope of welfare provision. Boushey et al. (2007) argue that the concept of social inclusion needs to move beyond America's limited poverty-based definition to a focus on creating policy that provides 'an inequality-based understanding of income and well-being, and build[s] understanding of social issues by naming a phenomenon that isn't adequately identified in the United States by existing terms' (Boushey et al. 2007: 4). Similarly, 'Vivir Mejor' (Live Better), Mexico's national social inclusion policy, developed in response to the financial crisis in 2008 (Global Extension of Social Security n.d.), is predominantly concerned with addressing poverty, labour force participation, and disparities in income and education.

Local area policies on social inclusion have been adopted within some countries, in some cases preceding national initiatives. For example, prior to 2007, when social inclusion became a key focus of national social policy in Australia, South Australia had adopted policies on social inclusion despite there being no national policy directive (Government of South Australia 2004, 2007). Similarly, some Canadian provinces have developed their own provincial-level policy in the absence of a national policy on social inclusion in Canada, although a report on the development of a national social inclusion policy was due to be released in December 2012 (Ogilvie 2012).

As Table 1.1 shows, a commonality across these policies on social inclusion is the focus on service provision. All the policies highlighted here have explicitly

Table 1.1 A summary of selected policies on social inclusion at the regional and country level

Scope	EU[a]	UK[b]	Ireland[c]	Australia[d]	New Zealand[e]	USA[f]	Mexico[g]	China[h]
Social exclusion	X	X	X	X	X	X		
Social cohesion/connectedness				X	X		X	X
Labour market participation		X	X	X	X	X	X	X
Education	X	X	X	X	X	X	X	X
Poverty	X	X	X	X	X	X	X	X
Welfare dependency		X						X
Income		X	X		X	X	X	
Pension rates								
Resources	X		X	X				
Safety and crime		X		X	X		X	
Rights	X	X	X					
Discrimination	X	X	X					
Goods	X	X	X					
Services (social, health or welfare)	X	X	X	X	X	X	X	X
Health inequalities		X	X	X				
Housing		X	X				X	
Transport		X	X					
Fuel poverty		X						
Digital inclusion		X						
Inequality (e.g. gender gap, income)		X		X			X	

Sources:
a European Parliament (2000a, 2000b), Commission of the European Communities (2005)
b Department of Work and Pensions (2008)
c Government of Ireland (2007)
d Australian Government (n.d.)
e Bromell and Hyland (2007)
f Boushey et al. (2007)
g Global Extension of Social Security (n.d.)
h Government of the People's Republic of China and United Nations Development Programme (2004).

targeted social, health or welfare services in order to address and combat social exclusion and improve social inclusion. Even though governments and international bodies may have positive intentions and aspirations in relation to social inclusion policy, and despite the importance of national and state-level frameworks, competing demands for finite resources means policy ends up being compromised. Thus, policies may have increasing applicability to the broader population, but potentially fail to meet the needs of those most excluded.

Socially inclusive policies

While policies on social inclusion at regional or national levels indicate commitment to improving the lives of the general public with specific targeting of those most at risk of exclusion, it is often argued that all policy should be socially inclusive (Popay et al. 2008). All policy should incorporate the principles of justice, equity and fairness, avoiding excluding particular socio-demographic population groups defined by characteristics such as gender, beliefs, culture, ethnicity, religion, or (dis)ability. The importance of socially inclusive policies was recognised by the EU in the development and implementation of the agreed social indicators and National Action Plan on Social Inclusion. However, evaluations of the social inclusion framework have demonstrated that these values have not underpinned the development of all EU policy (Cancedda and McDonald 2011). In Chapter 4, Crisp and Ross consider the issue of socially inclusive occupational health and safety policy for sex workers. Although occupational health and safety policy is intended to provide workplace protection to all workers regardless of occupation, Crisp and Ross demonstrate its frequent failure to do so in the case of commercial sex workers. They argue that policies and practices which actively promote protection, rather than regulate unsafe behaviours, are not only more socially inclusive but also more effective.

Mental health is one area where considerable effort has been undertaken to ensure policies are inclusive. For example, England's National Social Inclusion Programme aims to inform and implement inclusive policy in the area of mental health, including community engagement, employment, education, housing, arts and culture, and leadership and workforce (National Social Inclusion Programme 2009). Similarly, mental health policy in Australia is concerned with education, housing and employment of those who experience poor mental health, and specifically aims to implement policy that is inclusive (Commonwealth of Australia 2008).

In 2009, the Australian Federal Government launched the Australian Public Service Social Inclusion Policy Design and Delivery Toolkit. The purpose of this toolkit was to provide an approach for the design and delivery of socially inclusive policy. The toolkit covers both policies designed primarily to meet the needs of the whole population and those that are focused on meeting the needs of specific disadvantaged groups (Australian Government 2009). This was claimed to be a fundamental shift in the way all major policies were designed and delivered by recognising the need for all policy to be socially inclusive 'from health to education through to infrastructure, the law, financial services and other economic areas' (Australian Government 2009: 1). Similarly, New Zealand has developed a step-by-step checklist for policy development or service delivery planning to work towards socially inclusive policy and practice (Bromell and Hyland 2007).

However, national guidelines for inclusive policy do not necessarily result in local or regional policies that are socially inclusive. Layton and Wilson (Chapter 3) demonstrate this point when they discuss requirements for effective policy in the area of disability, drawing on the Victorian Aids and Equipment Programme which provides assistive technology in the state of Victoria in Australia. The authors posit that effective policy should be based on the principles of human rights, equity, and capability to promote inclusion rather than a rationing approach, which only serves to perpetuate social exclusion for those who are already marginalised.

Given the complexities and difficulties in designing and enacting truly socially inclusive policy, there can be a tendency for policy makers to ascribe exclusion to individuals' problematised behaviours rather than to problematic social structures and relations (Bacchi 2007); for example, government approaches to illicit drug use (Bletsas 2007). In Chapter 2, Barter-Godfrey and Shelley discuss the issue of conscience clauses in health policy, with a particular focus on reproductive health. They point out the challenges posed by trying to find appropriate policy solutions that respect the individual values of professional staff while at the same time not compromising the delivery of services to different population groups.

Inclusion in policy making

Perhaps one of the most basic and integral aspects of social inclusion in regards to policy is public participation in the policy making process. Without participatory policy development one has to question whether or not any policy can be fully inclusive. As discussed earlier, Arnstein's ladder of citizen participation (see Figure 1.1) offers a continuum of public participation from the least participatory to the most inclusive. The Universal Declaration of Human Rights' (UN 1948) and the International Covenant on Civil and Political Rights (UN 1966) both make explicit references to one's right to participation in civil activities and decision-making processes. Public or citizen participation is a right that aims to involve those potentially affected by or interested in a decision. Thereby, those who may be affected by a decision have a right to be involved in the decision-making process with the view that their involvement will influence the decision-making process and outcome.

In 2001, the Organisation for Economic Co-operation and Development (OECD) released ten guiding principles for open (transparent, accessible and responsive) and inclusive (inclusion of diverse citizens' voices) policy making designed to assist governments in strengthening their policy performance and service delivery. After evaluation and review, these ten guiding principles were updated in 2009 and now include: commitment; rights; clarity; time; inclusion; resources; coordination; accountability; evaluation; and active citizenship (OECD 2009).

A commitment to inclusive policy making is found in many countries, including Australia, Canada, France, Germany, New Zealand and the UK (OECD 2009). For example, inclusive policy making has been demonstrated in Wales as a way of interrogating policies and practices to ensure that consideration is given to 'advancing equality of opportunity, eliminating discrimination, harassment or victimisation, and promoting good relations' (Welsh Assembly Government 2010: 1).

One population for whom considerable attention has been given to inclusive policy making is young people. The United Nations Convention on the Rights of the Child, which came into effect in 1990, promotes the rights of young people, including their right to participate in all decisions that affect them (UN 1989). The inclusion of young people in policy decision-making is now firmly on government agendas internationally. However, it has been argued that this engagement with young people has been primarily around youth-centred issues rather than broader issues of public significance such as housing and transport (Tisdall et al. 2008). Further to this, the extent to and ways in which young people have been engaged in policy making have varied considerably. Vromen and Collin (2010) provide an interesting Australian-based analysis of the ways in which young people have been and can be engaged in policy making from the perspectives of young people themselves in addition to those of policy makers. They highlight conflicting views between the policy makers and young people, with young people arguing for less formalised ways of contributing than those being offered by policy makers. Similarly, Macpherson (2008) argues that, while the social exclusion policy agenda in the UK has incorporated active participation for young people, the focus of this participation has tended to be on 'reducing problematic behaviour rather than exploring positive engagement of young people in decision-making settings' (Macpherson 2008: 361).

Practising inclusion in service design

We turn now to inclusion in service design, covering the different fields within health and welfare services, and highlighting some of the key factors behind successful inclusion in design. Calls for inclusion in health and welfare service decision-making are found at international, national and local levels, and WHO (2003) identifies this as an essential ingredient of democratic and accountable health systems. The *Global Standards for the Education and Training of the Social Work Profession* note the importance of the 'involvement of service users in the planning and delivery of programmes' (IASSW and IFSW 2004: 5). Examples of the way this has been taken up nationally in different contexts are provided in Table 1.2. We now examine practising inclusion in service design in terms of overall governance, followed by specific services, and then inclusive environments and universal design. The chapters within Part 3 of the book are all exemplars on inclusion in the design of specific services, and are introduced within that section below.

Overall governance

Despite the proliferation of different organisational structures and processes implemented in different places to include service users and/or carers within the overall governance structures of health and social welfare services, there is only a limited amount of research that has examined the experience of the service users and/or carers involved. In the research that exists, two different types of governance structure can be distinguished. The first uses a wide variety of different kinds of representative structures, some elected, some not, but all

Table 1.2 Contrasts in mandates for inclusion in service design

Country	Mandate
Australia	• Federal level policy (DOHA 1998) • State-level frameworks or reference group reports (NSW DoH 2001; QH 2006) • Territory reference group report (NT DoHCS 2004) • Federal-level policy and strategies on mental health services (Common wealth of Australia 1992; DOHA 2002, 2004)
UK	• *Local Voices*, national policy initiative (NHS Management Executive 1992) • National Health Service (NHS) Plan (HMG 2000) • NHS Cancer Plan (DoH 2000) set a specific target that by 2001 cancer networks should take account of the views of patients and carers when planning services. This represented a considerable challenge, given the findings of a study by Gott et al. (2000) published in the same year as the cancer plan. Gott et al. (2000) found that, although user involvement was seen as important by both cancer service users and staff, there were significant differences in views on the scope of involvement and who should be involved. They also found considerable suspicion and hostility between users and service staff. • NHS-related legislation: Section 11 of the Health and Social Care Act 2001 (HMG 2001); and the NHS Reform and Health Care Professions Act 2002 (HMG 2002)
Scotland	• *Patient Focus and Public Involvement* (PFPI) policy initiative (Scottish Executive 2001, 2004) • Statutory requirement for direct involvement of patients and the public for NHS Boards (Scotland Bill 2004). This applies to all levels, understood to range from individual care planning up to major service redesign. Steps were also taken to ensure monitoring of progress. • Reporting requirements for Boards – yearly using a Patient Focus and Public Involvement (PFPI) self-assessment framework (Scottish Health Council Workplan 2006). Scottish Health Council, established in April 2005, responsible for monitoring achievements against PFPI performance standards jointly with Quality Improvement Scotland.

essentially working within a framework based on inclusion of representatives within traditional meeting or committee processes. In contrast, the second is where a variety of different ways of eliciting views – involving separate structures or processes – is used with the resultant views then fed into the planning/design process. The first type of structure has been associated with only limited success, and with a wide range of barriers and constraints, while the second has yielded more promising outcomes. A number of specific studies are considered below.

Milewa et al. (2002) studied NHS primary care groups and trusts in three districts in the UK to explore perceptions about partnerships for involvement. They found that managers and health professionals exercised considerable influence in comparison to patients and citizens; however, in the variation across the three districts studied, they identified some potential for increased lay influence through the development of advocacy coalitions. North and Werkö (2002) also examined consultative and participative processes in primary care groups/trusts in England, comparing them to the local budget holders for health services in Sweden, local councils and municipalities. Based on a review of the literature, they identified considerable activity among English NHS primary care groups and trusts; positive outcomes from this were often not present or were not known, and they concluded that participation is limited to consultation. In Sweden, initiatives were more limited in number to just a few councils. One distinctive approach in Sweden was the use of study circles (created using already existing adult education networks that are supported by government grants) to debate health care matters and to feed into deliberative processes. In the counties using this approach some 3–5 per cent of the total population participated, although those participating were not a representative group: older people and women were over-represented. In only one Swedish local council was there sustained channelling and use of citizens' views as a result of this approach. Important factors identified by North and Werkö as underlying these findings included political cultures, institutional arrangements, and the complexities in health care planning. Neither of these studies included any detailed examination of the experience of those participating or outcomes for participants.

Coad et al. (2008) presented a limited evaluation, based on a single workshop, of the working of a youth council at an acute hospital trust in the UK. The council consisted of a diverse group of 17 young people (aged 11–18 years), who contributed to a wide range of design activities in connection with hospital services and related research. The council was facilitated by the trust's Patient and Public Involvement facilitator, as was the evaluation workshop. Youth council members reported increases in self-esteem and confidence, and contrasted the way they felt taken seriously in the youth council compared to in society at large. The role of the facilitator was identified as particularly important in the positive outcomes reported.

Brooks (2008) explored a patient and public council created within an acute hospital in the UK. The council was set up by senior nursing staff as part of a locally initiated patient and public participation strategy. The study identified a number of tensions created as council members attempted to get their own issues onto the agenda but were resisted by the (nursing) chair of the council. There were also initial difficulties in the relationship between nursing staff and council members. Interestingly, it was the inclusion of a rather different type of process (based on a recommendation from the research team) that allowed council members to narrate their own experiences and use these as a basis for building a future agenda for action that significantly impacted on nursing staff views. Brooks (2008) concluded that real change, consequent on participation through means such as a council, requires change in the expectations of professionals about their relationship with service users. Similarly, Leung (2008), studying welfare organisations in Hong Kong with varied client groups, including older people, people with mental health issues, families, young people, people with substance misuse issues, and people with visual impairment, identified service providers' discomfort with the discourse of accountability to the service user. He concluded:

> the institutional inclusion of welfare service users into a discursive space is a necessary but not sufficient condition for the realization of a mandate of accountability to the welfare service users, unless the power dynamics in the due process of the users' involvement is properly confronted.
>
> (Leung 2008: 543–4)

Farmer et al. (2010), exploring barriers to the inclusion of older people's views in service design in remote rural Scotland, expressed a closely related conclusion in identifying:

> tensions that result from a misfit between the way communities live and the ideology and methods driving management and policy making. If the voices of local people are to truly be incorporated in service design, then the first step is to acknowledge that rural citizens have a distinct and legitimate perspective that aligns with their desire for quality of life in sustainable communities.
>
> (Farmer et al. 2010: 282)

Finally, in terms of more recent studies examining various forms of governance boards, Chessie (2009) explored the early experience of citizen governance boards in Canada's health service, and Gauld (2010) explored elected district health boards in New Zealand. Chessie found the Canadian boards deficient in 'real' engagement (understood as reaching the upper levels of Arnstein's ladder), and Gauld identified problems including: low voter turnout; failure to achieve minority representation; and constraints affecting the ability to achieve representation of different communities. Gauld concluded that boards have only a limited role to play in promoting participation, and need to be supplemented with other methods.

We now turn to examples that worked with diverse ways of eliciting involvement, illustrating the very diverse range of methods that can be used to foster inclusion in service design. Firstly, Nimegeer et al. (2011), drawing on work trialled in remote areas in Scotland, reported on the use of a planning 'game' that uses a number of types of cards to allow community members to express priorities and design preferences in a way that is directly usable by health service managers. The game combines the priorities of the community (including their experiences of using services) with existing service data. It can be used by groups of community members alone or mixed groups of community members and service managers. Their study of using this resource in different ways led them to conclude that the game needs to be embedded in ongoing processes. A game was also successfully used as a method of involvement with service users with serious mental illness in a residential service setting in the UK to elicit their views on the design and refurbishment of their environment (Fitzgerald et al. 2011). The researchers concluded:

> The serious game format enabled the bridging of significant barriers to service user involvement because of its flexibility, inclusivity and familiarity. As a result, this paper recommends it as a meaningful, useful and fun way to engage services users in potentially threatening, complicated and possibly boring service development.
>
> (Fitzgerald et al. 2011: 322)

Fletcher et al. (2011) describe a study into the views and experiences of children and young people with regard to hospitals that was carried out as part of an ongoing commitment to the reconfiguration of children's services and the development of a new undergraduate children's nursing programme in the south of England. The use of a draw and write/tell technique successfully involved children from pre-school age upwards. Murray (2012) discusses the Disabled Children and Young People's Participation Project that was established by Barnardos (Northern Ireland) in 2002 to explore ways of involving children and young people with disabilities in decision-making processes within Children's Services Planning of the Health and Social Services Board. Over 200 young people have participated in its ten years of existence. Participation is via peer group workshops or one-to-one activities, and there is also a project advocacy group. Communication involves specialist information technology (IT), music, drama and digital media, and those who have been successfully involved report empowerment. Murray notes that there are significant requirements for both resources and facilitation to enable these outcomes.

Inclusion in specific services

Another avenue for inclusion in service design is at the level of specific services, and, as already noted, mental health, cancer, HIV/AIDS and disability are all areas where a wide variety of different initiatives exist. The successful examples that exist demonstrate that inclusion can be achieved with a variety of different groups of people who have traditionally been excluded. As with the preceding section, the most successful inclusion initiatives are those based on diverse methods that move away from 'representation' or membership at meetings or in committee structures.

In relation to mental health services, the social movements created by service users and carers have resulted in the adoption of formal mechanisms for inclusion in many places. In Australia, 2002 data showed some type of formal mechanism to incorporate consumers' views was in place in 89 per cent of mental health services, and consumers or carers were present in local executive decision-making structures in 61 per cent of services (DOHA 2004; Whiteford and Buckingham 2005). One form of involvement is as a 'consumer consultant', which has been used successfully in Australia, and for a much wider range of functions than solely service design (Middleton et al. 2004). In New Zealand, Gawith and Abrams (2006) reported that consumers and carers were active in contributing to strategy, policy and service development, both nationally and locally. Such increasing opportunities for inclusion, be it advocacy, advice or input, in service provision have not been without challenges, including resourcing, staff resistance and user representativeness, as Whiteford and Buckingham (2005) demonstrated in Australia, Crawford et al. (2003) in the UK, and Mowbray et al. (1998) in the USA.

In terms of successful initiatives, Janzen et al. (2006) described a longitudinal study of four mental health consumer-run self-help organisations in Canada. They found staff and members of the four Consumer/Survivor Initiatives had participated actively in system-level activities, including community planning, public education, advocacy, and action research. These activities had some important outcomes: perceptions of the public and mental health professionals about mental health or mental illness improved; and, there were positive changes in service delivery practice, service planning, public policy, and funding allocations.

The Californian mental health system's use of stakeholder-driven planning was explored by Cashin et al. (2008), based on an analysis of 141 programmes in 12 county community services and support plans. They concluded that the innovative approaches to recovery-oriented services generated successfully involved consumers and family members in service planning and delivery, as well as building community partnerships that have created new opportunities for consumers to meet their recovery goals. Mechanisms used included paid and board positions, as well as attention to improving cultural competency in the workforce, and strategies for community collaboration. They noted the diversity in strategies they found, and concluded that this diversity is required.

The experience of a group of mental health service users in Northern Ireland involved in the Public Initiative for the Prevention of Suicide – Greater Shankill Bereaved Families Rights Group, supported by the Participation and the Practice of Rights Project is analysed by McMillan et al. (2009). Policy change was advocated for, using a human-rights-based approach that empowered participants. A participatory, 'bottom-up' approach was used to set human rights indicators and benchmarks defined by group members themselves. Focusing on just one issue, follow-up care, McMillan et al. (2009) demonstrated how the group was able to bring about change on this issue across Northern Ireland. This was done through the implementation of a simple service innovation, a card on discharge containing details of the next appointment, which enhanced service users' feelings of connection to services. McMillan et al. emphasise the range of activities the group undertook in order to achieve this change and, in particular, how the group worked outside the existing government-designed consultative structures that were regarded as unable to deliver change. This brings us to an important finding that reoccurs across much of the research, namely that flexibility in methods and processes of involvement is extremely important in ensuring that diverse groups are enabled to be included, as the work considered next also illustrates.

The Delphi method is a process that facilitates group consultation, with the aim of finding common agreement between experts, on topics of uncertainty (Rowe and Wright 1999; Hasson et al. 2000; Meyrick 2003; Okoli and Pawlowski 2004). The process is carried out over a number of rounds; after each round, results are summarised and fed back for further elaboration of views, aiming to identify, by the end of the process, statements expressing areas of consensus and areas about which there is no consensus. Delphi methods have proved useful in a range of settings, bringing together the views of 'experts by experience' with 'experts by profession' around various design tasks, for example: the development of guidelines for caregivers of people with bipolar disorder (Berk et al. 2011); and therapeutic and treatment interventions for domestic and sexual violence and abuse (Itzin et al. 2010a, 2010b). The methods have the advantage of being able to place the different sources of expertise on an equal footing through the anonymity of feedback in the different rounds. In some cases the method has been used with users alone; for example, Efstathiou et al. (2008) explored health care users' priorities for cancer care in Greece.

Yet another example of innovative methods is found in Burgess-Allen and Owen-Smith's (2010) study of local alcohol service review in England. They compared mind mapping with traditional thematic analysis, and their findings suggest that the use of a mind mapping approach to managing qualitative data can help achieve meaningful participation from service users and families in situations characterised by limited resources.

Hubbard et al. (2007) reviewed 28 studies of involvement of people affected by cancer in UK policy and planning, highlighting resources and changes in attitudes as prerequisites. While 12 studies claimed success in terms of positive impact on policy and planning, this was based on perceptions of those involved rather than any other evidence in 11 out of the 12 studies. Six studies reported positive effects of involvement on the people with cancer, including empowerment and finding the experience personally therapeutic. However, most of the studies reported a limited socio-demographic range of people involved, excluding key groups such as people who are socially deprived, minority ethnic groups, older people and younger people.

In relation to services for drugs and alcohol, three comparatively recent studies, two in Australia (Bryant et al. 2008a; Treloar et al. 2011) and one in Ireland (King 2011), found relatively limited achievement in terms of effective inclusion. Bryant et al. (2008a) reported that, although consumer participation activities were not uncommon in Australian drug treatment services, existing activities were largely low-involvement activities, or activities concerned with providing information to or receiving information from consumers. They also reported that consumers largely lacked knowledge of participation opportunities, and many were unaware of complaints systems. In analysing the reasons lying behind the disappointing results, both Treloar *et al.* (2011) and King (2011) identified problems with resourcing the initiatives adequately and the need for education and training for all involved, plus, importantly, attitude change on the part of professionals involved.

All three of the chapters in Part 3 on Practising Inclusion in Service Design take place within specific services and they all illustrate the use of new forms of information and communication technology to support inclusion in different ways. In Chapter 5 Pollock and Taket describe how flexibility in use of methods was necessary to ensure each individual service user in three very diverse service groups had a real opportunity to participate. In Chapter 6, Stagnitti et al. describe the variety of processes and new ways of working introduced into the primary school setting that helped foster inclusion, including the use of Kaizen groups (student leadership groups), based on ideas that originated in Toyota's drive for worker involvement in quality improvement (English and Hill 1994). Finally, in Chapter 7, Goldingay and Stagnitti describe how inclusive service design for young people with learning disabilities who exhibit behaviours of concern can be achieved through the use of innovative play-based approaches.

Inclusive environments and universal design

One important part of service design is the physical environment in which services are delivered or activities take place, including a wide range of community-based facilities and settings, as well as individuals' homes. The notion of universal design, the adoption of design practice that emphasises designing for use by diverse users, also serves to reduce resource requirements at a later stage to accommodate inclusion of diverse groups in terms of access to, and use of, particular spaces and facilities. Accessibility of facilities from which services are provided remains a key challenge to promoting inclusion. Buildings that require special adaptation to accommodate diverse users, and where these adaptations result in separated zones and entrances, are stigmatising and foster exclusion. Universal design represents an attempt by the design community to start with the notion of designing for diversity and to move away from copying accessibility features from codes, guidelines, and standards. This latter practice often results in 'code minimums' being applied in a manner that is separate and different from 'normal' design, and is not really 'equal'.

The Center for Universal Design (1997) sets out seven principles for universal design:

1. Provide equitable use.
2. Flexibility in use.
3. Simple, intuitive use.
4. Convey perceptible information.
5. Provide tolerance for error.
6. Require low physical effort.
7. Size and space for approach and use.

Catlin (2008) described the use of intensive design events (charrettes) involving members of the disability community in Chicago, as well as experts by profession (architects and accessibility). Catlin (2008) also identified that universal design need not cost more in terms of building products. Crews and Zavotka (2006), using literature from the USA and other high-income countries, explored the value of universal design in meeting the needs of the growing numbers of frail elders living in the community, and enabling them to remain in the community for far longer, without the need to move home. Price et al. (2004) presented an interesting case study of a state-wide community education programme on universal design in Ohio. In this, the collaborative partnerships achieved between educators, outreach professionals, students, and a community retail chain succeeded in raising both interest in and awareness of universal design changes that enabled older adults to age in place.

The notion of universal design applies to products as well as the built environment. De Couvreur and Goossens (2011) considered how community-based rehabilitation provides a useful context for innovative design of assistive technology by users and therapists, which can be shared increasingly easily through the internet to allow others to benefit also. They point out the possibilities of the internet assisting in getting designs manufactured, and discuss different cases of 'co-design', where clients with disabilities work in a team with a caregiver, a student of industrial design and a student of occupational therapy (and others as appropriate) to design and make something that helps the person with a disability in an activity of personal value to them. They describe how a 'design for (every) one' framework can support such co-design projects using case studies from Belgium and The Netherlands.

There are a number of examples where universal design has been used to promote social inclusion, including in higher education in Australia (for example, Hitch et al. 2011), accessibility for people with disabilities in New York (Myhill et al. 2008) and services for older adults in Texas (Dumbaugh 2008). Dumbaugh conducted a literature review of older adults' travel-related needs, abilities and preferences in order to move beyond the inevitable segregation that occurs for older adults (Dumbaugh 2008). The importance of the notion of universal design is clearly illustrated by Taket et al. in Chapter 11 in terms of the isolation faced by frail older people in the community brought about by lack of mobility, influenced strongly by the built environments in which they live.

Practising inclusion in service delivery

Staff attitudes and knowledge have often been identified as a barrier to achieving inclusion in service design, and different ways of addressing this have been identified. We first consider the literature on various forms of inclusive professional practice. Following that, we consider involvement of service users in training and education, and one approach towards addressing the barriers posed by staff attitudes and knowledge. A second approach seeks to include service users as employees within the system in specially designated posts, and this is also considered below.

While a service can be designed using inclusive principles, how it is delivered is crucial. There has been a proliferation of different terms used to refer to such inclusive practice. Within disability services and occupational therapy, terms such as person-centred approach, person-centred care, person-centred practice and person-centred support have been used, with yet a further set of variants with the word 'client' replacing 'person' (for example: McCormack and Collins 2010; Carnaby et al. 2011).

Anti-oppressive practice

There is an extensive literature on providing services in an inclusive manner, which is sometimes described as 'emancipatory practice', 'human rights practice', 'anti-discriminatory practice' and/or 'anti-oppressive practice' (Cemlyn 2008). Much of this literature has emerged from social work in the UK (Wilson and Beresford 2000; McLaughlin 2005) and predominantly involves practitioners working with individuals and communities who are the most marginalised members of society (Lavalette and Mooney 2000). Such an approach begins with the acknowledgement that individuals or groups are marginalised:

> An anti-oppressive practice model . . . examines differences used to set apart individuals or groups from one another. The people or group become excluded and marginalized by the dominant society that benefits from the group depicted as undesirable.
>
> (Hines 2012: 24)

Hence, anti-oppressive practice begins with the recognition that service users may have experienced oppression as a result of individual, organisational, cultural or social factors, which limits their ability to realise their full potential. Consequently, rather than reinforce existing sources of oppression, practitioners may need to advocate for, and challenge this oppression on behalf of, and in conjunction with, service users. This in turn requires practitioners to recognise the power imbalances between themselves and service users and seek to implement joint decision-making processes as to what responses should be undertaken to enhance wellbeing for the service user (Hines 2012). Nevertheless, it is important that practitioners do not 'perpetrate just what they are trying to avoid: grouping, sorting and "othering" marginalized individuals rather than listening carefully to what diverse, intersecting groups of individuals within their multiple communities identify as central issues and priorities' (Hudson 2012: 168). It is also critical that professionals recognise the limits of joint decision-making, for example when working with involuntary clients, including those with mental health issues who may be subject to legally mandated treatment orders (Campbell and Davidson 2009). There is a tension that needs to be negotiated, however, in ensuring that joint decision-making does not derogate from the professional's responsibility for assessing and managing risks while also clearly respecting the preferences of individuals, carers and families (Alaszewski 1999; Morgan and Hemming 1999; Munro 2010).

As mentioned previously, in many areas of health and welfare practice, there has been a growing recognition of the need for client or service user participation in decisions which affect them. However, as Furlong describes in Chapter 8, the relationship between service users and professionals is critical, and needs to be characterised by practitioners respecting and promoting the agency of those they are working with, and supporting them when they make courageous decisions. Nevertheless, this does not mean professionals can take a passive role. Those they work with may be unaware of the oppression or exclusion they are experiencing, or may be aware of it but have no idea as to how it can be challenged. Therefore, getting service users to the point at which they can engage in joint decision-making may require extensive preparation (Hines 2012).

Anti-oppressive practice challenges traditional paradigms that emphasise differences and boundaries between practitioners and those they work with (Martinez-Brawley and Zorita 2011). In her analysis of interviews with ten Canadian social workers, Hillock (2012) concluded that workers who identify themselves as 'other' are more likely to be able to identify experiences of oppression in the narratives of those they work with. Rather than being detached objective observers of social phenomena, Strier and Binyamin have argued that Israeli anti-poverty services

> . . . must be staffed by workers capable of developing emotional, intellectual and moral involvement with issues of poverty. The principle of involvement implies working at high levels of intensity, acting under conditions of ambiguity for extended periods of time and persevering even if there are no quick results.
>
> (Strier and Binyamin 2010: 1919)

Working with the most marginalised members of the community is frequently emotionally exhausting and demoralising. In addition to receiving adequate personal support, an important mechanism to retain practitioners working in an anti-oppressive framework is legitimising, within their job descriptions, the challenging of policies that marginalise segments of the populations (Jones 2012). Without such a commitment to promoting human rights, anti-oppressive practice can readily become tokenistic (Wilson and Beresford 2000; Cemlyn 2008) or merely aspirational (Hines 2012). Sung–Chan and Yuen–Tsang (2007) have discussed that, even though a group of Chinese social work students moved from identifying the problems of unemployed women as due to individual deficits, to recognising societal factors which contributed to their unemployment, actively redressing these societal factors did not necessarily occur.

While a focus on interpersonal relationships is a necessary component of anti-oppressive practice, it remains necessary for the structural inequalities that marginalise individuals and groups to be challenged (McLaughlin 2005). Rather than assuming issues are due to deficiencies in an individual which can be remedied by some form of intervention, anti-oppressive practice recognises the strengths of individuals and communities and seeks to explore how these can be used to challenge structural inequalities that underpin the need for services (Strier and Binyamin 2010). Hence, in addition to working with individuals, empowerment of service users may be further enhanced through facilitation of groups which provide social support and encouragement for members of excluded groups to gain strength to challenge their exclusion (Hines 2012). Lennon et al. provide an example of this in Chapter 10 when they describe a community service organisation in Australia that supports sex workers and aims to build their sense of social connectedness.

Working as an anti-oppressive practitioner requires skills in critical analysis. Additionally, it has been suggested that a '. . . critical and informed focus on human rights can be a further potentially powerful tool . . . in seeking to contribute to resistance to oppression, collective solidarity and the promotion of emancipatory change' (Cemlyn 2008: 238). Nevertheless, the effectiveness of an anti-oppressive approach on its own may be insufficient in multicultural communities, and there is a growing awareness of the need for practitioners to be culturally competent (Cemlyn 2008). Makhoul et al. make this point in Chapter 9 in their case study involving psychotherapy in Lebanon with individuals whose sexual orientation or identity is other than heterosexual. Cultural competence has been raised as an issue both in pre-qualifying education in the UK (Parrott 2009) and in ongoing professional development of qualified workers in New Zealand (Hair and O'Donoghue 2009).

Inclusion in the workforce

Inclusion of marginalised or disadvantaged groups in the health and social welfare workforce has been viewed as a route to increasing inclusion in the domain of service use, and to increasing the accessibility and acceptability of services to such groups. This has particularly been the case in terms of mental health services (Cleary et al. 2011; Ostrow and Adams 2012), but is also found in other health and social welfare services, such as services for people with disabilities

(Kemeny et al. 2011; Steel and de Witte 2011), cancer services (Cotterell et al. 2011), HIV/AIDS services (Tenthani et al. 2012), prevention and management of chronic diseases (Henderson et al. 2011) and health promotion (Cook and Wills 2012; South et al. 2012). While most of the coverage in the academic literature is within high-income countries, there are some interesting examples from low- and middle-income countries, demonstrating the widespread applicability of these approaches. One such example is Tenthani et al. (2012), who explored the use of expert patients in antiretroviral treatment provision in a tertiary referral hospital HIV clinic in Malawi. Their study identified that expert patient involvement added value to the services, and the expert patients felt valued by patients. A second example is that of Holland et al. (2012), who notes the growing moves towards inclusion of marginalised groups within service delivery in countries such as Nepal, Cambodia and Indonesia, and in particular the challenges posed by the post-conflict context. Participation of service users in service provision can also be seen in terms of increasing access to the domain of employment, not only in the range of professional posts, but also in terms of the creation of distinct consumer-led service organisations and/or the creation of new posts/roles in the system. Each of these represents a different route to moving beyond the simple dichotomy of service user/provider.

Inclusion in the workforce into specially designated posts (rather than participation in workforce in the usual range of professional roles) has received particular attention. The names given to such positions/post-holders vary considerably: peer worker, lay worker, user advocate, expert by experience, peer support specialist. As McLaughlin (2009) demonstrates, many, if not all, of these terms can be problematic and unable to do justice to the complexities of the relationships involved; a consequence of this, we argue, is the need for those involved to reflect critically on the terms in use and whether they are satisfied with the positionings implied by their use or whether they should be changed. As yet, there is only limited research exploring the experiences of people in this group. Mowbray et al. (1998) explored success in extending involvement into service provider roles, and identified the wide range of benefits this can bring, although emphasising that careful preparation is necessary to bring these about. In the UK, the Commission for Social Care Inspection (CSCI), now the Care Quality Commission, has developed an extensive 'experts by experience' initiative within its functions (CSCI 2007a; CSCI 2009). CSCI's own evaluations of the use of 'experts by experience' in inspections of care homes (CSCI 2007b) and domiciliary care (CSCI, 2007b) provided strong endorsement for their inclusion, although some, for example Scourfield (2010), have questioned whether the experts by experience have found their involvement to be empowering. Cook and Wills (2012), researching lay health trainers in the UK, found they experienced a considerable amount of ambiguity in their role, and they had more autonomy and success in engaging the community when they were located in organisations more embedded in the community than within the NHS itself, illustrating the constraints imposed by the governance context.

Training and education

Repper and Breeze's (2007) systematic review of service user participation in organisational development in health care identified 38 different studies examining participation in health worker training; over half of these reported on the initiatives involving mental health service users, but only two reported on carer involvement. Their conclusions highlight a number of studies in which service users found benefits (including increases in confidence, self-worth and empowerment), as well as benefits to students. They also identified the need for careful preparation, support and resources, including remuneration. Five further studies, not included in Repper and Breeze's review, highlight other successful initiatives. Happell and Roper (2003) report on the use of a 'consumer consultant', employed as an academic staff member of the Centre for Psychiatric Nursing Research and Practice in Australia, for training postgraduate psychiatric nursing students. Service users and carers were successfully involved in training mental health workers in the UK (Simpson and House 2002), and in social work education in England (Anghel and Ramon 2009). Fallon et al. (2008) reported on work involving young people in the design of a post registration module entitled 'The Adolescent with Cancer', using methods such as 'Post-it ideas storm' 'diamond ranking' and 'dot voting'. Mckeown et al. (2012) looked at service user and carer perspectives on the value of involvement in practitioner education, finding benefits in three different areas: a more positive sense of self; social and relational benefits; and the value of stimulating change.

Arguably the most extensive requirements for service user involvement in professional education are those which were mandated for providers of social work education in England. These specify that service users should be involved in all aspects of social work education, including selection of students, curriculum design, preparation for practice learning placements, provision of placements, and assessment of students and quality assurance, in addition to being involved in teaching. However the means by which this should occur was not specified (Levin 2004). For example, in respect of selection of students, three-quarters of social work education providers involved service users in some aspect of student selection in 2004–5, ranging from roles not involving direct contact with applicants, such as devising the interview schedule and shortlisting of applicants, to having direct contact with applicants, such as participation in selection interviews (Manthorpe et al. 2010). Service user participation in assessment has also varied, and this much more likely to occur in services provided to adults than to children (Moriarty et al. 2010).

Practising inclusion in community life

The health and wellbeing of individuals and groups can be enormously enhanced by their participation in community life (Wenger 1999; CSDH 2008). Community life is not just defined by place of residence; rather, individuals participate in, or identify with, a range of different communities defined by common interests, activities and/or values. Community life includes social and leisure activities, as well as participation in education, in paid and unpaid work, and through civic participation. Despite the right to participation enshrined in the Universal Declaration of Human Rights and other human rights instruments, the last half-century has seen a number of oppressive regimes worldwide, with associated conditions of corruption, poverty, and lack of participation and voice in political, cultural and social life. This section explores social inclusion and participation in community life, across different contexts and population groups. We do this through examining four different, though overlapping, bodies of work that have addressed social inclusion in the domain of the community life: community development and participatory development; participatory governance; community self-help; and, finally, neighbourhood renewal or regeneration.

Community development and participatory development

There are many definitions of community development, but the basic concept was described by the United Nations, in an early elaboration of article 55 of the charter of the UN, on economic and social progress and development (UN n.d.: para 61): 'Community Development [is] . . . a process creating conditions of economic and social progress for the whole community with its active participation and the fullest possible reliance upon the community's initiative'.

Blair (2008) traces the origins of community development to work in India following the conclusion of the Second World War. Community development has been a focus of considerable attention within social work (Ife 2002), health promotion (Minkler 2012) and development practice (Cornwall 2006) globally. Pawar (2009) reviews community development practice throughout Asia and the Pacific, arguing that the four values or principles of human rights, self-reliance, self-determination and participation can provide the basis for effective sustainable community development practice, despite the considerable challenges posed by many socio-political governance systems. O'Leary et al. (2011) provides an overview of the different roots of asset-based approaches to community development, identifying roots in all global regions.

One particularly important influence on community development is found in the work of Paulo Freire, the Brazilian educator, philosopher and theorist. Freire observed those who oppress, 'exploit . . . and fail to recognize others as persons' (1990: 41). For over 50 years Freirian education, also sometimes referred to as 'popular education', 'anti-oppressive education' or 'empowerment education', has played a critical role in achieving social change in Latin America (Kane 2001). More recently, Wiggins' (2011) systematic review of popular education for health promotion and community empowerment found popular education effective in enhancing empowerment and achieving health. However, the *relative* effectiveness of popular education, compared to traditional education, in increasing health knowledge and changing health-related behaviour remains to be examined (Wiggins 2011).

Participatory development centres on the inclusion of people who are affected by the development process as planners in that process. Arimoto (2012) describes an early participatory rural development programme implemented in Japan in the 1930s that helped foster the adoption of cattle raising and crop diversification. According to Binswanger-Mkhize et al. (2010), Bangladesh and India first implemented programmes that advanced community roles in development in the 1940s. Cornwall (2006) traces a number of different roots of participatory development stretching back into the colonial period. The participatory development approach became widely used in the 1980s and 1990s, arguably as a response to globalisation and neoliberal development policies (Mohan 2001). It was taken up by organisations such as the World Bank (World Bank 1994) and the Asian Development Bank (ADB 1996). The approach is often particularly associated with the work of Robert Chambers and the Institute of Development Studies in the UK (Chambers 1983).

Community development and participatory development have both pioneered the use of a diversity of methods for involving people in matters relating to community life. Rapid Rural Appraisal and Participatory Rural Appraisal (Chambers 1994) represent a family of approaches that draw on insights from Paulo Freire's work, together with that of Orlando Fals-Borda, the Colombian sociologist who was one of the founders of participatory action research, discussed further in the section on research later in this chapter. The emphasis of these approaches is on moving from professionals being 'on top' to professionals being 'on tap', emphasising the importance of professionals acting as facilitators. Action methods refers to a group of different approaches that emphasise diverse ways of exploring and understanding different situations through various forms of action and reflection (rather than just verbal articulation and discussion) with a view to deciding how to change things for the better. Sociodrama (Fox 1987; Sternberg and Garcia 1989) is one US-born tradition, based in Jacob Moreno's psychodramatic approach to psychotherapy (Fox 1987), while Augusto Boal, the Brazilian director, artist and activist, influenced by Freire's work, created the Theatre of the Oppressed to facilitate the identification and investigation of different possible strategies for action (Boal 1998).

Boal's work has also been drawn on in other countries. For example, in the UK, a commissioned report for the Department of Transport, Local Government and the Regions and the Economic and Research Council (ESRC) Cities Initiative identified ongoing inter-ethnic tensions in urban areas, together with a ghettoisation of ethnic minorities into deprived urban areas, and culminating in riots in 2001 (Amin 2002). Amin notes that Boal's Theatre of the Oppressed approach has a key role to play in unravelling deeply held prejudices. He cites examples of effective work in Marseilles, France, and South Yorkshire, England. In particular, enactment of controversial issues enables 'inter-ethnic and intergenerational understanding' (Amin 2002: 14) and is a way to rehumanise those who have been marginalised and excluded. In the USA, Sadler (2010) has used Boal's Theatre of the Oppressed to engage college students in a dialogue about social justice, privilege and equity. She notes that universities struggle to be truly inclusive of under-represented student groups, an issue considered in Chapter 12 by Crisp and Fox.

The literature on participatory development is extremely large, and views on its desirability and effectiveness vary. Cooke and Kothari (2001), for example, offer a critique of participation as 'the new tyranny' in development thinking, while Hickey and Mohan (2005) offer a very different view, identifying its possibilities for creating social transformation. Participatory development has often been criticised for being tokenistic in the actual levels of participation achieved. There is a smaller but growing literature on the evaluation of participatory development. One particularly helpful review by Gaventa and Barrett (2010) is considered in the concluding section of this chapter. The Asian Development Bank undertook an evaluation study (ADB 2003) of capacity building and participation activities in 22 projects and other activities in 2000 and 2001, concluding that the costs of participation were small compared with the gains.

Participatory governance

Both community development and participatory development are usually associated with the most local level in society. However, the notion of participation has also been taken up at other levels, across the entire spectrum from local to national and international. 'Participatory governance' is the term often used to refer to participation across this entire spectrum (Osmani 2008), with others using the term 'participatory democracy', dating particularly from the various programmes and initiatives set up to support development of democracy in Latin and Central America from the mid-1980s onwards (Blair 2008).

Lack of transparency in decision-making, leading to corruption and lack of trust between state officials and citizens, has been identified as a key block to participatory governance (Malena 2009). As a result, Transparency International set up their first Advocacy and Legal Advice Centres in 2003, and now over 50 countries have such centres, including countries in South America and Eastern Europe (Transparency International 2012). These centres have raised citizens' awareness of corruption and assisted them to address it by promoting dialogue between citizens, institutions and government officials (Malena 2009).

The political will (Malena 2009) for both the governors and the governed to engage in dialogue is another key factor in successful participatory governance. Around the world, a number of initiatives have worked to promote such dialogue, but found a number of barriers to doing so. For example, in Tajikistan, local governments were significantly under-resourced following the collapse of the Union of Soviet Socialist Republics (USSR) and subsequent civil conflict (Holloway et al. 2009). Lack of integrity, accountability and transparency were problems identified in work with local civil society organisations in Kenya and Tanzania (Holloway et al. 2009). Strategies to address these problems included improving the motivation of authorities to involve citizens in joint decision-making. To achieve this, effort was made to show how collaboration could benefit those in power, including being voted back into power.

One specific manifestation of participatory governance is the Participatory Budget, a particularly successful example dating from 1989 being that of the city of Porto Alegre in Brazil (Blair 2008). Other examples of this practice have been found in other metropolitan areas such as São Paulo (Hernandez-Medina 2010) and in also in rural Zimbabwe (Mumvuma 2009). Hernandez-Medina (2010) observed that, in São Paulo, a new way of talking about inclusion in community life has occurred, and now 'participation in decision-making is not only a right, but is also instrumental in achieving greater effectiveness in the implementation of public policies' (Hernandez-Medina 2010: 512). Thus, in São Paulo, Participatory Budgets involve the inclusion of citizens in the production and implementation of public policy, so that decisions are made in the interests of all, especially those experiencing poverty. A similar movement has been noted in rural regions of Zimbabwe, where a number of strategies have been adopted in order to promote 'transparency, accountability and local economic development, as well as improve the well-being of local citizens' (Mumvuma 2009: 159).

The linking of participatory development in particular, and participatory governance more widely, to human rights has occurred in a number of ways, with the use of specifically rights-based approaches to development programming (Jonsson 2003) and debates amongst international development agencies about rights-based approaches and their value (Silva 2003; Nyamu-Musembi and Cornwall 2004; Davis 2009). Miller et al. (2005) explore the links between human rights and participatory development, arguing that these have much to learn from each other. In particular, Miller et al. (2005) call for a more holistic understanding of the concepts of power and empowerment and the links between them, arguing this would help to bridge the gaps between development, participation, and rights, and would lead to more effective processes of social change.

Neighbourhood renewal

For many people, one of their key communities is defined by their place of residence, and the importance of the built environment and housing to health and wellbeing cannot be overstated. The existence of enormous geographically patterned inequalities in material resources has led to a variety of initiatives to try and address these, while at the same time promoting social inclusion, health and wellbeing. Sometimes, as in the Healthy Cities movement (Rydin et al. 2012; de Leeuw 2012), this has occurred at the city level, while in other cases, such as neighbourhood renewal (Klein 2004; Thomson et al. 2009) and urban regeneration (Glasson and Wood 2009; Colomb 2011), efforts are concentrated at a much smaller spatial scale, targeting the most disadvantaged localities. The precise composition of such initiatives varies from place to place, but as well as improving the physical environment, social amenities, and employment opportunities, some also aim to increase pride in and sense of community, including feelings of safety and connectedness. A number of jurisdictions have responded to this through neighbourhood renewal projects, including the UK and Victoria, Australia (Klein 2004; Shield et al. 2011).

The aim of neighbourhood renewal in Australia and the UK is to investigate the complex interrelation between 'local sources of health inequality' and to intervene by 'transforming poor housing, creating employment opportunities, improving education, rejuvenating local economies, reducing crime, and building social capital' (Klein 2004: 110; Neighbourhood Renewal 2010). We note that the term 'neighbourhood renewal' is not always used in this way. In Brussels and Montreal, for example, neighbourhood renewal is considered a process of relatively wealthy groups buying into deprived areas, upgrading the dwellings and hence the social status, and thereby ejecting the more disadvantaged people out of the area (Van Criekingen and Decroly 2003), a process referred to as 'gentrification' in the UK and Australia. These initiatives are carried out in the interests of those already privileged, and promote further exclusion of those already disadvantaged. They therefore fail to acknowledge and build on the potential capacities inherent within the neighbourhood.

While successful examples of renewal or regeneration schemes do exist, many schemes have been criticised for only achieving tokenistic levels of participation and falling far short in adequately resourcing the community capacity building required to achieve any more meaningful inclusion that does not perpetuate, or even worsen, social inequities (Jones 2003; Maginn 2007; Agger and Larsen 2009; MacLeavy 2009; van Bortel and Mullins 2009; Pollock and Sharp 2012). The critique offered identifies the importance of recognising the complexity of community life and the power relations within it, as well as how these are constrained by actors and factors outside the community itself, and responding to these in the decision-making and governance processes involved in regeneration (Jones 2003; Taket and Edmans 2003; Agger and Larsen 2009; van Bortel and Mullins 2009; Pollock and Sharp 2012).

Community self-help

As mentioned earlier, Freire and others have stressed the importance of enabling disenfranchised citizens to take the initiative to address their oppressive circumstances. One mechanism by which citizens can do so is via community-based self-help and support groups. For example, Kingsnorth et al. (2011) describe a parent peer support group in Toronto, Canada, for parents of children with special care needs. These parents, who were suffering isolation and stress from caring for their teenagers with physical and/or developmental disabilities, initiated the group themselves. Through participation in the group, parents recognised their own expertise, and were able to take some ownership of the processes that affected them. They gained 'validation and comfort' (Kingsnorth et al. 2011: 837) from the group that they did not receive from paid professionals, and sought information about participation, inclusion and citizenship. Chapter 14 by Gill et al. also describes a self-help group established by parents of teenagers who have high functioning autistic spectrum disorder

(ASD). This group was set up in response to ongoing isolation experienced by the teenagers, and was inspired by a similar group that one parent had observed on an exchange visit to Sweden. In addition to providing support for these, often isolated, teenagers, the group also acted as a source of support for the parents. Also, in Chapter 13, Hanna and Moore discuss a community-initiated and sustained multicultural women's friendship group in Melbourne, Australia, which offered peer support and companionship to potentially excluded older women from a range of ethnic groups.

Another example of self-help and support is found amongst people with disabilities in the European Centre for Excellence in Personal Assistance (Mladenov 2012). This movement was initially begun by people with disabilities in America, but spread to Sweden to found the Stockholm Co-operative for Independent Living. Two rallies were organised by this group, one in Bulgaria and one in Strasbourg, to advocate for funding to provide community-based personal care assistants for people with disabilities. Having the funding support to hire personal assistance had a very empowering effect for those receiving these services, as it liberated them to live in the community and empowered them to choose who worked with them and how (Mladenov 2012). A similar emphasis on the need for ongoing financial and political support to ensure the success of self-help initiatives was noted in Germany by Geene *et al.* (2009), where a preference for decentralised systems at local levels led to a number of self-help initiatives which were supported by professional services.

Practising inclusion in research

In this section we consider the design and execution of socially inclusive research and provide examples of how inclusive research practice can be achieved. As with practising inclusion in the other domains discussed in this chapter, practising inclusion in research means involving under-represented population groups or individuals/communities that are vulnerable, marginalised, or disadvantaged. Within a research context, this also includes groups considered 'hard to reach' or groups that are frequently overlooked or omitted from the research agenda, as a consequence of sampling or analysis units chosen. Examples of such groups are: people or communities of a particular ethnicity; older people; children and young people; socio-economically disadvantaged people; people from sexual minorities; people with disabilities; and women without children. This section will consider in more detail why socially inclusive research is important, the practice of inclusion at all stages of the research process, and participatory research approaches.

Why is socially inclusive research important?

In an era of evidence-based practice, rigorous research underpins multiple facets of health and social care practice: it informs the development and evaluation of inclusive policy, service design and delivery, and illuminates the practice of inclusion in community life. However, the extent to which research informs inclusive policy varies; for example, Jørgensen (2011) compares the research–policy nexus in Sweden and Denmark, and concludes that Swedish social science researchers have shaped agenda-setting and inclusive migration and integration policy, whereas in Denmark research has been used more selectively to justify particular policy in this area.

In order to provide robust evidence to drive socially inclusive practice, research methods themselves must be socially inclusive. For example, research that excludes certain population groups from participation due, for example, to language barriers, may produce results that are not transferable to the omitted populations. As discussed in previous sections, research should be sufficiently inclusive of the perspectives of service users in order to design and deliver appropriate and effective services. For example, Read and Maslin-Prothero (2011) have reported two case studies from the UK which illustrate the realities of conducting nursing-related research with service users and carers (in this case people with disabilities and older people) in order to inform service design. Based on their reflexive research practice and drawing on Fox et al. (2007), they provide practical examples of implementing six evidence-based recommendations for user and carer involvement in health and social care research: mutual respect and partnership working; organisational support; time; effective communication; financial support; and accessible and meaningful information. Illustrating the nexus between inclusive research methods and inclusive service delivery in social work, Mitchell et al. (2009) have drawn on their experiences of research in the UK with children with disabilities to make recommendations on how best to involve the views and perspectives of this often excluded population group in social care processes (and how to embed these skills in social work education). They suggest using a range of communication tools, spending time with and learning how to communicate with children with disabilities, and valuing non-traditional forms of data and types of knowledge. Disciplines such as market research have also acknowledged the need to consider meaningfully the views of potentially excluded groups, and have reflected on ways in which this inclusive research practice might be achieved. For example, Stevenson (2011) has developed guidelines for incorporating the views of people with mental health issues into mainstream market research, including provision of a safe and supportive environment for focus-group participants and ensuring appropriate moderator training. The success of the consumer movement in mental health in putting service user or consumer involvement in research on the political agenda in many countries is reflected in the recently published *Handbook on Service User Involvement in Mental Health Research* (Wallcraft et al. 2009).

Practising inclusion across the research process

Socially inclusive research involves practising social inclusion at multiple stages of the research process: generation of the research question, methodology and design, sampling and recruitment, data collection, and data analysis/interpretation of findings. Individuals or groups can be excluded at each of these stages. For example, certain groups may be excluded deliberately from sampling, such as the well-documented gender bias against women in medical research (Holdcroft 2007); excluded indirectly because of inequality in access to research participation, for example by a failure to provide culturally competent or linguistically appropriate research materials such as information, consent procedures, data collection tools or techniques; or marginalised in the analysis and interpretation of results and their translation into practice due to selective privileging of professional or academic expertise. To illustrate inclusion at various stages of the research process, the chapters in Part 6 of the book are now considered alongside examples of contemporary inclusive research practice from the international literature and from a range of health and social research disciplines.

In Chapter 17, Foster and Freeman examine the processes of obtaining informed consent in inclusive research. They discuss research carried out amongst older, socio-economically disadvantaged African migrants in the UK, and reflect on how traditional 'formal' research consent procedures may increase the likelihood of these groups being excluded from research. The authors suggest that other forms of consent, such as implied consent, can increase inclusion of marginalised and under-represented groups in research.

Chapter 18 by Graham considers the practice of inclusion in epidemiological research question identification and data analysis. Childless women have been shown to experience multiple forms of social exclusion, including exclusion from the population health research agenda, and in Chapter 18 Graham discusses the research methods necessary to ensure inclusive and robust representation of this often overlooked topic in research. Given the increasing prevalence of childlessness among female populations in high-income countries and the significant negative associations between childlessness and social health and wellbeing, Graham's recommendations to increase the visibility of childlessness in research are timely and pertinent internationally.

Participatory approaches to research

Research methods that have at their core an emphasis on inclusive practice across all stages of the research process have proliferated in recent years as the inclusivity of methods involving a research 'subject' have been questioned. For example, Dominelli (2005) reflected on the use of grounded theory methodology within a feminist orientation to research the experiences of young mothers in care in the UK, and concluded that these research techniques positioned participants as subjects and curtailed their full inclusion in the research. In comparison, participatory approaches such as community-based participatory research (CBPR) prioritise the collaborative involvement and agency of the traditionally 'researched' community (Minkler and Wallerstein 2008). Such research approaches are increasingly common across a range of health and social care disciplines, and span a variety of study designs, having been used in experimental, intervention and evaluation studies, and in studies using a range of qualitative approaches, including innovative forms of data collection such as photovoice (see Minkler and Wallerstein 2008; Catalani and Minkler 2010). For example, in the medical research field, it has been recommended that CBPR move from the 'margin to the mainstream' (Horowitz et al. 2009: 2633, considering the example of research in cardiovascular health).

A systematic review of CBPR studies concluded that intervention studies using this approach were effective in promoting community health (Salimi et al. 2012). Similarly, de las Nueces et al. (2012) carried out a systematic review of CBPR approaches to enhance clinical trials of ethnic minority groups. They found that 'trials examined a wide range of behavioural and clinical outcomes, [and] such trials had very high success rates in recruiting and retaining minority participants and achieving significant intervention effects' (de las Nueces et al. 2012: 1363). The multisite 'translational community trial' approach has also been proposed as a means of incorporating CBPR principles in the translation of interventions established through randomised controlled trials to a real-community context (Katz et al. 2011).

As discussed earlier in this chapter, inclusive research practice can underpin the development of inclusive services and their delivery. For example, participatory research approaches have been shown to be useful in the context of mental health service delivery in the USA (Alegría et al. 2011) and reconfiguration of mental health day services in the UK (Bryant et al. 2010). CBPR can also be used to effect policy change, for example policy to eliminate or reduce health disparities (Israel et al. 2010). CBPR has also been employed extensively in social work research and policy development: for example, Balffour (2011) discusses how CBPR can be used to address rural social (and health) disparities via research partnerships between social workers and rural communities.

In Chapter 15, Grieb et al. explore how CBPR approaches can be used to foster social inclusion in the context of HIV prevention and health promotion. Their research was carried out in the USA, where CBPR has gained 'national prominence' (McKenna et al. 2011: 387), particularly in relation to addressing health inequities and disparities between population groups (Wallerstein and Duran 2010). The vulnerable population conceptual model (Flaskerud and Winslow 1998) understands vulnerable populations as 'social groups who have limited human capital, are of low social status, or lack health care access, and consequently . . . have higher risks for morbidity and premature mortality' (Wang-Letzkus et al. 2012: 257). Wang-Letzkus et al. (2012) used this model to frame their reflections on carrying out culturally competent CBPR with older diabetic Chinese Americans and recommend:

> (a) identifying an accessible community and key persons within the community, (b) obtaining interest and support from the identified communities, (c) using the expertise of community advisors, (d) establishing a culturally sensitive caring partnership, and (e) establishing ownership by sharing research findings with the community.
>
> (Wang-Letzkus et al. 2012: 257)

Also from the USA, Panapasa et al. (2012) discussed using CBPR with community-based organisations and faith-based organisations (FBO) in the Pacific Islander American Health study and concluded 'FBOs represent a valuable resource for community-based participatory research (CBPR) data collection and for effective interventions' (Panapasa et al. 2012: 58).

Chapter 15 by Grieb et al. is representative of a very large volume of CBPR studies that work with community-based organisations, and by doing so, succeed in including previously 'hard-to-reach' groups in health research. They present three case studies in which the CBPR approach has been employed with vulnerable communities in the USA – African Americans, youth, and sexual minorities – and discuss how academic–community partnerships can provide opportunities for communities at risk of social exclusion to play an active and empowering role in the research process and in the shaping of HIV prevention strategies and health promotion agendas.

There is also a large body of emancipatory and participatory research in disability studies. For example, from the USA, Hassouneh et al. (2011) have described a number of practical strategies that can be used to overcome the challenges in conducting fully inclusive and participatory intervention research with people with disabilities, for example in relation to training and funding. Delman (2012) has summarised key recommendations for carrying out successful participatory action research (PAR) with young adults with psychiatric disabilities, including mentoring for the young adults by more experienced researchers. Lorenzo (2008) carried out a PAR project with women with disabilities in South Africa to mobilise for public transport to enable their equitable workforce participation, and Milner and Kelly (2009) used a PAR approach with vocational service users in New Zealand to examine social inclusion and community participation for people with disabilities. Rights-based emancipatory disability research has also been discussed in the context of Australian social work (Stevenson 2010). In Chapter 16, Wilson and Campain reflect on their experiences as lead researchers in an inclusive research process with people with intellectual disability in Australia, and consider the importance of acknowledging and recognising the key role played by social relationships in carrying out inclusive research, a lesson applicable to the international context.

In addition to the examples above, participatory approaches have been used with a wide variety of other potentially excluded population groups globally, and there is a large body of literature reporting and examining the use of such approaches. For example, an international review of CBPR studies with children and adolescents (Jacquez et al. 2012) concluded that there were overwhelming benefits to partnering with youth in research. Prilleltensky (2010) has advocated PAR approaches to increase child wellness and social inclusion; and Ataöv and Haider (2006) have used PAR with street children in Turkey to facilitate their meaningful participation in research, inclusion in public space, and empowerment. At the opposite end of the age spectrum, Doyle and Timonen (2010) have recommended the use of CBPR in gerontology. Hayashi et al. (2012) have used CBPR as an effective research approach with a vulnerable population group of drug users in Thailand, and Ahari et al. (2012) have reported successfully using health-related PAR with highly socio-economically deprived communities in Iran. O'Neill et al. (2005) used PAR with refugee children and families to address educational needs and explore issues of social justice and social integration. Fenge (2010) reflected critically on the use of PAR with older lesbians and gay men in the UK, recommending the approach as empowering and promoting inclusion. However, Fenge also cautioned that researchers should remain aware that 'voices can be silenced as well as enhanced by participatory methodologies' (Fenge 2010: 891). One example is the possibility that group members whose views vary from the majority may feel unable to participate.

Participatory research approaches have also been used to facilitate equitable research partnerships between professional or academic researchers and indigenous peoples in colonised countries internationally. For example, from Canada, Koster et al. (2012) have reported on the application of CBPR in partnership with the Nishnawbe Aski Nation and on the benefits to the community when researching 'for' rather than 'on' them. Wesche et al. (2011) outlined their experience of CBPR on food security led by the Vuntut Gwitchin First Nation and the multiple positive outcomes and applications of the research. From the USA, Mohammed et al. (2012) provide reflections on effective CBPR techniques when conducting research in partnership with an indigenous community in the Pacific Northwest. They describe the process of developing a data-sharing agreement and qualitative data collection guide that met the needs of both academics and tribal members, and describe 'a process of negotiation that required: (i) balancing of individual, occupational, research, and community interests; (ii) definition of terminology (e.g., ownership of data); and (iii) extensive consideration of how to best protect research participants' (Mohammed et al. 2012: 116). In Chapter 19, Barter-Godfrey et al. reflect on their experience, as white academics, of carrying out participatory health-related research with members of Australian Aboriginal communities. They describe how inclusive research approaches can provide an environment that fosters community empowerment and reconciliation and has the potential to address the multiple forms of social exclusion and disadvantage experienced by Australia's indigenous peoples. Insights from this chapter are applicable to the practice of inclusive research in other countries in which indigenous peoples experience the 'colonial legacy of multiple deprivations' (Johner and Maslany 2011: 150).

Barter-Godfrey et al. (Chapter 19) describe their training of, and collaboration with, community researchers from the Australian Aboriginal population. The importance of research capacity building in enabling inclusive and participatory research has also been emphasised elsewhere, for example by Kwon et al. (2012), when reflecting on community empowerment training when carrying out research with community-based organisations from the Asian American, Native Hawaiian and Pacific Islander communities in the USA. Such research capacity building in indigenous or any other potentially marginalised communities increases the likelihood of genuinely inclusive research to be generated and practiced by and with such communities. Barter-Godfrey et al. (Chapter 19) also describe how their project collected, analysed and disseminated research data in socially and/or culturally inclusive forms; again, this principle and practice are applicable to research in other contexts and populations. For example, when carrying out a CBPR project with indigenous peoples in Canada, Christensen (2012) used research storytelling as a method by which the research outcomes could be communicated and disseminated in a culturally congruent manner.

Achieving successful social inclusion

Looking across the range of different initiatives that have aimed at including service users, their families/carers, and/or the wider community in policy, service design or delivery, what can be said about the success of these in achieving inclusion and their effects on services and the individuals involved? A number of systematic reviews or syntheses of research provide some partial answers. The earliest of these, by Crawford et al. (2002), examined studies of involving patients in the planning and development of health care and identified many case studies. Evidence from these showed that involvement can contribute to a range of changes, including increased service accessibility and improvements in the attitudes of organisations and their staff towards consumers. Most interesting here perhaps is the finding in seven of the 31 studies they reviewed of increased self-esteem in those involved; no studies reported decreased self-esteem, although two studies did report dissatisfaction on the part of those involved. Many studies did not look at the effects of involvement on those who participated.

Nilsen et al. (2010) reported a systematic review of methods of consumer involvement in developing health care policy and research, clinical practice guidelines and patient information material. They limited their review to randomised control trials and found six studies involving 2123 participants; they assessed these as having moderate or high risk of bias. They concluded there is moderate-quality evidence that involving consumers in the development of patient information material results in material that is more relevant, readable and understandable to patients, without affecting patient anxiety. This 'consumer-informed' material can also improve patients' knowledge. When setting priorities for community health goals, very low-quality evidence was found that telephone discussions and face-to-face group meetings engage consumers better than mailed surveys; different priorities were also found with different methods.

Preston et al. (2010) examined 37 studies in their review of links between rural community participation and health outcomes. They found some evidence of benefit of community participation in terms of health outcomes, although they identified only a few studies at higher quality levels of evidence. Tempfer and Nowak (2011) reported a systematic review of consumer participation in organisational development in health care. Unfortunately, this review did not examine the consumer experience of involvement. They identified 467 studies including five systematic reviews describing various participation projects, using a variety of methods/processes including: workshops, citizens' panels, focus groups, citizens' juries and consultation meetings. They found no discernible trend favouring a specific method. Only six studies included outcome assessment: three judged the outcome as successful, two as negative, and one multi-project study reported 'very successful' project assessments in 24 per cent of the projects. In 18 studies, the level of consumer participation was described as 'informed' in two, 'advisory' in 14, and 'decision-making' in only two; this indicates that the majority of initiatives are certainly not acting at the highest rungs on Arnstein's ladder (see Figure 1.1), and the category 'advisory' may well extend down into the lower rungs. They identified a number of factors associated with project success: adequate resourcing; partnerships with well-developed consumer organisations; advanced project logistics; small-scale projects; and adequate internal and external communication.

Of particular interest in terms of its global coverage, Gaventa and Barrett (2010) explored the outcomes of citizen engagement through a systematic meta-analysis of 100 researched case studies of citizen engagement in 20 different countries; most of the cases were from low- and middle-income countries. They examined four different types of outcome: construction of citizenship, including both knowledge and sense of agency and empowerment; strengthening practices of participation; strengthening the responsiveness and accountability of states; and, finally, developing inclusive and cohesive societies. They found positive outcomes in relation to each of these different types of outcome, although not uniformly across all cases, the overall ratio of positive to negative outcomes being 3 to 1. Their findings point to the relative importance of associations and social movements compared to institutionalised fora for participatory governance, and to the need for multiple strategies of engagement. Interestingly, no simple linear relationship between level of democratisation and level of positive outcomes was found; instead, the highest incidence of positive outcomes related to social inclusion and cohesion were in the weakest and most fragile democracies, many of which are characterised by recent histories of conflict or violence.

Finally, and this time focusing particularly on low- and middle-income countries, Mubyazi and Hutton (2012) examined a number of reviews, primary publications and the grey literature, examining community participation in health planning, resource allocation and service delivery. Their conclusion sounds a note of caution, identifying that, although community participation is a concept that is widely promoted, few projects/programmes have demonstrated its practicability in different countries. In many countries, they found the level of participation to be very low, with control remaining with elites or politicians, with professionals dominating the decision-making processes.

Reading across these reviews as well as the earlier parts of this section offers the strong conclusion that considerable flexibility in the methods by which people are involved is required (see also Taket and White 2000; Picard 2005; Mayo and Rooke 2006). Earlier sections noted the value of methods such as action methods, sociodrama, and photovoice, which include non-verbal forms of representation, and as Taket and White (2000) identify, these methods can help to subvert the usual operation of power and privilege, facilitating those often silenced in being heard. Recent and continuing developments in information and communication technology have increased the feasibility of inclusion in a wide number of settings and domains (Zambrano and Seward 2012). Some methods have been specifically developed for allowing participation at a distance, and in a way so that individuals can contribute views unhampered by perceptions of their personal power or prestige. One example of this is the Delphi method, discussed in the section on service design above. Catalani and Minkler (2010), in their systematic review of the use of photovoice in health and public health find that, particularly among highly participatory projects, photovoice appears to contribute to an enhanced understanding of community assets and needs and to empowerment.

One important factor is individuals' willingness to be involved in policy, planning, service delivery or research. Here a number of studies indicate that it cannot be assumed that all are equally keen to participate, even if offered an appropriately supported chance. Abelson et al. (1995) found significant differences between groups in the community in terms of willingness to be involved, desired roles and representation in the case of devolved decision-making on health care and social services in Ontario, Canada. Participants, perhaps especially in light of understanding the complexity of the decision-making involved, tended to defer to traditional decision-makers (elected officials, experts and the provincial government), and favoured a consulting role for interested citizens, for example at town-hall meetings. Allsop and Taket (2003), studying opportunities offered for participation in a primary care service development in the UK, found that service users believed there *should* be a high level of user or local community participation. However, most people were only prepared to involve *themselves* in planning in a very limited way. Allsop and Taket (2003) argue that the apparent contradiction between in principle support for user involvement but reluctance to become personally involved is probably explicable in terms of the perceived costs and benefits for the individuals concerned, in the context of other demands and priorities in their lives. Bryant et al. (2008b) report similar findings in their study of Australian drug treatment services. They identified consumers who indicated they did not want to participate, expressing beliefs that it was 'not their place' to be involved and that they lacked the required skills. Similarly, McGrath (1989) found that carers of people with an intellectual disability in Wales were keen to participate in planning for their child's future, and believed there *should* be carer input into area plans; however, 63 per cent had little interest in *personally* contributing at area level.

Perhaps the most detailed examination of willingness to participate is provided by Litva et al. (2009), who explored lay perceptions of user involvement in clinical governance in the UK. They reported that different groups of lay people varied both in their desired role and in their preferred type of involvement in different aspects of clinical governance, as summarised in Table 1.3.

Table 1.3 Preferred role and type of involvement for different groups

	Improving and assessing services	Dealing with poor performance	Education and training
Citizens	Role: Citizen Type: Overseeing	Role: Citizen Type: Overseeing	No desire to be involved
Patient user group 1	Role: Citizen Type: Partnership	Role: Citizen Type: Partnership	No desire to be involved
Patient user group 2	Role: Citizen Type: Informing	Role: Citizen Type: Overseeing	No desire to be involved
Health interest groups	Role: Advocate Type: Overseeing	Role: Advocate Type: Overseeing	Role: Advocate Type: Partnership
Frequent users	Role: Consumer Type: Informing	Role: Citizen Type: Overseeing	No desire to be involved

Source: Litva et al. (2009).

There also seems to be an increasing focus on the value of recognising human rights as a basis for inclusionary practice. Examples of this have been discussed in earlier sections of this chapter. Most recently there are the World Psychiatric Association's recommendations (Wallcraft et al. 2011), including respecting human rights as the basis of successful partnerships for mental health. This is taken up in a number of the chapters in this book: Chapter 3 by Layton and Wilson on policy design and people with disabilities; Chapter 5 by Pollock and Taket, on inclusive service development, provides a detailed example of such an approach, based on the recognition of the right of each individual to determine the life they want to lead; and the work described in Chapters 6 (Stagnitti et al), 7 (Goldingay and Stagnitti), 9 (Makhoul et al), 17 (Foster and Freeman) and 19 (Barter-Godfrey et al) can also be seen as strongly rights-based.

A number of the studies discussed above have used approaches based in action research, participatory action research, participatory research and CBPR as a basis for involving various 'hard to reach', disadvantaged, excluded or marginalised groups in service design, and such approaches have been considered in the section on inclusion in research. The participatory approach followed in the work described in Chapter 5 by Pollock and Taket, involving both service providers and service users, produced very important changes in the beliefs and attitudes of the service providers and other stakeholders involved.

The importance of language is illustrated by the careful use of the term 'expert by experience' together with 'expert by profession' in Itzin et al's Delphi study (2010b). The choice of words was deliberate in trying to subvert the traditional power relationships between those who experience violence and abuse and those who provide services. This served to empower the experts by experience that participated in the Delphi process used (personal communication) and gave them confidence to express their views. The specific chapters illustrating this most explicitly in the current book are: Chapters 5 (Pollock and Taket), 8 (Furlong), 9 (Makhoul et al), 13 (Hanna and Moore), 17 (Foster and Freeman) and 19 (Barter-Godfrey et al).

One challenge a number of authors have referred to is that of achieving ongoing inclusive practice, not limited to one-off initiatives, but instead part of ongoing processes. Chapters 5 and 6 present organisation-wide approaches, with widespread participation from staff as well as service users, as one way of surmounting this challenge. They are in two very contrasting settings: Chapter 5 discusses a non-governmental organisation (NGO) providing community services across the state of Victoria in Australia, whereas Chapter 6 is located in a single primary school in the same state. Gaventa and Barrett's (2010) findings about the need for multiple strategies point to the advantage of embedding specific initiatives in wider work at different societal levels.

Reading across the findings from these diverse reviews, together with the material in the earlier sections of this chapter, offers some clear messages of guidance to those concerned with practising social inclusion. We close this chapter and the first part of this book with the following list of factors required to achieve authentic inclusive practice:

* authentic, trusting relationships;
* subjecting the political and economic *status quo* to critical scrutiny and a willingness to challenge it;
* analysis of power relations in the socio-economic–political–cultural context concerned and a willingness to work to change these;
* clear rights-based and anti-discriminatory framework for analysis;
* flexibility and adaptability in terms of methods or processes;
* carefully choosing language to support the above;
* resourcing and support for inclusive practice.

Part II

Practising inclusion in policy

2   Conscience clauses

Your right to a conscience ends at my right to safe, legal and effective health care

Sarah Barter-Godfrey and Julia Shelley

One of the challenges of socially inclusive policy is the appropriate, ethical and effective inclusion of one group whose interests and values are in diametric opposition to another group's needs. In health policy, 'conscience clauses' have been inserted into policies to accommodate health professionals for whom certain procedures are morally untenable, despite these procedures and/or drugs being legal and medically safe, as well as fulfilling patient/client demands and needs. At present, these clauses pertain almost uniquely to sexual and reproductive health; however, extending clauses into other fields, such as adoption, euthanasia and journalism, has also been initiated. This chapter provides an introduction to the use of conscience clauses, which are then re-examined using three standards – liberty principles of harm; the zero sum; and the judicial–philosophical principle of 'my rights end where yours begin' (or in its original form 'the right to swing your arm ends at the other man's nose') – with comment on ways policy can be simultaneously inclusive and protective of population wellbeing.

What is a conscience clause?

A conscience clause is a protection of an individual professional who refuses to carry out an aspect of their job on the basis of their moral or religious view of that task; and protection for organisations which refuse to provide particular services as part of the organisation's mission (Wicclair 2009; Pope 2010). Those provided protection include individuals such as doctors, nurses and pharmacists, as well as health insurance companies and health care organisations. As the notion of a company or organisation having a 'conscience' may be problematic, the term 'refusal clause' is sometimes used interchangeably to sidestep that issue.

Historically, conscience clauses were provided to protect individuals and service users within large powerful systems; for example, to permit parents to withdraw their children from religious instruction in schools, even Church schools (Education Act 1870, in Marcham (1971); Education (Scotland) Act 1872, in Scotland (1972)), or to permit parents to refuse a smallpox vaccine on the basis of conscience (Vaccination Act 1898, in Durbach (2002)). In its contemporary form, conscience clauses were established in the USA as part of abortion reform, when legalising abortion provision from 1973 onwards was weighted against the individual health care provider's option to refuse to perform abortion services (Flynn 2008; Hull 2010). Partly, clauses were included to appease opponents of abortion. However, it was also a pragmatic decision to recognise that, as abortion had been hitherto illegal, some medical professionals could have entered the profession in good faith, willing to perform all required duties but unwilling to perform abortions. To avoid ruptures in the workforce, a conscience clause permitted individual professionals to opt out and refuse to provide abortions. Since then, conscience clauses have grown in number, scope and severity, and extended to include the conscience of organisations (Rovner 1997; Sonfield 2008a, 2008b).

Why are conscience clauses being inserted into policy?

The rise of and growth in conscience clauses has emerged in response to three social processes. Firstly, a decentring of reproductive health care, with greater access to safe, medically approved reproductive and contraceptive care that can be distributed through GPs, pharmacies and non-prescription ('over the counter') medications, has led to widening social engagement with health care options. Secondly, this has been accompanied by 'concern' that these changes are uncomfortable for some professionals and service providers, as seen in a 'backlash' against increasing access and use of reproductive services (Gomperts 2002; Guttmacher Institute 2011). There are also 'slippery slope' concerns that suggest increasing access to reproductive services is the first step towards un(der)regulated cloning, trans-species reproduction, the creation of cyborgs, and euthanasia or assisted suicide. So, there are now more options, of which a greater number are asynchronous with traditional practices, which are available across a greater number of settings, and out of which potentially controversial issues may arise. Thirdly, an increasingly 'risk-averse' medical profession has shifted towards models of accountability with greater 'built-in' protections (Bell et al. 2011; Chamberlain 2011). Of these, opt-out clauses legitimise refusal to provide services and to resist controversial requirements emerging from new or newly available medical procedures.

In the field of health care, ideal conscience clauses adhere to core principles of balancing the professional's refusal with the patient's health needs, including the requirements that: 'Health care professionals must provide all patients with accurate and unbiased information, prior notice of professionals' objections and timely referral in cases of refusal, and medically indicated care in an emergency' (Sonfield 2008b: 19). In this model, conscience clauses permit refusal to provide a service, but do not permit the professional to obstruct the patient from accessing that service elsewhere, and the professional remains responsible for facilitating that referral and access. A model of ideal conduct is generally reflected in the UK General Pharmaceutical Council's (GPC) guidance on conscience clauses for pharmacists who wish to refuse to provide emergency contraception. The GPC, which is the industry regulator for pharmacists in the UK, states that '[the pharmacist] must make sure that if your religious or moral beliefs prevent you from providing a service, you tell the relevant people or authorities and refer patients and the public to other providers' (GPC 2010). The guidance further states that if a service is withheld, the referral to an alternative provider must be timely and not prevent the patient from accessing effective care.

Not all demands for conscience clauses lead to policy opt-out choices. In the UK, exemptions to equal rights provisions in the field of adoption were not provided in the Equality Act 2007 (HMG 2007) after considerable debate during the construction and passage of the bill. Adoption agencies that receive public funding can no longer refuse to place children with same-sex couples on the basis of their gender – agencies that do not wish to comply with this regulation cannot have public funding, and some agencies have chosen to lose funding rather than comply. The trend in the UK has also been to disallow refusal clauses in situations where service providers, including foster parents and social workers, are expected to provide information on sexuality, so that homosexuality must be placed as a legal, valid and morally acceptable sexual identity and orientation. Similar issues have been created by the introduction of a civil union for same-sex couples: services should not, in their provision of services, discriminate between same-sex couples in civil unions and opposite-sex married couples.

The recent trend in the UK has been for minimal use of conscience clauses, and a preference for refusal rather than obstructionist styles of exemptions. In contrast, in the USA conscience clauses are shifting towards having fewer provisions for ensuring timely referral or responsibility for ensuring access to the requested service or medication. Instead, there is a move towards conscience clauses that permit the professional to obstruct the patient from receiving care, not merely refusing to provide it oneself (Sonfield 2005; Buerki 2008; Wernow and Grant 2008; Bradley 2009). This creates a system where individuals refuse to *collude* with the activity as well as refuse to directly participate in it, thus disrupting access to requested services or procedure.

Conscience clauses in health policy can emerge in conflict with other principles of policy drafting. Evidence-based policy is based on principles which include: decisions based on high-quality, replicable and consistent evidence; the accommodation of the needs and preferences of the client; and evaluations which demonstrate that the policy is economically effective and sustainable. Conscience clauses, in contrast, are highly individualised, focus on the preferences of the service provider and are driven by evaluations that cannot be measured objectively. Conscience clauses can, therefore, be seen as politicised rather than evidence driven, and can be shaped by the political will and context of a policy environment. For example, a generic conscience clause in Poland's Medical Code of Ethics, written in 1991 at the time of establishing a post-Soviet state, translates into English as '"a physician can withhold health care services which are not in agreement with his conscience," but must make a referral elsewhere where there are "realistic possibilities of obtaining such health care"' (Nesterowicz 2001, in Mishtal (2009: 163)). This was produced ostensibly to protect the conscience of individual practitioners, but in consequence set up a systemic lack of access to otherwise-legal procedures, once a critical mass of practitioners opted out of providing services. In the period coming out of communism, individual rights were a relatively new and unformed cultural phenomenon in Poland, and as such were less rigorously protected by policies written during that post-Soviet phase (Mishtal 2009), so that the political climate which was unused to supporting citizens' rights helped to produce a code of conduct that favoured the practitioners' systems and structures over the individual patient.

There is a substantial overlap between religious beliefs and notions of and claims to define 'morality', and religious organisations may also be influential in the establishment and proliferation of conscience clauses. In the UK, where the head of state is also the head of the national religious institution (the Queen is the Defender of the Faith and Supreme Governor of the Church of England), fewer conscience clauses have been required, and, for example, the national educational curriculum has been less challenged for its placement of secular introductions to religious instruction and teaching of science compared to the USA. By contrast, in the USA, the special status afforded to religion 'immunises' religious beliefs against state interference or governance (Ellis 2006), and thus forms a justification for the presence of conscience clauses in government-mandated service policies. However, this also occurs in the context of the constitutional separation of church and state. There has also been much greater proliferation of conscience clauses at a state level in the USA compared to the UK, rapidly increasing in the last decade (Guttmacher Institute 2012). Although the 'special status' of religion has not changed constitutionally in that time, there has been momentum towards restricting access to reproductive and sexual health care for women on the basis of religious or conscience arguments. The relationship between religion and governance is therefore not straightforward, and in practice is mediated by other political and cultural factors. Further, claims to morality and conscience positions within any religion, as well as between different religions and denominations, may be contested (for discussion of the changing views on abortion within Catholic teaching, see O'Brien (2008)). Conscience clauses therefore emerge in response to social and cultural pressures, rather than to accommodate any one specific universal standpoint or belief.

Outside of health and social care settings, there has also been some call for the use of conscience clauses to protect journalists. The National Union of Journalists (NUJ) suggests a revised approach to the conscience clause, where journalists would be protected for doing their job in adherence with a code of conduct, and resisting pressure or direction to break that code. The NUJ has proposed a motion that: '[a] journalist has the right to refuse assignments or be identified as the creator of editorial which would break the letter of the spirit of the Code [the Press Complaints Commission code of conduct]. No journalist should be disciplined or suffer detriment to their career for asserting his/her rights to act according to the Code' (NUJ at the Levesen Inquiry 2011, reported in *The Guardian* (2011)). This is a very different approach, where the protection is being demanded for those who uphold all legal and approved parts of their profession, rather than seeking to opt out of professional expectations, and demonstrates one of the possible future directions of conscience clauses.

Inequalities in conscience clauses

Conscience clauses represent a pivot of competing positions, claims and responsibilities. As with many issues where groups with different social status and power come into conflict and compromise, conscience clauses are not necessarily sites of equality. Four points can be identified where the construction and practical effects of such clauses facilitate or are associated with social inequalities: gender and sexual identity, religious affiliation, institutional status, and socio-economic status.

Conscience clauses tend to be introduced *by* institutions that are predominantly male (e.g. parliament, medical governing bodies) *for* professions that are predominantly male (e.g. medicine and medical services), and typically in domains of female reproductive health care (e.g. abortion, sterilisation, contraception). Non-approval of conscience clauses has tended to be in fields in which female labour is more visible, such as foster care, adoption and medical receptionists or administrators (Dyer 1988; Roshelli 2009). The spread and burden of conscience clauses is therefore not equal across gender identities and roles. There is a lack of clarity in some instances of whether a conscience clause is about the refusal to perform a particular service (e.g. sterilisation) or to perform a service for a particular population (e.g. assisted reproduction for lesbian-identified women) (Roshelli 2009). This is particularly acute in domains of services provided to people who do not identify as heterosexual and cis gendered. Inequalities based on lines of gender and sexual identity are at particular risk of being reinforced through conscience clauses.

Conscience clauses generally require a strong, coherent commitment to a religious or moral belief to be demonstrable. Some forms of faith and doctrine are more readily documented and acceptable than others (Nelson and Dark 2003), and thus not all consciences are equally protected. Conscience clauses favour those with the most power, those in institutional positions of authority, with 'only infrequent consideration of the potential impact on patients and haphazard adoption of any concomitant obligations' (Sonfield 2009: 6), so that power inequalities in professional settings are amplified in the performance of refusal of otherwise-approved services.

The effects of refusal and obstructive conscience clauses in health care do not affect a population evenly. Rural and remote areas are more burdened, where geographical spread and population density make accessing more than one service less feasible; and low socio-economic status women are even more likely to be burdened by the effects of refusal and obstruction in rural or underserved communities (Green 2005; Teliska 2005; Day 2008). Given the potential for social harms, perhaps we can re-purpose an old slogan, and suggest that conscience clauses should be safe, legal and rare. In the following sections we consider how the notion of safety can be constructed in policy, through the lenses of the zero sum, liberty and the boundaries of competing rights.

The problem of the zero sum

In describing conflict and decision-making, contentious outcomes can be described in terms of their 'sum'. Zero sum is a description of a scenario where a gain for one person or 'side' results in a loss for the opposition (a score of +1, a win, co-occurs with a loss of −1, thus having a 'sum' of zero). This sets up different standpoints in direct competition with each other. However, many points of human and civil rights are *not* zero sum – it is possible for both sides to 'win' or not lose out, leading to a 'positive sum' (Cohen and Burg 2003). The provision of rights or access for one group does not necessarily prevent another group from doing the diametrically opposite activity or belief. One of the problems of the rhetoric of conscience clauses is the setting up of health care access as a zero sum moment, for example, allowing women to access abortion services will (in a zero sum model) harm the religious beliefs of people who oppose abortion. There may also be a zero sum moment set up between competing harms.

Conscience clauses are at least in part based on the principle of protecting people with conscientious objections from being harmed spiritually; it is not simply that they 'don't want to' but that carrying out an activity would be detrimental to their wellbeing. In this model, religious people are considered to have a burden of eternal soul and/or a duty to a higher purpose, which may be harmed by doing immoral or forbidden acts, so that the request to, for example, pass across a box of contraceptive medication prescribed by a doctor for a designated patient, is potentially harmful for a pharmacist whose religious beliefs prohibit providing contraception. The potential that a sexual assault victim may undergo further stress, humiliation and physical risk by having emergency contraception refused, obstructed or delayed through referral, is set up in direct competition to that of the pharmacist, in a zero sum moment: whose harm is the greater, whose harm should be protected? Finding the limits of each party's rights, and working out where to fairly set the pivot point between two sides, is an ongoing challenge of inclusive policy. One approach which appears promising in resolving these issues, and moving away from zero sum and competitive models, is the principle of 'my rights end where yours begin'.

The right to swing your arm ends at the other man's nose

The origins of the phrase 'my rights end where yours begin' came from the temperance and prohibition movement in the USA in the 1880s (although earlier versions may have existed colloquially but are undocumented). John

Finch, in his role as chairman of the National Prohibition Committee, used the following rhetoric in an 1882 speech: "'Is not this a free country?' 'Yes, sir.' 'Have not I a right to swing my arm?' 'Yes, but your right to swing your arm leaves off where my right not to have my nose struck begins.'" (Finch 1887: 128). The general principle was re-told in various speeches in the temperance movement, as recorded in Mary Woodbridge's biography:

> Neither in law nor equity can there be personal liberty to any man which shall be bondage and ruin to his fellow-men. John B. Finch, the great constitutional amendment advocate, was wont to settle this point by a single illustration. He said, "I stand alone upon a platform. I am a tall man with long arms which I may use at my pleasure. I may even double my fist and gesticulate at my own sweet will. But if another shall step upon the platform, and in the exercise of my personal liberty I bring my fist against his face, I very soon find that my personal liberty ends where that man's nose begins."
>
> (Woodbridge 1895: 239)

These early uses drew on contemporary notions of harm and liberty, echoing the work of utilitarian philosophers, including John Stuart Mill and Jeremy Bentham. Mills' Liberty Principle posited that the only legitimate use of power (as regulation, intervention or coercive prevention) to circumscribe a person's activities and choices was in the prevention of harm occurring to others (Mill 1858/1991). In these terms, one was at liberty to believe and act in any way one chose, up to the point that that choice became harmful for others; and, conversely, that legal governance was entitled to limit that choice to prevent harm accruing to others. Legal commentators took up the notion in the 20th century, applying the principle to wider issues of liberty, democracy and judicial decision-making, and by the 21st century 'my rights end where yours begin' has become one tenet of contemporary feminist writing (McEwan 2007, 2011; Laurakeet 2011).

For conscience clauses, we can apply two assumptions: that social goods are *not* zero sum (it is possible for individual rights to be protected without detriment to others') and that the pivot between the liberty of one person and another can be identified, so that each are protected to the fullest extent until that protection becomes harmful for the other (the rights of one person ends at the rights of another, without infringement).

The first implication of this is that an obstructionist-style conscience clause, where the professional disrupts the patient's access, is untenable. The assertion of the pharmacist's liberty to not provide contraception (which may potentially harm his or her wellbeing) cannot be extended to preventing contraception from being accessed (which would have the consequence of infringing on the patient's wellbeing). The obstructionist model of conscience clauses therefore fails both assumptions: it maintains a zero sum, where the pharmacist is only protected from harm if the patient does not receive contraception, and fails to limit the pharmacist's liberty at the point where it infringes on the patient's liberty. In contrast, the refusal–but–referral model may allow for a non-zero sum outcome, where the pharmacist does not provide contraception but the contraception is still provided.

Widespread conscience clauses, even those that pass the non-zero sum requirement, may also fail the balance of liberties requirement. To ensure that both parties have their liberty fairly protected, refusal conscience clauses would need to be carefully constructed to ensure that the right to refuse is weighted with a responsibility to refer, and that referrals must be timely and not lead to harm or failure of care. The burden of the refusal should be carried by the person refusing, such as taking steps to maintain a referral register, calling ahead to check that another professional will fulfil the requirements and are able to do so, and clearly displaying both their intention to refuse *and* their commitment to refer to ensure coverage of access. Thus the harms of refusal should not accrue to the patient who is legitimately seeking service. It is essential that the effects of conscience clauses, which allocate choice to institutions and people with institutional power, do not subordinate the autonomy of the individual service-user (McLean 2010).

It may be also helpful to consider a temporal element to conscience clauses. In the early spirit of conscience clauses, it was necessary to accommodate people who had joined the profession in good faith, agreeing to carry out all of the tasks demanded, but who found themselves newly in conflict with their professional requirements. Future clauses could be selective so that they only apply to professionals already in the profession at the time of the change in policy. Given that entry to medicine and health care is rarely an instantaneous decision, this may need to include a lag period, to accommodate those entering shortly after a policy change. This would allow professional expectations to adapt to new requirements, and gradually phase out objections, so that people who are unwilling to provide a service can simply choose not to join the profession that provides that service. Selective coverage of opt-out clauses may also support easier referral, where junior partners not covered by the refusal clause could take up the referrals and not feel obliged to sustain their senior partner's objections. Finally, selective coverage would reinforce the notion that opt-outs are exceptional and not routine, and keep a check on the normalisation of refusal.

Conclusions: inclusion and 'opt-outs'

The construction and use of conscience clauses has the potential for social harms, the reinforcement of social inequalities, and a failure to care for people in vulnerable and dependent positions. However, models of conscience clauses that allow for forms of opting out of service provision in ways that do not cause harm for others can be created. Here we have identified three principles that can be used impartially to evaluate conscience clauses and to support inclusive and equitable balance of diversity in health policy. Firstly, construct the scenario in non-zero sum terms, to allow for shared gains; secondly, find the pivot point between one position and another or others by establishing the point at which one's liberty infringes or harms another; and, thirdly, place the burden for the refusal with those who hold institutional power rather than the people who are dependent on them. Although each case for a conscience clause will need to be evaluated on its own merit and circumstance, working from a position of 'my rights end where yours begin' has the potential to support both inclusion and protection in public and health policy.

3 Practising inclusion in policy design for people with disabilities

Natasha Layton and Erin Wilson

This chapter examines the ingredients required for effective policy in the area of disability. Effective policy should foster the inclusion of people with disabilities as citizens and the full realisation of their human rights. This chapter draws on an analysis of Victorian State government assistive technology (AT) programme policy, in Australia (Layton et al. 2010). This research surveyed 100 Victorians with disabilities in order to identify their current and desired use of AT (aids and equipment), environmental modifications and personal care, together conceptualised as an 'assistive technology solution' (AT Collaboration 2009). The methods included an online survey, designed to be accessible to a broad range of people with disabilities utilising AT to communicate. This was supplemented by a small case study sample who participated in an interview series. The research had substantial involvement of people with disabilities at the design, recruitment and dissemination phases. AT policy is a useful lens through which to view effective policy for people with disabilities, as there is significant critique of the existing policy framework (see, for example, KPMG 2006; Pate and Horn 2006; Wilson et al. 2006; Summers 2010). The arena of AT has been demonstrated to greatly improve the lives of people with disabilities in a wide range of areas (Layton et al. 2010). This chapter reviews key concepts from the literature relating to policy for marginalised groups (including disability-specific literature) and goes on to identify the core ingredients necessary to align disability policy with the aspirations and experiences of people with disabilities. The analysis concludes that existing disability programme policy, at least in the arena of AT, is underpinned by a rationing approach to social inclusion, causing people with disabilities to ration their inclusion activities and fundamental life needs.

Understanding of disability

For people with disabilities to be served effectively by policy, they must be affirmed as humans and citizens of value, with the entitlement to the same full life as other citizens, and worthy of government policy and expenditure towards these ends. A number of key ideas underpin such an approach and are absent from the instrumental end of policy in Australia. Specifically, we refer to programme guidelines, i.e. the point at which higher level policies are translated into practice and deliverables in the form of tangible resources and supports. While policy concepts related to marginalisation will be discussed later, we first need to identify the understanding of disability that is necessary as the foundation for effective policy.

The World Health Organization (WHO) offers a widely accepted current conceptualisation of disability (WHO 2001) that acknowledges the role of impairment and the social, physical and attitudinal environment, or *milieu*, in creating disablement (Bickenbach et al. 1999; Scherer 2005). This nuanced understanding of disability has emerged from a long and contested history. Among other models, disability has been defined and understood in relation to the disciplines of medicine and rehabilitation, with their focus on individual pathology (Swain et al. 2004; Thomas 2007). Critics argue that this focus on individual impairment has also 'established and reinforced notions of the boundaries between normalcy and aberrance in Western society' (Albrecht et al. 2001: 13). This focus has translated into discourse and policy, and results in an approach that 'dis-enfranchises a large segment of society by making them permanent objects of social beneficence, a status that few, if any, members of our society would wish to occupy' (Pope and Tarlou 1991: 245).

In contrast, a crucial element of contemporary disability theory is the belief that people living with disability can and should participate in the full range of life activities along with the rest of the human community, despite the reality that life with disability may present 'predicaments' due to functional limitations and the lack of supports or accommodations (Lutz and Bowers 2005; Shakespeare 2008). This understanding posits disability as just 'one dimension of human diversity' (Arneil 2009: 235). In everyday life, disability is differently constructed for each individual according to their impairment effects, the barriers and facilitators within the environment, and the availability of resources to facilitate participation.

It is governments that are tasked with collecting and redistributing finite resources based on society's moral priorities (Sen 1999) as part of the broad social contract underpinning any community. How to allocate finite resources has been the subject of longstanding enquiry in fields such as economics and political science; however, these disciplines are noted to have partial and limited views of the issue of disability (Cummins 2005; Arneil 2009; Kimberlin 2009). In theorising the effects of economic and political circumstances upon society, the idea of the rational citizen has been taken as a reference point. The rational citizen is assumed to be capable, independent, and therefore able to exert agency within, and benefit from, the economic opportunities of the day (Arneil 2009). This normative assumption regarding the essential nature of 'man' is flawed in that it neither encompasses human diversity (Patston 2007; Megret 2008), nor the interdependency which characterises life for people living with disability (Nussbaum 2003). It fails, for example, to encompass individuals whose cognition or mobility precludes 'rational choice' (Arneil 2009). Such a view also causes the disability community to ask: 'Is our social contract, and our deepest imagining of our polity and its political institutions, prem-ised on the figure of able-bodied citizens?' (Goggin and Newell 2005: 142). Crucially, the moral priorities (Sen 1999) of society that influence policy and resource distribution have been based on these ideas about 'normality' and ableness, significantly influenced by medical and rehabilitative models of dis-ability, which has resulted in the continued exclusion and devaluing of people living with disability (Oliver 1990; Corker and Shakespeare 2002).

To address this exclusion, notions of human rights have received prominence in the definition and understanding of disability. Such an approach gives peo-ple with disabilities an equal entitlement to human rights as all other members of society. Human rights principles are articulated in a series of international conventions and charters, and accompanied by monitoring and compliance tools with which to critically evaluate a polity's performance (UN 2010). They cover various areas of freedom, such as economic and political rights, as well as the specific rights of certain minority groups, such as the rights of refugees, chil-dren and, most recently, the Convention on the Rights of Persons with Dis-abilities (CRPD) (UN 2006). In the language of human rights, the individual is primarily a rights bearer, and these rights may either be upheld, or fail to be realised, either partially or in full. In this paradigm, society's moral priorities are redirected to concepts of human rights, including those for people with dis-abilities. As Australia is a signatory to the CRPD, the human rights enshrined there become a moral priority for Australian disability policy.

Human rights legislation also proffers directives regarding steps toward the realisation of rights. While some rights are absolute, for example freedom from torture, others are deemed to require progressive realisation, often in recog-nition of their resource implications for governments. The principle of pro-gressive realisation refers to a situation where governments (or 'State Parties') must make progress towards human rights goals, and where retrogressive steps are avoided (Megret 2008). The CRPD, for example, directs State Parties to 'undertake and promote the full realization of human rights' (UN 2006: Article 4 Point 1), by taking measures 'to the maximum of its available resources . . . with a view to achieving progressively the full realization of these rights' (UN 2006: Article 4 Point 2). Additionally, the CRPD identifies denial of needed supports as an act of discrimination. The nature and extent of needed supports is articulated in the concept of 'reasonable accommodation', defined as 'necessary and appropriate modification and adjustments not imposing a disproportionate or undue burden, where needed in a particular case, to ensure to persons with disabilities the enjoyment or exercise on an equal basis with others of all human rights and fundamental freedoms' (UN 2006: Article 2).

The entitlements enshrined within these conventions resonate deeply with the experience of people living with disability in terms of aspirations and, in many cases, the failure to attain them (Goggin and Newell 2005; National People with Disabilities and Carers Council 2009). The contemporary under-standings of disability discussed above, place disability as one aspect of all human experience where 'ability–disability is a continuum' constructed by environments in which all humans live (Bickenbach et al. 1999: 1182). As equally valued members of human society, people with disabilities are rights bearers, and society is required to provide needed supports to overcome, as well as dismantle, the barriers that construct disability. This set of ideas requires that understandings of disability and the moral priorities underpinning policy must now change.

Understanding key components of policy for marginalised groups

Just as understandings of disability and citizenship are fundamental to constructing inclusive policy, so too are understandings that capture the experience of marginalisation. At present, in Australian society, people with disabilities, as a population, remain marginalised and disadvantaged (ABS 2003; National People with Disabilities and Carers Council 2009), and inclusive policy needs to adequately recognise and address this state (Disability Investment Group 2009).

Literature in social science and economics explores key concepts for identifying and understanding marginalisation. Such understandings underpin the design of effective policy for addressing marginalisation, as well as decisions about the allocation of resources. Three of these key concepts are summarised briefly below, and later discussed in relation to Victorian disability policy.

Marginalisation

Understanding the meaning and experience of marginalisation is critical to designing effective policy to address it. In broad terms, the notion of marginalisation is defined through concepts such as social exclusion, poverty, deprivation and quality of life, the definitions of which are all contested in the literature. These are discussed briefly below in order to identify some of the dimensions of marginalisation that disability policy should encompass.

Poverty and income levels have traditionally been a significant marker of marginalisation and disadvantage. Saunders et al. (2007: viii) define poverty as 'a situation in which someone's income is so inadequate as to preclude them from having an acceptable standard of living. It exists when people's actual income is below a poverty line'. They go on to argue that poverty, on its own, provides insufficient detail with regard to the living conditions and experiences resulting from this situation, and propose two additional concepts: deprivation and social exclusion. Deprivation is defined as 'an enforced lack of socially perceived essentials' (Saunders et al. 2007: viii). Social exclusion, by contrast, focuses on participation and occurs 'when individuals do not have the opportunity to participate in widely practiced social and economic activities' (Saunders et al. 2007: viii), also referred to as 'participation poverty' by the Australian government (Senate Community Affairs Reference Committee 2004: 2.4). This suite of concepts highlights the need for effective policy to meet needs relating to income levels, standard of living, access to essential items, and participation in social and economic activities.

Levels of disadvantage and marginalisation have also been understood in terms of health status and health-related quality of life. In particular, social policy has utilised the measure of health-related quality of life to assist in quantifying the extent of benefit resulting from a social policy, programme and funding allocation. Health-related quality of life refers to that part of quality of life that may be affected by a person's health status (Oldridge 1996), encompassing such areas as independent living, relationships, mental health, coping, pain and the senses (Hawthorne et al. 1999). Benchmarks of health-related quality of life exist for the broader population (Monash University 2010), against which to compare the indices for marginalised groups.

Equality, equity and conversion handicap

Multiple dimensions of the experience of marginalisation, discussed above, result in unequal opportunities to realise human rights on an equal basis across all members of society. We have already established that human rights instruments, such as the CRPD, require that people enjoy rights on an 'equal basis' with others (UN 2006). Equality infers that people should be treated as equals (Jones 2009) and implies equal allocation of public resources, which, at face value, may be seen to be fair and reasonable. However, all people are not in equal situations, and effective policy design incorporates attention to the need for differential levels of resourcing. A core concept in this arena is that of equity.

The notion of equity recognises that a range of factors, such as the presence of impairment or the lack of financial resources, may lead to unequal need and unequal capacity to address that need (Culyer 1995). As Sen (1999: 70) describes, 'what use we can respectively make of a given bundle of commodities, or more generally of a given level of income, depends crucially on a number of contingent circumstances, both personal and social'. The impact of disability here is noted to be a significant source of variation between incomes and the real 'advantages – the well-being and freedom – we get out of them' (Sen 1999: 70). Sen refers to this problem as 'conversion handicap', identifying that it occurs when more resources than usual are required to achieve an outcome, due to the presence of impairment (Kimberlin 2009). Effective policy incorporates the notion of 'vertical equity', which recognises that steps must be taken to ensure equitable access to resources is provided to those with 'unequal need' (Culyer 1995; Ong et al. 2009). These steps require a recognition that individuals require 'different treatment to arrive at a similar result or outcome', a concept known as 'complex or positive equality' (Rioux and Riddle 2011: 44). In this way, effective policy enables differential, rather than 'equal' or same, treatment in order to provide services and resources appropriately targeted to meet differing needs and contexts.

Capabilities

A related key concept in the understanding of marginalisation and disadvantage is that of 'capabilities' (Nussbaum 2003; Sen 2009), referring to 'what people are actually able to do and be' (Nussbaum 2003: 33). This approach proposes that, in order to further understand inequality between people, 'one must consider not just each person's resources and rights but each person's ability to use their resources and exercise their rights' (Kimberlin 2009: 38). This recognises the link between a person's own characteristics, the resources available to them and what they can individually achieve with these. Nussbaum (2003) argues that a capabilities approach requires government to explicitly focus on how to enable people's capabilities to function, in any domain, by both the direct provision of supports as well as ensuring there are no impediments to capabilities being enacted. Taking a capabilities approach 'directs government to think from the start about what obstacles there are to full and effective empowerment for all citizens, and to devise measures that address these obstacles' (Nussbaum 2003: 39). This directly links to a human rights approach and reasonable accommodation requirements. Nussbaum argues for 'effective measures to make people truly capable' of enacting their rights (Nussbaum 2003: 35), which requires policy and government action that directly addresses the multiple elements in society that limit individuals' capability.

Using the notions of marginalisation (as a multidimensional experience of disadvantage); of equity (as equalising the life chances and opportunities of marginalised groups with the rest of society) and of capabilities (the potential to achieve given the right supports), we now turn to the case study of AT in Victoria with these concepts in mind, to explore both exclusionary and inclusive policy.

Case study of assistive technology policy in Victoria

High-level policy documents in Australia embed contemporary disability rights and appear to adopt the 'moral priorities' of the CRPD. The Commonwealth Government's National Disability Strategy (2010–2020) is expressly aligned with the principles of the CRPD (UN 2006), and outlines the intent of all Australian governments (State and Federal) to maximise the potential and participation of people with disabilities (Commonwealth of Australia 2011). As well as aligning with human rights principles, high-level policy recognises the importance of key supports, such as AT, to the maximisation of individuals' capabilities. A growing body of literature (summarised in Layton et al. 2010) shows that AT contributes significantly to a range of life outcomes for people with disabilities, including social and economic participation. Given the established importance of AT solutions, it is not surprising that the CRPD includes 16 mentions of these as components of rights entitlements (UN 2006), including promoting their availability and use (Article 4). Elements of AT solutions are also embedded within several of the six core outcome areas of the National Disability Strategy (Commonwealth of Australia 2011).

However, beneath these larger policy frameworks sit the actual service delivery mechanisms (or programmes) designed to enact policy intent and, at this level, problems with policy to support people with disabilities become clear. Programmes for the provision of AT in Australia differ for each state, but overall have been described as an '*ad hoc* and uncoordinated patchwork' of over 100 programmes across three levels of government (Summers 2010: 1), split according to eligibility, category of AT, as well as area of use (for example, work or school). The Victorian programme for AT provision provides a useful example of exclusionary policy, at the service-delivery level, for people with disabilities.

The Victorian Aids and Equipment Program (VAEP) is the key funding source designed to provide AT to community-dwelling Victorians. The stated purpose of the VAEP is to: 'Provide people with a permanent or long-term disability with subsidised aids, equipment, vehicle and home modifications to enhance independence in their home, facilitate community participation, and support families and carers in their role' (DHS 2010a: 5). Programme guidelines provide a list of 'approved' equipment, and home and vehicle modifications, alongside subsidy rates or maximum payments for each item. Subsidy rates represent an average allocation of 60 per cent of the actual cost of each item. As a result, virtually all recipients (91 per cent) are required to make a co-payment for items (Wilson et al. 2006). Applicants experience long wait times averaging seven to eight months for needed equipment, and procedural guidelines restrict some eligible items to a 'once in a lifetime' funding allocation (Wilson et al. 2006). From a resourcing perspective, the latest government review of the VAEP reported substantial underfunding (KPMG 2006), with unmet need estimated to require a doubling of the annual budget to be fully addressed (Coalition for Disability Rights 2006).

The experience of people with disabilities using AT solutions and the relevance of the VAEP were investigated in *The Equipping Inclusion Studies* (Layton et al. 2010). Participants confirmed that the use of a wide range of AT solutions made a significant difference in their lives, acting as enablers to overcome impairment effects and barriers to inclusion. The 100 survey participants described over 900 instances of activity and participation, enacted across a wide range of life domains, enabled by elements of AT solutions such as mobility devices and information and communication technologies (ICT). These elements were repeatedly seen to be effective in more than one life domain. AT solutions were a key support in terms of people with, often severe, disability enacting their lives in ways consistent with the areas of human endeavour reflected in the CRPD. For example, studying at tertiary level by deaf–blind individuals and those with quadriplegia and locked-in syndrome (using ICT devices); running a web-design business from home for a bedfast individual (via the use of an adapted bed and workstation); and joining the local dog club by an individual with ataxia (via use of a rough terrain powerchair). Similarly, the denial of needed AT solutions was found to be a significant barrier to life participation. Key themes regarding denied participation resulting from lack of AT covered a wide range of life areas and essential life items (Table 3.1). The

Table 3.1 Areas of participation denied due to unmet need for AT solutions

Themes identified by participants	Percentage of response
Travel more freely; get out and about; get to things	22
Be more productive; get a job; get more done	13
Have a life; 'freedom to do what I want to'	12
Recreation; 'go to things that I only dream about at the moment'	11
Less frustration; increased sense of coping; increased confidence	10
Socialise; participate; communicate; have a say; be involved; change relationships for the better	9
More independence and choice; autonomy	9
Spend more time away from home and out in the evenings	6
Safety	5
Holidays	3
Exercise	1

provision of AT solutions was directly shown to increase participation as well as health-related quality of life.

A key finding was the overlapping and interdependent use of elements of AT solutions. The majority of participants (66 per cent) used a combination of AT devices (aids and equipment), environmental interventions and personal care to make up their individualised AT solution. Only 2 per cent of participants used a single element such as aids and equipment. Participants' individualised AT solutions were found to comprise an average of 13 elements (including devices, environmental modifications and personal care) including, on average, eight AT devices. In addition, all participants identified unmet need for elements of AT solutions, averaging an additional five elements per individual, in order to fully meet life participation needs. This overall level of requirement has significant implications for inclusive policy design.

Despite the benefits of AT and the need for multiple AT elements, participants experienced significant barriers to accessing this resource. Analysis of the programme guidelines identified that subsidy rates now average just 66 per cent of the actual cost of AT, although this can be as low as covering an average of only 28 per cent of the cost of home modifications (Layton and Wilson 2010). In addition, the VAEP subsidises a very limited list of AT devices, reflecting just 13 per cent of recognised AT devices on the market (ISO 2007) and excluding multiple AT device categories (such as stand-up wheelchairs and recreation devices), despite their relevance to the aims enshrined within the CRPD and National Disability Strategy. Overall, respondents reported currently using 386 devices that are not eligible for VAEP subsidies, 32 per cent being information and communication technologies, and 9 per cent being mobility devices. Significantly, the VAEP explicitly excludes many items considered to be more generic in nature, such as mobile phones, computers and other non-disability-specific items, despite their affordability and effectiveness in meeting need. Participants described contacting multiple alternate funding sources (including philanthropists) to find the funds to top up the subsidy shortfall or to fund ineligible items. Participants frequently could not afford these co-payments nor find adequate alternate funding, and thus went without AT (and the participation it enables).

The ingredients of inclusive policy for people with disabilities

The analysis of the VAEP highlights several factors that contribute to the exclusionary effect of this policy. These assist in highlighting some of the core ingredients of a more inclusive policy approach.

Policy must be designed to achieve outcomes valued by the target population

The research focused on 'whole of life' outcomes, as defined and referenced in documents including the International Classification of Functioning (ICF) (WHO 2001) and CRPD (UN 2006), and as directed by people with disabilities involved in designing the research project. As discussed above, participants reported that AT enabled the achievement of outcomes in all life areas. In addition, elements of AT solutions were repeatedly seen to contribute to outcomes in more than one life domain. The lack of AT led to failure to achieve outcomes in a wide range of human rights and life areas. The results demonstrated that people with disabilities do indeed aspire to full and varied lives, and AT solutions are key resources to achieve these.

By contrast, the narrow parameters of the VAEP (focusing on independence and a narrow range of participation) serve to limit the life activities and capabilities of people with disabilities in ways contrary to both the named aspirations of people with disabilities themselves, as well as the moral priorities of human rights conventions. Life outcomes are also constrained by the substantial restriction of identified equipment eligible for funding. Whole fields of life are omitted from approved VAEP funding (such as recreation and leisure), with participation being only narrowly supported in other areas (for example, less than 20 per cent of AT devices for personal mobility listed in the international standard (ISO 2007) are reflected on the VAEP Equipment List). The CRPD provides the scope of life outcomes expected for and valued by people with disabilities. Policy must now focus on supporting the achievement of these.

Policy must be designed to match the demographics and requirements of its target group

Megret argues that, unless the disadvantage, particularly the poverty, of people with disabilities is explicitly recognised in policy, then it 'is quite possible to accord full civil and political rights to persons with disabilities, while effectively disenfranchising and silencing them through the maintenance of policies which ignore the particular situations and needs of persons with disabilities' (Alston, quoted in Megret 2008: 265). In this way, policy must be explicitly designed in response to demographic and other data that speak to experiences and levels of disadvantage and marginalisation.

Participant data identified the multiple dimensions of disadvantage and marginalisation that affected the levels of need of people with disabilities (Layton et al. 2010). Participants had high rates of unemployment (74 per cent) and low incomes, with 67 per cent reporting their income as being under $21,600 per annum. Most respondents (75 per cent) were dependent on government pensions or allowances as their main source of income. The health-related quality of life of participants was found to be far lower than that of the broader population, averaging less than half that of the norm for the Australian population (0.32 compared to 0.80). In relation to their level of social exclusion, participants named multiple incidents of denial of participation and human rights across all life areas. Rationing, choices and trade-offs regarding social inclusion were evident in the data, particularly trading lower-order activities for those that participations perceived as more fulfilling. For example, one participant reported, 'I give up having washes so I can get out', and another stated, 'I have one shopping afternoon to live my life per week'.

Despite these experiences of disadvantage, the VAEP policy pays no attention to this context. The VAEP targets a disadvantaged population and requires substantial co-payments, which become multiple in nature given the number of AT devices required by each individual. There is no recognition of the additional barriers to and costs of participation for this group, which function as a conversion handicap. Its design as a subsidy programme, with no co-payment contribution caps or safety nets of any kind, suggests no interest in making needed AT solutions affordable. Similarly, as discussed above, there appears to be little real commitment to enabling the participation of people with disabilities in all life areas.

A key policy design mechanism to address marginalisation is the application of the notion of equity (discussed above), via the recognition that unequal need will require unequal levels of resourcing in order to equalise opportunities for participation or attainment of capabilities. Given the presence of impairments, significant elements of disadvantage (including poverty), as well as disabling attitudinal, structural and environmental factors, a clear argument exists for the application of equity concepts to the VAEP policy design. Colgan et al. (2010) demonstrated the need for a two- to three-fold equity weighting in calculating quality of life improvement for *The Equipping Inclusion Studies* cohort. The equity principle here recognises that comparatively more resources are needed to achieve outcomes for this group than would be needed for other populations.

Policy must be designed to deliver what works in order to meet need

The Equipping Inclusion Studies (Layton et al. 2010) presents evidence of the diverse needs of individuals with disability and the plethora of AT solutions they use to meet these. The three elements of AT solutions (equipment, environmental modifications and personal care) were found to be key and inter-dependent ingredients of meeting people's needs. The vast majority of partici-pants utilised multiple elements of AT solutions as part of a 'suite' designed to fit their context. In contrast, AT policy focuses largely on one element of this suite, aids and equipment, with limited attention to environmental modifica-tions, and no acknowledgement of the evidence for the multiplicity of ele-ments needed, nor the critical interdependence of these in order to be effective. A policy that subsidises one element of a required AT solution, but pays no attention to the others required to make this element effective, is an exclusion-ary and ineffective one.

As part of the suite of AT, participants listed a wide range of AT, going well beyond the narrow confines of identified equipment eligibility. The VAEP 'approved' equipment list represents a tiny sample of the internationally under-stood taxonomy of AT devices, with many useful solutions simply unfunded. Furthermore, participants identified a high demand for 'generic' items such as laptops and mobile phones. These remain ineligible for funding despite their value as a base for more specialised applications. Such an approach denies fund-ing to many elements that are most effective and affordable.

This policy approach appears to be aligned with understandings of disability based on the medical model, in which valued and 'legitimate' interventions are those involving specialist and clinical approaches to impairment only. By contrast, there is evidence of the range and effectiveness of AT solutions which should form the basis of policy design. This denial of effective supports neces-sary for achieving broad life capabilities can be understood as discrimination and a breach of human rights.

Conclusion

The literature establishes that effective policy for marginalised groups should be based on understandings of marginalisation (as a multidimensional experience of disadvantage), of equity (differential resource levels to reflect differential need) and of capability (the potential to achieve given the right supports). These are clearly missing at the level of policy implementation (i.e. programme guide-lines) in relation to AT funding in Victoria. It is also important to look at the underpinning definitions and beliefs about the focus group of policy intent, in this case, people with disabilities. In current AT policy, people with disabilities are not inherently valued as equal citizens with equal rights to life participation and living standards. Instead, their participation is expected to be limited, is not of particular social value, and is therefore not worthy of extensive resourcing. As a result, disability programme policy in Victoria, Australia, is underpinned by a rationing approach to social inclusion, where it is required that people with a disabilities continue to ration their inclusion activities and fundamental life needs. In order to foster the inclusion of people with disabilities, policy needs to be premised on understandings of universal human worth and rights, and to support outcomes towards these ends.

4 Practising social inclusion through regulation

Occupational health and safety for commercial sex workers

Beth R. Crisp and Michael W. Ross

Introduction

Occupational health and safety provisions are a factor which many contemporary workers take for granted, particularly when their work places put them at risk of injury or illness. However, despite sometimes being regarded as 'the oldest profession', the occupational health and safety needs of commercial sex workers or prostitutes have largely been ignored, except in relation to sexually transmissible infections (STIs). Rather, as is argued in this chapter, provisions that have the potential to reduce the health and safety risks of this occupation group have tended to be by-products of other efforts, such as attempts to reduce levels of STIs in the wider community. Consequently, recognition of a broader range of health and safety issues for commercial sex workers have until recent years received scant recognition except from sex workers themselves and others closely aligned with the industry. Indeed, the European Agency for Health and Safety at Work (2003) has noted that the needs of commercial sex workers tend to be overlooked by occupational health and safety and other employment regulations.

Before outlining a range of health and safety issues that need to be recognised in respect of this group, and suggesting some reasons why their needs have been ignored, let us first consider why occupational health and safety is an issue which should be firmly on the social inclusion agenda. Social exclusion has been described as a denial of civil rights that citizens might reasonably expect (Room 1999), which arguably include adequate health and safety regimens in the workplace. Furthermore, typically policies and programmes to promote social inclusion do so by promoting social cohesion and/or by enhancing the resources of the poorest and most disenfranchised groups in a society, most commonly through employment and welfare programmes (Bhalla and Lapeyre 1997). Hence it is has been proposed that:

> . . . to achieve social inclusion would require policies and programmes that . . . provided pathways into employment for the unemployed and secured basic rights and conditions from the employers, including a minimum wage, trade union representation, to promote economic integration . . .
>
> (Sullivan 2002: 508)

Social inclusion policy initiatives in countries such as Australia and the UK are one approach to promoting social inclusion. However, at times this has resulted in exclusion being attributed to individual choice rather than recognising the failure of social structures (Bletsas 2007). Furthermore, the heavy and competing demands on initiatives of this type are such that efforts are most likely to be concentrated efforts on areas of policy that have wide application rather than on the very specific needs of a relatively small number of people (Provis 2007).

Public policy typically emerges in response to issues which have been identified as problematic, or potentially so. When policy options are presented, typically each is based on differing assumptions as to what the underlying problem is that needs be addressed. If only one option is presented, it should not be assumed that there are not other representations of the problem, as it may well be that other viewpoints have not been considered or have been silenced. As such, policy solutions can readily legitimate and privilege particular sectors of the community and fail to recognise the needs, or even the existence, of other stakeholders (Bacchi 2009). Hence, this chapter, which explores a range of policy responses to the occupational health needs of commercial sex workers, provides a case study on how policies can be framed to promote social inclusion.

Occupational hazards

Although, as already noted, the occupational health and safety needs of commercial sex workers tend to be overlooked, it is not because they are negligible or do not exist. Sex work itself can have a negative impact on health, and sex workers may be exposed to unsafe working conditions. Also, sex work may attract workers who have health issues, including poor mental health and drug use (Seib et al. 2009b).

In a review of occupational health and safety in commercial sex workers, Ross et al. (2012) have noted that occupational health and safety issues in commercial sex workers – male, female and transgendered – have been ignored and commercial sex workers have been at the mercy of moral and legal agendas. In addition to the stigma associated with sex work, there are policing risks and risks of extortion where the activity is illegal, violence from clients, risks associated with specific settings of work and with achieving protection in those settings, higher levels of alcohol and drug use, STIs and strain injuries associated with sex work, and the relative absence of health and safety interventions for commercial sex workers. Regulation (in a positive rather than a punitive sense) and a recognition that commercial sex workers are worthy of protection by recognising them as deserving of protection, is one way of practicing social inclusion and providing a measure of social justice.

Policy initiatives which aim to promote health for commercial sex workers typically recognise STIs (Scott 2005), and pregnancy for females (Sanders 2004), as occupational risks. However, focusing primarily, or only, on sexual health may lead to a range of other occupational hazards not being acknowledged, including violence, harassment, bladder problems, stress, depression, alcohol or drug addiction, latex allergy (Groneberg et al. 2006), musculoskeletal injuries (Alexander, 1998), having money stolen by clients, and being forced to have unprotected sex (Plumridge and Abel 2001). Such injuries may be chronically disabling or result in death.

While studies of commercial sex workers report often higher lifetime rates of STIs than found in the general population (e.g. Seib et al. 2009a), it cannot necessarily be assumed that these infections are acquired through their work (Lee et al. 2005). The risks, however, vary considerably; for example, one Australian study found the prevalence of sexually transmitted bacterial infections to be 80 times greater among illegal street workers than their counterparts who were working legally, always used condoms with clients and were subject to monthly screening (Loff et al. 2000). Condoms may not be consistently used with clients (Fang et al. 2008), and, even when used universally by female sex workers when engaging in vaginal intercourse, use during oral sex was much less likely, and oral sex can also result in transmission of bacterial infections such as gonorrhoea (Linhart et al. 2008).

Along with STIs, there is a high prevalence of violence experienced by commercial sex workers (Elmore-Meegan et al. 2004; Gilchrist et al. 2005). It is not uncommon for sex workers to be coerced or threatened by clients with guns and knives (and occasionally crowbars and baseball bats), leading to consequences such as rape, sexual acts that the sex worker would not ordinarily want to perform, threats of death by strangulation or stabbing, and abduction. In addition, risks may not necessarily be limited to clients, as commercial sex workers who are believed to carry large amounts of money or drugs may be targeted for robbery (Bletzer 2003). Commercial sex workers may also be at an increased risk of violence from the police (Mayhew et al. 2009), long-term and regular partners (El-Bassel et al. 2001), and neighbours and community members (Mayhew et al. 2009).

Mental health issues are also common. In their study of commercial sex workers from nine countries (Canada, Colombia, Germany, Mexico, South Africa, Thailand, Turkey, the USA and Zambia), Farley et al. (2003) found that prostitution was multi-traumatic, and that close to 70 per cent of the women surveyed about their current and lifetime history of sexual and physical violence met the criteria for post-traumatic stress disorder. This relates to a high prevalence of violence and abuse (Bletzer 2003), as well as homelessness, substance misuse and a lack of control over interactions with clients (Vanwesenbeeck 2005). The incidence of suicidal thoughts and suicide attempts almost doubled for sex workers who reported coercion compared with those who were not coerced (Wang et al. 2007), and those who have had traumatic experiences prior to commencing sex work, such as childhood sexual abuse, are particularly vulnerable in respect of their mental health (Månsson and Hedin 1999).

Alcohol and drug use are not infrequently associated with sex work, either because the nature of the work leads to self-medication, or because sex work is a relatively easy way to obtain money to finance a drug habit (Plumridge and Abel 2001). However, the specific context of sex work may also require commercial sex workers to consume alcohol (Fernández-Esquer 2003), and alcohol or drug consumption may place sex workers at greater risk of unsafe sexual encounters with clients (Clatts et al. 2007; Wang et al. 2007).

Sexual acts may also cause repetitive strain injury if performed repeatedly. Musculoskeletal conditions reported by commercial sex workers include injuries to the wrist, arm and shoulder due to repeated hand jobs; jaw pain as a result of repeated fellatio; knee pain from working in a crouching position; foot problems relating to standing or walking in high heels; and back problems related to dancing or walking in high heels, or working on inadequate massage tables or beds (Alexander 1998). Repeated consecutive vaginal or anal intercourse may also cause trauma (Bletzer 2003), particularly with inadequate lubrication.

The health risks to commercial sex workers are often exacerbated by the legal context in which the sex occurs, particularly if it is illegal. Soliciting, engaging in, or agreeing to engage in prostitution; loitering with intent to commit prostitution; living off the earnings of prostitution; encouraging or promoting prostitution; crossing state lines for the purposes of prostitution; and operating or managing a prostitution business or renting premises for that purpose, may be criminal offences for both female and male sex workers (Alexander 1998). There may be the additional risk for male sex workers in settings where sex between males is illegal or highly stigmatised (Okal et al. 2009). Fear of arrest can have a number of health consequences. For example, street sex workers may spend less time negotiating safe sexual practices in order to reduce their visibility to law enforcement personnel, with the result being a higher exposure to STIs (Seib et al. 2009a) or them not carrying condoms, which may provide evidence of their occupation (Alexander 1998). Fear of legal sanctions also results in sex workers who have experienced crimes against them not being prepared to go to the police, either because they believe that the police will not take their complaints seriously (Hawkes et al. 2009; Lorway et al. 2009) or because they may be arrested themselves (Alexander 1998).

Despite the very real risks to health, commercial sex workers may have limited access to appropriate health services. Mainstream health services are frequently incapable of responding appropriately to those whose sexual health needs or sexual practices are perceived as unconventional or atypical (Taket et al. 2009b). For illegal immigrants, who form the majority of commercial sex workers in some countries, their precarious legal situation may render them unwilling or unable to access health services, resulting in STIs remaining undiagnosed and untreated (Folch et al. 2008).

A legitimate occupation

One explanation for the marginalisation of the occupational health and safety needs of commercial sex workers is that prostitution is not regarded as a legitimate occupation. However, this is certainly not due to it being a form of work employing small numbers of people. In fact, arguably, in many countries there are substantial workforces that need protecting. Some years ago it was estimated that there were at least 8000 sex workers in New Zealand (Plumridge and Abel 2001), a country which then had a population of around four million people (Statistics New Zealand, 2010). With no suggestion that the proportion of New Zealanders employed in commercial sex work is significantly higher than in other parts of the world (see Plumridge and Abel 2001) and may in fact be much lower than in other countries (Elmore-Meegan et al. 2004; Dandona et al. 2006), the numbers of people who work in the industry are far from negligible.

As it is clearly not lack of numbers of persons involved that fails to render sex work being regarded as a legitimate occupation, another possibility is that the nature of the activity is not considered to be work (Barnard 1993). Although most societies have proscriptions concerning who can engage in specified sexual behaviours, being sexually active, at least during some period of one's life, is considered normal. Consequently, the distinction between persons who are sexually active outside societal norms and those engaging in prostitution has often been blurred. Historically, the 'promiscuous amateur' was considered impossible to distinguish from a 'normal' woman, and 'prostitution' has included a wide range of sexual behaviours outside heterosexual marriage, including cohabitation of unmarried couples. Not until the late 19th century was the commercial transaction for sex considered an integral aspect of prostitution (Scott 2005).

A further consideration is *whom* commercial sex work is considered to be an occupation for, irrespective of whether it is deemed an appropriate form of work. Among single women in many countries, those who were from poor or working class backgrounds were far more likely to be regarded as engaging in prostitution than those from wealthier backgrounds if they were sexually active or perceived as being so. This included young women who had been sexually abused (Mahood and Littlewood 1994; Abrams 2000; Abrams and Curran 2000).

Prior to the 20th century, discourses on prostitution focused almost entirely on female sex workers. Commercial sexual contact between men was usually not recognised as prostitution but rather as unnatural or inappropriate behaviour (Scott 2005). As with female sex workers, experiences of poverty, homelessness, hunger and powerlessness may be critical factors that facilitate men's entry to commercial sex work (Lorway et al. 2009). However, the stigma and fear of sanctions associated with being either a male sex worker (Minichiello et al. 1999) or a transgendered sex worker (Harcourt et al. 2001) can differ from those experienced by their female counterparts, and result in a reluctance to publicly identify as being employed as a commercial sex worker or use health services (Harcourt et al. 2001).

Another key issue in respect of whether commercial sex work is considered an occupation, and therefore work in which occupational health and safety issues must be addressed, concerns the nature of the workplace. Where commercial sex work is not illegal but subject to regulation, the workplace may be readily recognisable as such. For example, it has been suggested that 'Indeed, the advent of licensed brothels in Queensland may have created a "disciplined" group working in a highly regulated environment where they are expected to arrive for shifts on time and dressed according to brothel guidelines' (Seib et al. 2009b: 477). However, for commercial sex workers who work in other venues (Withers et al. 2007), work in their own homes (Scott 2005) or on the streets (Seib et al. 2009a), not only is the likelihood that their place of work is not necessarily recognised as a workplace, but the risks may be far higher than for those working in licenced premises. Hence, although controlling brothels may be perceived to be an 'economical' way of policing prostitution (Scott 2005: 87), there remains a need to distinguish between legislation that seeks to protect sex workers and that which controls the activities which occur inside a brothel.

The prevention of immorality

Historically, one of the key strategies to promote the health and welfare of those deemed to be engaging in prostitution or at risk of entering such work has been some form of rescuing and incarceration of young women (Mahood and Littlewood 1994; Swain 1986), with the stated aim being the prevention of immorality. Often known as 'Magdalene' asylums, these institutions locked sex workers away from the community in order to reform their sense of morality, and became a common response in Western Europe, Australia and elsewhere. Such highly punitive regimens were seen as good for both the individual and the wider society. In some places, rather than waiting to rescue those who had already commenced working as prostitutes, significant deterrents were put in place against contemplating this form of work. For example, in 19th century France, this took the form of registration by the police of women entering brothels. Women seeking registration were required to undergo a medical examination, and were asked questions by a panel about their social situations and reasons for entering prostitution (Scott 2005). Both rescuing and deterrents continue to this day in many places. For example, in India,

> One popular method is to 'rescue' sex workers by force, thus reducing the exploitation said to be characteristic of the sex industry, and then to offer the rescued workers alternative sources of employment or relocation to place of origin. Methods to restrict entry, such as a ban on trafficking women and girls, would be a natural accompaniment of this approach. In practice, groups that consider sex work as immoral are likely to favor both forcible removal of sex workers and restraints on entry into sex work, so that it is not always clear whether the policy stems from the desire to impose a particular moral perspective or to improve the well-being of sex workers.
>
> (Mistra et al. 2000: 95)

A more recent approach, which is less punitive, but ultimately underpinned by an ethical imperative, involves an appeal to sex workers to be 'good' citizens. However, as with previous attempts to prevent immorality, improved health and wellbeing for sex workers is positioned as a consequence rather than the main objective:

> Responsible strategies, presented as humane, economical and efficient, have become the chief line of defence against HIV/AIDS. . . . The objective regarding female or male prostitution is not longer to rehabilitate individuals so that they might assume 'normal' (productive, heterosexual etc.) lives. Nor is it to eradicate prostitution by targeting either its supply and demand. Instead, the objective is less ambitious. Rather, the existence of prostitution has been accepted within governmental discourses which have sought to improve the conditions in which prostitution is practiced. Those who identify as prostitutes are not expected to aspire to be 'normal' members of the community. They should, however, aspire to be 'good' prostitutes. Being a 'good' prostitute means different things in different contexts, though it may generally be understood as to be a hygienic and socially responsible subject. Nowadays, this means being a 'professional' prostitute as opposed to an 'amateur' or public prostitute.
>
> (Scott 2005: 238–9)

As such, the health needs of commercial sex workers are only important in that they may have an impact on the health of the wider community, which is deemed to need protecting.

Protecting the community

Historically, if individuals cannot be protected through persuasion not to engage in prostitution, this has resulted in attempts to ensure that commercial sex work does not have a negative impact on the wider community. For example, it has been suggested that

> Australian prostitution law reform in the past 50 years has generally been driven by perceived 'associated nuisance' aspects of the industry, such as criminal involvement, drug and alcohol abuse, official corruption, and loss of neighbourhood amenity.
>
> (Harcourt et al. 2005: 121)

A key aspect of protecting the community has been efforts to prevent the transmission of STIs through contact with commercial sex workers. For example, Prussia established regulations in 1792 prohibiting prostitutes from working in particular districts and making it compulsory for them to attend weekly medical examinations. This led to a clear distinction between registered and unregistered prostitutes, with unregistered workers being blamed for the spread of venereal diseases (Scott 2005). France and Britain were among other countries which instituted regular medical examinations during the 19th century, with denial of the right to work for those found infected and imprisonment for those refusing to attend examinations as legal sanctions which could be applied to commercial sex workers (Scott 2005). Interestingly, we are not aware of any attempts to licence the clients of commercial sex workers, which could subject them to regular testing and potentially protect a wider population, including their non-commercial sexual partners in addition to sex workers. We nevertheless note that, unlike in most countries where it is those who sell sexual services who are liable to be prosecuted, since 1999 in Sweden, and 2009 in Norway and Iceland, it is illegal to purchase sex (Ross et al. 2012).

In some places, the regulation of commercial sex workers was not necessarily to protect the whole community but rather key sectors. For example, in 1860s India regulation of prostitutes was essentially a measure to limit the spread of syphilis and gonorrhoea among the more than 60,000 British troops who were stationed there. During this period, the incidence of STIs among prostitutes was said to be resulting in more than 200 admissions annually for every 1000 members of the military, and it has been suggested that 'In short, restraints on local women were preferable to checks on troops, even though the latter would indubitably have been easier to enforce' (Levine 1994: 597).

Notions of protecting communities continue to this day. For example, persons considered to have either directly or indirectly benefitted from the proceeds of prostitution within the past 10 years are barred from visiting the USA according to the restrictions specified in the Immigration and Nationality Act. Importantly, such restrictions include commercial sex workers who have worked in countries where prostitution is not illegal (Williams, 2010), and may be based on an unfounded assumption that immigrant sex workers are more likely to be infected with STIs than are local workers. For example, a Catalan study of over 350 immigrant female sex workers found that the prevalence of STIs was consistent with the wider population of sexually active young people in Catalonia (Folch et al., 2008). In Argentina a study comparing STIs in immigrant and non-immigrant female sex workers found that rates of syphilis and hepatitis C were actually higher in the Argentinean sex workers, whereas hepatitis B prevalence was higher among the migrant sex workers (Bautista et al. 2009).

Health-promoting workplaces

Regulatory provisions that have the potential to reduce the health and safety risks have tended to be by-products of other endeavours, such as regulations that provide disincentives for workers to enter or remain working in the indus-try, or attempts to reduce the levels of STIs in the wider community. Such approaches can reinforce the marginalisation of commercial sex work and increase the vulnerability of commercial sex workers to injury or illness, rather than protecting them from work-related harm. Hence, while commercial sex work remains illegal or highly stigmatised, and sex workers have good reasons for wanting to avoid contact with law enforcement agencies, a purely regulatory approach to promoting the health and safety of commercial sex workers is likely to be ineffective.

More socially inclusive approaches to health promotion that have the explicit aim of promoting the health and safety of commercial sex workers are likely to be both more effective and less stigmatising. For example, Rickard and Growney (2001) used a peer education approach to sex workers in London, with a short (28 minute) audio cassette that involved stories from other sex workers about selected key safety issues and sex worker approaches to it. The evaluation found that all but one of 15 sex workers who participated in a pilot study aimed at improving occupational health felt they had learnt something. In particular, the peer education materials were regarded as credible and likely to be engaged with by sex workers, who commented on the practical advice and sensible suggestions relating to safety and vetting of 'dodgy punters'. Several participants also made their copies of the cassette available to sex workers who were not part of the study.

In addition to working directly with sex workers, health promotion efforts for sex workers who are 'employed' need to engage with the relevant 'gatekeepers' (i.e. the owners and managers of establishments were sex is transacted on a commercial basis) to create supportive workplace environments. Where there are supportive 'gatekeepers', who articulate health promotion messages to workers, condom use becomes normative and is more likely, and there are fewer perceived barriers to condom use (Yang et al. 2005). A supportive management may also be more likely to enforce regular health checks, including testing for STIs. Nevertheless, although this may be health promoting for individual sex workers, the commercial benefits to venue owners and managers of having healthy workers should not be underestimated (Withers et al. 2007).

It is important to recognise that the health issues for commercial sex workers employed in premises may differ significantly from those who work for themselves 'at home' or who work on the streets or in other public places, and it should not be assumed that measures suitable for one group will be adequate with another (Plumridge and Abel 2001). Nevertheless, it may be worth encouraging lone workers to explore how they may adopt working practices that many employed sex workers may take for granted, such as not working alone and being part of a network that shares information about high-risk situations and clients (Bletzer 2003).

Conclusion

This chapter provides a case study exemplar as to why the emergence of social inclusion policies may be inadequate in promoting the health needs of some groups who experience significant social exclusion, such as commercial sex workers. This chapter also demonstrates that, while social policy has the potential to positively influence the occupational health and safety of commercial sex workers, frequently this has occurred as a consequence of other measures, e.g. initiatives which aim to prevent the spread of STIs in the wider community. Bacchi's (2009) approach of identifying the social problem that policies are responding to, understanding why this option has been favoured and whose needs are promoted and neglected as a result of this, provides a useful framework for exploring how policies promote inclusion or exclusion for segments of the community, particularly those who have historically been excluded. It should be recognised that policies and practices which actively promote protection rather than regulate unsafe behaviours are not only more socially inclusive but also potentially more effective. Critical reflection as to what policy measures are actually tackling will be essential if policy measures are to effectively promote the occupational health and safety of frequently excluded groups such as commercial sex workers.

In suggesting that policy measures have the potential to promote occupational health and safety among commercial sex workers, we are conscious of criticisms that we are not being realistic. Certainly, it is easier to promote occupational health where sex work occurs in licenced premises, but we do not believe it to be impossible in other contexts. We have long seen the health and social benefits of adopting harm-reduction approaches to the spread of STIs and the impact of substance misuse. This has involved adopting new moral paradigms in which addressing the health and welfare needs of socially excluded individuals and groups is considered more important than preventing so-called immoral behaviours (Crisp and Barber 1997). Practising social inclusion with commercial sex workers may require a similar approach, with policies aimed at ensuring the safety of workers is paramount, despite prostitution being morally reprehensible to many in the wider community. This is likely to require policy makers to take courageous stands supported by evidence, rather than ignore an issue which is only seen to affect a small and marginalised group in society (de Leeuw et al. 2008).

Part III

Practising inclusion in service design

5 Inclusive service development

Exploring a whole-of-organisation approach in the community service sector

Sarah Pollock and Ann Taket

Introduction

This chapter discusses the participative process used to involve service users and families in service development. It is based on work the authors undertook in a large, multi-sector community services organisation (CSO) in Melbourne. Through this process, the organisation hoped to increase service user autonomy, understood as 'how much control you have over your life – and the opportunities you have for full social engagement and participation' (Marmot 2004: 2). The chapter demonstrates that participatory approaches to service development can simultaneously increase participants' sense of control over their lives and align service development towards outcomes that service users and families identify for themselves.

Participatory practice in the context of service development

The approach described in this chapter draws on the tradition of pragmatic pluralism focused on dialogue and action (Rorty 1989; Ulrich 1998). According to Ulrich (1998), engagement in processes of shared meaning-making and action enables citizens to develop the competencies for active participation in processes that affect them, provided that multiple methods of communication are included which work for them. He also highlights the need to develop practices of collaborative critical reflection, implemented in the everyday context of service delivery, in order to lift the constraints that systems place on individuals. Communication processes should also liberate individuals from discourses that diminish their experiences, values and beliefs (Rorty 1989).

The focus of much participatory service development work has been with programme staff as participants and directed at improving utilisation of evaluation findings or the empowerment of staff in relation to their own practice development. The involvement of people using services, where it is mentioned at all, tends to be confined to the data-collection stage of evaluation. Some recent community-based participatory research projects have successfully taken up the challenge of involving community members and/or service users in all parts of service development (Earle-Richardson et al. 2009; Neuhauser et al. 2009).

The organisational context

Wesley Mission Victoria (Wesley) is a large multi-sector CSO providing around 50 different services to people from over 100 sites across Victoria. Its programmes include some that are unique to Wesley, for example Resilient Kids (RK, see Table 5.1) and those that are also delivered by other CSOs in Victoria, Australia, such as funded facilitation for individual support packages (ISPs, see Table 5.1).

Social inclusion is at the centre of all Wesley's activities. The organisation has developed a policy that frames the socially inclusive approach it takes to all its work. The Social Inclusion and Belonging policy, adopted in 2009 (Wesley Mission Victoria 2009), outlines an organisational framework that focuses on development at multiple levels, from individual to societal. As defined in the policy, Wesley's approach emphasises the importance of each individual having choice about, and control over, how they live their life. The policy is based on the idea that each individual has the right to determine the life he or she wants to lead. The service development process described here is a key strategy within this policy.

The participatory approach was selected because it gave service users and families a voice in determining the best ways to provide services and supports that would assist them to live lives of their choosing. As participants in such a process, service users and families would have a role to play in making decisions that would inform the future service delivery, extending their role from being solely a service recipient. The process gave them the key role in identifying important outcomes for the service they receive and deciding how to evaluate the achievement of these as a basis for identifying how the service should develop.

The work initially took place within three Wesley services, with an overarching governance structure to ensure applicability at the whole organisation level. A team of three staff was drawn from Wesley's research unit, staff within the organisation but with no direct service role. Led by the first author, the team set up and facilitated the participatory process, and then executed and reported the resultant evaluations. The process was formative and action-oriented in that it sought to understand how the service was working whilst evaluation was being conducted. The researchers fed findings back into the service delivery context, and staff made changes to practice and service development along the way. To give just one example from the ISP, service users were unclear about their entitlement to receive assistance in between the regular reviews of their package. This was resolved by the addition of a paragraph to the end of review letter setting out the assistance and how to access it, coupled with a more responsive system for phone messages recorded from service recipients. The participatory process was also pluralistic, accepting that there are multiple perspectives and interpretations of a shared context that are equally valid. The process brought together a broad range of people with an interest in the service, including service users and their families, Wesley service delivery staff and managers, and personnel from relevant areas of government departments funding the

Table 5.1 Description of services

	Funded facilitation for individual support packages (ISPs)	Resilient kids (RK)	Wesley Aged Care Housing Service (WACHS)
Service users	People with a disability (intellectual, physical, psychiatric) who have an ISP (funds allocated to them for disability-related support)	Children whose families have experienced homelessness and who are receiving services from a family violence or homelessness service provider	People over age 65 who have a long-term history of mental illness, substance abuse and/or homelessness
Service type	Facilitators work with the individuals to help them develop a plan for how they will use their ISP	Weekly therapeutically oriented groups for children to help them explore their experiences of homelessness and develop appropriate responses	Accommodation and support within a low-care setting, in two-, three- and four-bedroom houses in a suburb in inner north-west Melbourne
Service focus	Enhancing individual capacity and independence	Healing from trauma and skills building	Maintaining independence
Duration of intervention	Facilitators are funded to provide 30 hours of assistance every 36 months (12 months in the case of degenerative conditions)	Groups run once a week during a school term. Children can attend multiple series of groups	People tend to remain at WACHS for many years, and only move on when they need higher level care or when they die
Contact between service user and service provider	Extensive: intensive contact for a short period of time, with long intervals between periods of service	Short-term intensive	Ongoing: residents have contact with staff on a daily basis
Funder	Department of Human Services (Victoria, i.e. state level)	Department of Human Services and philanthropic sources	Department of Health and Ageing (federal agency)
Scope of service	Also provided by other CSOs	Unique to Wesley, and developed at a time when there were no specific homelessness services for children	The model is unique, although low-care residential support is offered by other care providers for the aged

service delivery, most particularly the Department of Human Services (DHS). To ensure applicability at whole organisation level, services were selected to ensure diversity in target groups, of interventions and activities involved and their locations within Wesley's functional structure. Table 5.1 provides a brief description of the three services.

A governance structure was established comprising specific reference groups and steering committees for each service, linked to an overarching group, chaired by an external person, the second author. Table 5.2 provides details of the composition and role of the various groups developed to govern and guide the work. A two-way feedback loop ensured that reference group business was reported to the steering committees, and vice versa. Progress of the work in each of the three services was reported to the overarching governance group, in order that they could consider the implications for the organisation as a whole in the context of the broader community services sector.

Work was conducted over a 20-month period, from late 2009 to the middle of 2011. The same general stages were followed in each of the three services, but with differences in response to participants' needs in relation to engagement and their advice about what the evaluation should focus on. The different stages in the work are summarised in Table 5.3.

Table 5.2 Governance structure

Group	Composition	Role
Community reference groups (CRGs) (one per service)	Service users and family members who self-selected to take part in this aspect of the project	Advice and guidance in relation to the involvement of service users and their priorities and interests
		Feedback on outputs
Management reference groups (MRGs) (one per service)	Wesley manager, coordinator and other staff as appropriate, representatives from government department involved	Advice and guidance in relation to service delivery and funding context
		Feedback on outputs
Steering committees (one per service)	All members of MRG and CRG	Endorsement of reports, including, recommendations from evaluations
Governance group (one, at whole-organisation level)	Wesley CEO and senior staff from external organisations, including other CSOs, peak body, university and Department of Health. Chaired by external person (second author)	Endorsement of outputs and recommendations
		Oversight of service development process at whole-organisation level
		Ensure applicability of the approach in broader community sector context

Table 5.3 Stages in the service development process

Stage	Content
Establishment	Researchers worked separately with the different groups of participants to get committed and comfortable engagement
Production of programme logics	Produced by each participant group separately (using individual and group interviews), then discussed in first participatory workshop, followed by modification by each participant group if required
Design of evaluation	Programme logics used to decide what data to collect, and how; surveys etc. designed and data collected
Analysis and interpretation	Initial analyses and interpretations discussed with participant groups separately in reference groups
Action planning, reporting and advocacy	Final interpretations of the findings and recommendations negotiated at second participatory workshop involving all groups for the service. Researchers then developed evaluation reports for each service, including action plans for practice and service development, as well as advocacy for policy change and development. Reports endorsed by steering committees

The establishment stage took around 4–6 months to build committed and comfortable engagement. In the next stage the researchers worked with participants through individual and group interviews to develop a programme logic (Kellogg Foundation 2004) for each of the three participant groups (service delivery staff, service users and government department officers). The programme logics identified the aims, key processes and desired outcomes for each service, and the underpinning assumptions that participants held about the context for the service and its delivery. This enabled each group to describe in their own terms the service, its place in their lives and priorities (the context), and what they sought from it.

For each service, two participatory workshops were held, the first of which was at the conclusion of the programme-logic stage. This workshop enabled participants to review and discuss the different views of the service, articulated in the three versions of the programme logic, and what it could or should be achieving. Workshop participants also identified the most important issues to focus on in the following evaluation stage. After the workshop, each group met separately to review their programme logic and amend it in response to what they learned from seeing and hearing other perspectives on the services.

The researchers developed a data-collection strategy in response to the outputs from the workshop and subsequent meetings with the reference groups. The data-collection strategy was endorsed by the steering committee for each evaluation, and implemented in the service context. The research team predominantly undertook the data collection and analysis, and initial findings were presented to the reference groups for consideration.

Final interpretations of the findings and recommendations were negotiated by all participants working together at the second participatory workshop. The researchers then developed evaluation reports for each service, including action plans for practice improvement, service development and systemic advocacy.

At the conclusion of the evaluations, all participants were invited to take part in an interview to discuss their experiences of being involved, what their participation meant to them, what had worked well and not so well, and what could or should be done differently in order to enable service users and families to take part in future service development activities. Participants had the choice to be interviewed by the first author, a Wesley staff member involved in the work, or by someone outside Wesley, the second author. So far, interviews have been conducted with 35 people involved in the work across the three different services. Interviewees included 15 service users and/or family members, 13 Wesley service delivery staff, three Wesley managers and four DHS officers. Drawing on the analysis of these interviews, in the sections that follow we first discuss the outcomes for service users relating to the participatory processes in terms of achieving inclusive service development, and then those aspects of the participatory approach that participants identified as being effective in securing their engagement in the projects.

The value of the 'big picture'

The researchers worked throughout with participants in separate and shared spaces to develop an understanding that could incorporate different ideas and experiences of the service and the context people saw it working within. In particular, the process set out to deliberately throw light on the users' views of the service, as this is the view that is most likely to be overlooked in a traditional service development project. Interview participants consistently reported the value of seeing alternative views alongside their own, referring to this expanded view as having a 'big', 'wider' or 'whole' picture of what they were setting out to evaluate. The 'big picture' does not try to draw together the different views, but allows them to sit alongside each other so that participants can reflect on their own and others' views and interpret these in relation to what matters to them.

Evaluation strategies were responsive to the 'big pictures' through the development of surveys and data-collection strategies that privileged the service user view. In the interviews, staff suggested that it was the combination of direct involvement with service users and families and outcomes data that reflected what users and families sought from the programme that was most impactful in terms of helping them understand how their programme was working. It ensured that consequent action planning could be oriented towards service users' needs and desires for their own lives.

Generally, there was a high degree of attunement between service users and service delivery staff in terms of working towards outcomes that service users and families value and seek. However, where differing ideas exist about the programme, the business of determining effectiveness is complicated. In the case of Wesley Aged Care Housing Service (WACHS), a variety of ideas about the programme emerged (non-traditional aged care, a housing programme within aged care), who its service users were (e.g. people who are homeless or with mental health issues, those with long-term disadvantage, those who do not fit into mainstream aged care) and what the focus of the intervention was (e.g. looking after people, prolonging their independence, providing a safety net). These differing ideas made it difficult not only to determine what outcomes constitute effectiveness, but also inhibited service development.

Seeing people in a different light

Service users frequently described themselves in the service delivery context as devalued and passive, people who need help and who have nothing to give back, and depict a system that focuses on their problems and what they lack. However, their reflections in the interviews on the participatory process identified that it had offered them other ways of being and other ways of thinking about themselves that were more active and agentic:

> I think that this is something that you don't think about when you're in the system and you're just this poor, disadvantaged, vulnerable . . . and there's so many labels . . . and you just fall into it . . . and you don't actually question . . . well, how is this helping me, or . . . is this actually supporting me, or is this actually making it worse. And I think in some ways, it was very empowering to be part of a group that was actually saying, well, was this helpful? Was this actually supportive? These were our intentions, did we actually get there? (Bella, Parent, RK – all names are pseudonyms)

In particular, development of separate programme logics legitimated service user constructions of the shared service context and offered possibilities that were generally not afforded to 'clients' in a range of professional discourses and associate practices:

> They are an important contributor in actually resolving some of those bigger issues. That's exactly how they should be recognised, and we don't do it enough. We don't use that expertise, that knowledge near enough. It's crazy.
>
> (Abbie, DHS officer, RK)

The process facilitated shifts in the way that service users saw themselves, and consequently how they acted within the service system. Adele, a parent in RK, said that when she came into contact with other service users and heard about their experiences, she realised that 'it wasn't just me', and that: 'It made me feel a bit differently about myself. It made me feel that this is a circumstance. This isn't me. This isn't who I am'. Likewise, Ursula, a woman in ISP, talked about hearing Ivan's story about how he had given up full-time work to look after his daughter who had an acquired disability, and who saw care as an opportunity to lead a new kind of life. As she listened, she reflected on her relationship with her own father who saw her as his 'disabled daughter', a label which she strongly rejected. Ursula's contact with Ivan allowed her to reaffirm her value as a person, regardless of her condition and the support she now required. Most importantly, she was able to develop an alternative understanding of the transformative potential of the relationships she had with those who cared for her, for them and herself.

There appear to be two aspects to this repositioning or re-envisioning. The first is that the individual's experiential knowledge is valued, and their reality viewed as legitimate and worthy of consideration. During the interviews, service users spoke about the importance of sharing their knowledge as an opportunity to give something back. This simultaneously placed them in a more reciprocal relationship with service delivery staff and the organisation assisting them, and enabled them to reframe their experience as something useful that might assist others in creating different possibilities for future development of services. Secondly, the broadening of the context to accommodate the organisational and system context within the lives of service users, rather than the other way round, had the effect of depersonalising their situation and shifting how the 'problem' of homelessness or disability (or, in fact, any need for support) is conceptualised from an individual to a social sphere.

There were practical outcomes for people from this combination of increased sense of self-efficacy and new knowledge. Some participants reported an increased sense of wellbeing and self-worth because they were taking part in something where they were useful and helping others. Others started to exercise greater control over their interactions with the service delivery system. In ISP, Finn, a man with autism and a mild intellectual disability, recounted how he had changed his service provider because he was not happy with the support he had been receiving. Hearing his story encouraged Wanda, also in ISP, whose son had a disability similar to Finn's, to approach her son's provider to negotiate changes in the supports he received.

These instances suggest that participation which combines the acquisition of new knowledge with an increased sense of self-worth can enable people to take action to construct lives of their choosing.

Effective processes

The chapter now turns to focus on the processes that participants themselves identified as effective in fostering inclusive participation. Processes were specifically aimed at working with multiple groups of participants and facilitating input from people who are usually left out of service development activities in the organisational setting. They were designed to surface and explore differing experiences of the context or 'problem' the service addressed and differing ideas about desired outcomes. This kind of dialogue required a platform of strong relationships between participants. This includes: the relationships within the research team; between the researchers and service delivery staff and managers; between the researchers and people in each of the participant groups; within the participants in the groups; and, finally, between groups.

Universal participation

In each programme, all current service users were invited to take part. Where appropriate, family members were also invited to talk about their experience of a family member using the service. Feeling welcome and feeling that each person had something useful to contribute mattered to participants. Drawing on previous experiences with hard-to-reach groups, and the knowledge of service delivery staff, the researchers used a range of strategies to create inclusive and welcoming environments in which to work with participants. These included having means of participation other than meetings, flexible meeting times, making sure people had transport to and from meetings, having welcoming and familiar settings and sharing food.

> Ah, it was like somebody cared. They took notice of . . . our family situation, and OK, yeah, well if you can't come to us, we will come to you.
>
> (Camille, Parent, RK)

Throughout the process, the researchers stressed that multiple knowledges, including policy, professional and experiential, were equally important and useful. For service users, having a process that acknowledged their specific expertise as well as their complex life situation contributed to the development of an inclusive process in which they felt valued as equal participants.

Allowing sufficient time for relationships to develop and, later, providing time for participants to consider and interpret findings in their own groups and together was also important in securing participation of diverse groups. While participants acknowledged that the process was lengthy, there was general agreement that the critical reflection and dialogue that brought about the richest learning and led to changes in the way people saw things and acted could not have been achieved in a shorter time frame.

Having different ways to take part

Different 'spaces' where groups could meet separately were highlighted as an important aspect of the relationship building that enabled participants to engage in meaningful and effective dialogue in the workshops. Service users and families placed high value on the separate group sessions, where they were able to get to know each other, explore experiences and issues, and gradually build an understanding of what was important to each of them individually and to them as a group. A staff member participant commented that the separate spaces allowed each group to concentrate on what was important to them before they engaged in dialogue with other groups in the workshops. They then came into the shared space feeling like they had a firm foundation, legitimated by the researchers (and thus the organisation) from which to negotiate around what they did and did not share or agree on. Participants reported generally that communication in the workshops was open and equitable, and they felt able to contribute and to listen to others.

Having a variety of activities was also effective in enabling broad participation and giving people a choice, and thus a sense of control, in relation to their participation. Researchers were flexible and responsive in relation to how people took part, and worked with individuals to make arrangements that suited them. There was no requirement for service users to commit to participating in a particular way, and individuals chose to move in and out of the process, depending on what else was happening in their lives. As work developed, a core group of service users for each service met consistently and formed the Community Reference Group, while others contributed at different stages.

Using accessible language

Although the evaluations relied on written and spoken English, the researchers worked with individuals to determine their communication needs and preferences, and, where possible, provided information in a variety of formats, including complex (fully detailed) and simple (overview of main points) documentation with opportunities to receive the same information face to face.

The attention paid to language was also very important. Where possible, the researchers used participants' own words to construct the programme logics and surveys used in the evaluations, and provided multiple opportunities to review and change language. This contributed to participants' sense of control over the construction of descriptions and their sense of self-efficacy as actors in a dialogic process of negotiating meaning within group contexts. At times, where no unified view emerged through dialogue, multiple versions remained, although all participants agreed to privilege service user views in the development of surveys. One example of this from ISP related to outcomes for families in a programme where supports are aimed at individuals, with the intention of building individual capacity. In one version, the only outcomes were those that related to the programme's impact on the individual. However, the service users and families included a number of outcomes about family support, sense of security and hope for the future. These were accommodated in the survey in the form of specific questions about the benefits experienced by package recipients' families.

Having the opportunity to describe things in their own words and on their own terms was important to service users in bringing their own particular reality into view. In the first participatory workshop in the RK programme, participants had a lengthy discussion about whether services provide 'help' (service users' preference) or 'support' (professionals' preference). 'Help' was important to service users because it stressed the personal relationship between the parents and the staff who assisted them, and brought to the fore elements of working together and caring, whereas 'support' was redolent of a professional discourse with more distant relationships and overtones of neediness and dependency. The professionals found this insight extremely useful to their practice.

Being involved in an ongoing process

Participants in all three groups said that involvement in an ongoing process rather than a single event or during data collection was important in fostering engagement and responsibility. The ongoing process also enabled people to move in and out of the evaluation as their life circumstances changed. Ongoing involvement of both service users and service providers included opportunities to review and modify process and outputs at every stage of the process. This also signalled accountability on the part of the organisation back to the service user and family participants, so that control was genuinely shared. The ongoing nature of the work meant that the researchers had to ensure that people were kept up to date with progress, regardless of their patterns of participation. Service users identified that accessible and regular information and updates assisted them in maintaining a sense of engagement over the course of the work, and to make decisions about which events to take part in.

Participants identified the importance of their involvement in the early stages of the work where the scope of the evaluation was determined. They placed high value on negotiating the outcomes they sought from the service prior to designing the evaluation. However, the openness and lack of pre-conceptualisation resulted in some confusion and uncertainty. This was particularly so for professional participants, who struggled to cope with the broad context for service delivery that service users identified. Some professionals initially expressed uncertainty about how to respond to problems that were beyond their immediate professional responsibility. As the evaluations progressed, familiarity and trust increased. A shared agreement developed on what different stakeholders could change and what was beyond their control and required advocacy in the longer term. Following this, the initial uncertainty and confusion in the professionals was replaced by a shared sense of control over the process.

Being linked to action-planning

It was important to all participants to be involved in something that they thought would be likely to actually make a difference. One family member in ISP remarked that being able to give feedback in an action-oriented process gave a sense of hope that he was unaccustomed to in his interactions with the service delivery system.

Service users were not naïve about the difficulties of achieving change in complex systems. What they wanted to was to have a voice at the table where decisions were made and actions planned, and to be part of the dialogue that would shape future action rather than simply being framed as part of the problem:

Doesn't mean that they're going to take it on board, but at least we got the opportunity to say something, to give back . . . and [the researcher] made me feel like I was a part of it, and I did get to have a say, so, I think it really does help when people take the time to wanna know what's going on and how things are helping.

(Camille, Parent, RK)

The role of the researcher

The core values, first and foremost were, that they gave people a voice . . . they gave people a voice.

(Vera, Family member, ISP)

You need someone that is outside of it to come in and ask some questions that you're not going to think of because you've just got your blinkers on and you're heading in one direction with what your role is and your job is.

(Helene, Staff member, ISP)

The two most important aspects of the researcher role identified by participants were the nature of the leadership they offered and the critical questions they posed along the way. The Social Inclusion and Belonging Policy, with its focus on bringing silent and silenced voices to the fore in decision-making processes, framed the researchers' work and the way in which they took up their role. Through regular research team meetings, the researchers developed a style of leadership that aimed to facilitate input and collaboration from all participants, and to be responsive to their needs and priorities as they guided the research process.

The researchers used their developing sense of the service and its broader context to formulate critical questions that allowed service users to step back from the immediacy of their experiences. This helped them reflect on what the service system was and was not providing them with in relation to what they sought for their own lives. As noted before, this critical reflection led some to ask for different responses from the service system, or take action to change their own lives. The questions also led service users and family members to reframe their experiences, which were often hard, as valued and valuable knowledge that could be useful to others in the future.

Conclusions

In many areas of community service delivery there are moves towards self-directed models of support, supported by client-centric service systems. However, there is a need to pay attention to how those people using the system will be involved in their development, instead of letting this be driven by government bureaucracies. Getting the involvement of service users right is key to providing services that meet their needs and work in ways that work for them, thus increasing the likelihood of effectiveness in terms of outcomes. This also enables a shift in the relationship between service users, providers and policy makers from one characterised by inequality and dependence to one characterised by equality, reciprocity and shared control.

Organisations wanting to involve service users in their service development activities will need to develop strategies that are consistent with their own governance structures, the services they provide and the communities they work with. The strategies and participatory process that we have discussed in this chapter may provide useful ideas to draw on, but is not intended to provide a blueprint. Based on our work with Wesley, we suggest the following guidelines can be helpful in this process:

1. *Ensure commitment to the process at the whole-organisation level.* The interviews reveal the emotional and psychological value to the individual of belonging without having to fight for a space, but finding that one's needs and requirements in terms of participation are accommodated in the organisation's processes. This sense of belonging cannot be fostered without whole-of-organisation commitment to giving service users a real role in its ongoing development, and the recognition that they are as valid a part of the life of an organisation as are the staff, board members and funders.

2. *Find ways to value and utilise the experiential knowledge of service users and families.* By combining the creation of spaces in which service users can contribute their specific knowledge of an intervention and its value in their lives with critical reflection on that and other, more dominant forms of knowledge, professional participants began to question accepted views of how things are. The process was effective in terms of illuminating professionals' understanding of how service users place the service in the context of their lives, and interpreting this in terms of service development. Additionally, professional participants came to appreciate service users as individuals, more capable than they had realised, and existing autonomously rather than as subjects of the service delivery mechanisms.

3. *Build relationships that challenge the professional–client discourse.* Acknowledging service user knowledge and placing this at the centre challenged the marginalised position generally afforded the service user voice in service development processes. This was a deliberate and conscious strategy on the part of the researchers leading the process, and was a topic of discussion in all three services. Organisations wanting to undertake participatory service development must be prepared to place the service-user view before their own, regardless of the implications of this in terms of action planning. Although this does not mean doing things the particular way service users want, it does mean being prepared to consider all possibilities, and negotiate ways forward on this basis. The key to operationalising this lies in the quality of relationships between participants, and a

preparedness to see beyond accepted professionally derived positions to new possibilities.

4. *Develop a model of leadership that is facilitative, responsive and transformative.* The researchers played a role that was critical to the success of the process. The model of leadership the researchers employed, and their position external to the service delivery team were key elements of this success. Ongoing supervision and regular team meetings enabled the researchers to critically reflect on their experiences in the process, remaining open to possibilities for transformation and change. These qualities of leadership emerged as being more important than the research skills that the research team brought, suggesting that organisations interested in employing this kind of approach could consider a role where the facilitator came from outside the service, but was not a researcher.

6 Increasing social cohesiveness in a school environment

Karen Stagnitti, Mary Frawley,
Brian Lynch and Peter Fahey

Introduction

Australian children who begin school at risk of failing are more likely to come from disadvantaged and lower socio-economical areas (AEDI 2009). A national population measure, the Australian Early Development Index (AEDI), has been completed with 95 per cent of Australian children as they enter school, and has found that 23.6 per cent of Australian children are vulnerable in one or more areas of development. Developmental vulnerability refers to children who score in the lowest 10 per cent of the AEDI checklist, which is filled in by their teachers using the domains of: physical health and wellbeing; social competence; emotional maturity; language and cognitive skills for school; and communication/general knowledge. Developmental vulnerability is compounded by socio-economic disadvantage, with 32 per cent of children living in the most socio-economically disadvantaged areas being developmentally vulnerable in one or more AEDI domains. Children who are developmentally vulnerable are at risk of failure in their schooling, and this has long-term consequences for lack of employment, poor health and wellbeing, and social exclusion from community in adulthood (Justice and Pullen 2003; Walker et al. 2005; Gagnon et al. 2007; Pungello et al. 2009).

This chapter is about how a school in a disadvantaged and socio-economically low area implemented a whole-school educational approach to increase social inclusion of the children and families within the school community and wider community. The school that is the focus of this chapter is introduced next, followed by the presenting issues in the school, which resulted in the school staff questioning their values and realising change was required within the school. The specific processes that were put in place to bring about change are then discussed, and the chapter concludes with considerations about the broader implications of the changes made within this one school. Within the story of the change process that occurred in the school, the two research projects that were carried out and their results, together with school data and teacher observations, are put forward as sources of evidence for changes noted in children's behaviour and children's and parents' social inclusion in the school.

School context

The focus of this chapter is a school called St. James Parish School, which is in Sebastopol, a suburb of a regional Victorian city in Australia called Ballarat. The school was established in 1956 by the Sisters of Mercy, and the school remains within the Catholic education system to the current day. Since 2000, St. James Parish School has been staffed entirely by lay people.

Sebastopol has one of the highest proportions of children in the local area who are developmentally vulnerable in emotional maturity (20.6 per cent) and social competence (18.6 per cent) (AEDI 2012). For comparison, nearby Buninyong (a small hamlet and more affluent than Sebastopol) recorded only 2 per cent of children having developmental vulnerability in these areas. Within the school community in 2010, 36 per cent of students came from the bottom quarter of the income distribution in the region (St. James Parish School 2011).

Presenting issues

Teachers at St. James were concerned about the low skill levels of children entering the school, particularly low oral language levels and social/emotional/behavioural issues. Following school entry, these low skill levels persisted for some time, despite various systemic supports with children continuing to achieve low levels on standardised academic assessments. Children were also frequently displaying disruptive behaviours. The pressure from the system to have children achieve at a higher level in a narrow set of literacy and numeracy outcomes was felt by teachers. Teachers felt pressured to do the same things 'better', and this adversely affected teacher attitudes and actions and compounded the presenting issues of children failing in school and being disconnected from school. For example, in 2007, with a school population of 147 children, there were 130 recorded behavioural incidents, of which 106 were serious (e.g. bullying, physical, non-compliance and consistent offending and rule-breaking). These incidents included 65 students (i.e. 44.2 per cent of students were involved as the perpetrators of serious behavioural incidents). Also in 2007, there were 48 students (32 per cent) out of a total of 147 students who, according to the Strengths and Difficulties Questionnaire (SDQ) (Goodman 1997; Hawes and Dadds 2004), were within the borderline/high-risk range for significant social and emotional needs. The SDQ is a short screening tool for children aged 3–6 years that gives information on a child's emotional and behavioural problems. This questionnaire is freely available for use by schools, clinicians and researchers (Youth in Mind n.d.). Alongside the SDQ results, teachers also observed that there were large numbers of students who exhibited low self-esteem, believed that they were unable to achieve at high levels, and were disengaged from learning. The staff could see that the permeating culture and self-esteem of individuals needed to change if the students were to be high achievers and socially connected at school and in life. It was time to both raise and change expectations of teachers and students.

A passion for possibilities!

Through a process of questioning and discerning a way forward (see Table 6.1) staff built the belief that, together in solidarity, they had the power and ability to make a real difference in the children's lives. Collective commitments to bring about positive, educational reform were made and espoused publicly, for example, through public speaking at conferences on educational reform within the Catholic school system. This public commitment firmed the resolve of the staff and helped hold them accountable to one another and to the school and wider diocesan educational community. They realised that a whole-school change was needed: 'We need a metamorphosis of education – from the cocoon, a butterfly should emerge. Improvement does not give us a butterfly, only a faster caterpillar' (Anon. n.d.).

Staff at St. James Parish School began to question the basic concept of teaching according to the principle that 'If a lesson works well for one child, it should be appropriate for all children, especially if the teacher taught the skills well'. Teachers also started to question the clinical 'test and fix' model, which still permeates so much of systemic educational thinking and practice. Their thoughts started to shift towards identifying what children really need to thrive and how to build their self-esteem. Staff identified that they needed to start acting seriously on the statements so readily espoused by teachers and found in school charters or schools' learning and teaching statements such as: 'Children learn in different ways', 'Children learn at different rates', 'Children's uniqueness is nurtured in our environment', 'We value the diversity between children', 'We nurture children's imagination and creativity'. Staff asked themselves a number of confronting, challenging and uncomfortable questions. Could they expect different results by doing the same thing 'better'? Why had their teaching become so regimented, inflexible and tied to timetables? What are they testing for and for whom? Are their kids failing or are they failing them? How is society changing? How does that affect their children? What does education look like elsewhere – in other schools and other countries? What are the abilities that impact on skill development? What do theorists say about how children learn best? These questions provoked staff to research various educational theorists and visit progressive schools so that they could inform their deepening understanding of what children really need to thrive at school. This eventually led to a significant change in teachers' fundamental paradigms about the role of education, and from there to a significant shift in teacher practice.

Bringing about a whole-school change

This section outlines the process that took place within the school as a result of the teachers' questioning about their core beliefs and practices. What happened resulted in a shift from a traditional classroom with tables and chairs and a timetable, to a play-based approach, where the physical set up of classrooms was changed and the teacher's role undertook a shift to become a facilitator of learning. Table 6.1 summarises these changes.

Table 6.1 Summary of changes made within the school from 2005 to 2011

Year	Concerns or actions	Changes/action
2005	Lack of student engagement, poor social skills, significant behavioural issues. Low academic performance of children	Professional development based on Dr Loretta Giorcelli's (1996) work on developing inclusive schools
		Professional reading focusing on inclusive education, including The Salamanca Statement (UNESCO 1994)
		Building teacher capacity through a focus on cooperative learning strategies
2006	Re-visioning for an inclusive, holistic understanding of children's development	New strategic plan launched incorporating a new vision and mission statement
	Children's academic scores were very low – of particular concern was increasingly low oral language ability of children entering school	Systemic support provided by CEO advisors focusing on academic abilities
	Students were disengaged from their learning and their community. High levels of bullying and anti-social, aggressive behaviour in children	Being consistent as a staff (behaviour management programs and intervention)
	Staff under pressure to perform 'better'	
	Doubts start arising about whether the current pedagogy is meeting the needs of our children	
2007	Extremely poor oral language skills of children entering school	Ongoing systemic support provided by CEO advisors focusing on academic abilities
	High levels of bullying and anti-social, aggressive behaviour in children	Work with speech pathologist on developing oral language capacity of children in Prep-2
	Staff under increasing pressure to perform 'better'	
	Increase in staff anxiety and feelings of inadequacy because of continuing low academic test scores	Implementation of the PATHS (Promoting Alternate Thinking Strategies) programme in Prep-6
	Increasing doubts about whether our current pedagogy is meeting the needs of the children. Meeting with Karen Stagnitti on ways to assess children's abilities	Visit to other best-practice schools in Melbourne

2008	Commitment to significant educational change – implementation of a developmental curriculum in Prep	Public commitment to change at a Catholic Zone Education Conference – a key moment for school staff
	Expanding recreational and play opportunities for students	Professional development of Junior Teaching Team
	Giving children choice in pursuing personal interests	Provide a range of elective club activities around children's personal interests
	Continued development of a shared educational vision and pedagogical understandings	Two classrooms embark on implementation of a developmental curriculum
	Meeting with Karen Stagnitti for discussions in preparation for research study	Visit to other best-practice schools in Melbourne/Geelong
		Staff and students adopted six key focus words – imagination, diversity, expression, relationships, reflection, discovery
		Continued professional reading, research, discourse and dialogue
2009	Whole-school approach to a developmentally appropriate curriculum	Implementation of a whole-school approach to a developmentally appropriate curriculum
	The physical, developmentally appropriate learning environment	Establishment of junior, middle and senior learning communities, where teachers plan and work in teams; co-teaching begins
	First research study comparison of children's play, oral language, cognitive development and social connectedness	Change to more holistic assessment and reporting practices
		Increase in complexity of play, social connectedness and oral language documented (Reynolds et al. 2011)
		Continued professional reading, research, discourse and dialogue
2010	Students establishing links to their own local community groups or organisations	Greater involvement with community both in and outside the school
	Aligning religious education practices to be compatible with the school's learning and teaching practices	Co-teaching throughout school

Table 6.1 Continued

Year	Concerns or actions	Changes/action
	Building teacher capacity to personalise the curriculum	Continued professional reading, research, discourse and dialogue
	Training in the Learn to Play (Stagnitti 1998) programme by Karen Stagnitti	Visit to other best-practice schools in Melbourne/Geelong
	Teachers planning and teaching collaboratively	Early Learning Centre redeveloped – from three individual, traditional classrooms into one open, flexible learning space
	Second research study – comparison of children's play, oral language, cognitive development and social connectedness	
2011	School review	Significant data collection, including community consultation with students, staff, parents and parishioners to provide feedback for review panel
	Development of new strategic plan	
	All Year 3–6 students in being connected to and being of service to their community	Introduction of Kaizen student leadership groups
	Further development of student independence and confidence	Even greater involvement with the local community in the life of the school
	Students being self-aware and self-regulating their learning	Students identify their own learning styles
	Home and school working collaboratively to support children's learning	Continued implementation and refinement of a personalised learning approach
		New reporting processes developed
		Continued professional reading, research, discourse and dialogue
		Visit to other best-practice schools in Melbourne/Geelong
		Review data indicated a high level of student engagement with learning in their school and a high level of connectedness to their local community

The rest of this chapter considers in more detail the process that the teachers undertook to bring about a school environment where children became engaged and connected to their community, bringing about a change in the school to achieve a socially inclusive connected environment between students and their community. The specific processes that are addressed are changes made to: core values, personalising the curriculum, use of ICT, voice/empowerment of the students, spirituality, community and co-responsibility, and sharing wisdom. These processes were all considered as the school changed its physical, social and emotional environment.

Core values

Teachers' ongoing professional reading, visits to other schools, professional development activities and challenging professional conversations at staff level resulted in the staff team beginning to develop a deep understanding of how children learn, of how the brain functions and the developmental stages of learning (see Table 6.1, the readings included: Edwards et al. (1998); Stagnitti (1998); Stagnitti and Jellie (2006); Wilson and Murdoch (2006); Sunderland (2007); Walker (2007); Doidge (2010); Planning with Kids (2010)).

Initially, one of the change strategies that staff implemented was to adopt some key words that would focus their efforts and hold them accountable to their vision of having every child socially connected and thriving at school. Along with a new appreciation of their school motto 'Christ is Our Light', the school community soon owned and utilised the energy and focus derived from the following words: imagination, diversity, reflection, discovery, relationships and expression.

As professional readings stimulated their thinking (e.g. Edwards et al. 1998; Beare 2001; Harris Helm and Beneke 2003; Sluss 2005; Stagnitti and Jellie 2006; Wilson and Murdoch 2006; Sunderland 2007; Walker 2007; Robinson 2009, 2011; Stagnitti and Cooper 2009; Doidge 2010), staff developed some basic but deeper shared understandings that informed their teaching practice. These foundational 'key tenets' are a work in progress as staff continue to explore and research best educational practice. Their key tenets are:

- A child assimilates new understanding into an already existing framework.
- Children develop higher order cognitive thinking by engaging with the collective.
- To develop competence, children must have a foundation of factual knowledge and understand this in the light of a conceptual/theoretical framework.
- Children need to be able to self-regulate their learning. This 'meta-cognitive' approach (i.e. thinking about thinking) enables children to realise their natural disposition and modulate it with scaffolded support. So, children need to be encouraged to think through how, what and why they are learning.

It was this theoretical knowledge that empowered staff, and even demanded them to have a paradigm shift in their thinking. The shift was from 'all children learning the same thing in the same way, at the same time with the same teacher in the same place', to 'all children learning from different people in different ways, at different times, in different places, at different rates and for different purposes'.

The staff realised that they needed to change their model of education, the environment and themselves, rather than to persist with forcing the children to change, to adapt, conform and fit in with their existing unchanging teacher-created environment. This change of focus and direction by teachers at St. James saw an almost immediate increase in children's enthusiasm for and engagement in learning, and consequently a huge increase in self-esteem and social connectedness. Many children who previously had a poor self-image now saw themselves as unique, strong, capable and independent contributors, and viewed others as unique and valued members of the community. Children were becoming self-directed independent thinkers and learners but, more importantly, they were realising the importance of thinking and acting interdependently in their school community. They now saw themselves as part of a community. Evidence for these observations was also captured in empirical measurements used in the school, such as the SDQ and the Insight SRC school data; for example, in 2011, only 7 per cent of children (that is 11 children) in the school scored within the borderline/at risk group on the SDQ.

Staff started to realise that the constructivist view of education (see, for example, views espoused by Vygotsky (1966, 1997)), that children construct the knowledge of their world and learn in an environment with competent peers and adults, was more closely aligned to their beliefs. They were keen to find out more about the Reggio Emilia philosophy of education (Edwards et al. 1998), which challenges the widespread view that each child is an empty vessel needing to be filled up with the teacher's wisdom. The Reggio Emilia view holds that children are strong and powerful and competent, creative and curious and rich in potential (Edwards et al. 1998).

At St. James, teachers decided that they really needed to find out and embrace each child's strengths and build on what that child already knew and was interested in discovering next. This also meant transforming the emotional environment so that diversity, and not conformity, was seen as a strength and celebrated. This now meant that all children were listened to, respected and valued for who they were and what they brought to the school community. Each child has a voice, is heard, acknowledged and responded to in a respectful and empowering, personalised way. Each child is also part of something bigger, is part of the collective that is the St. James Parish School learning community.

As well as the emotional environment, the physical environment at St. James has been transformed and is now organised to cater for different learning and working styles. The space is no longer tables and chairs lined up in order, rather each classroom is a space divided into flexible, contemporary and functional learning spaces with plenty of nooks, prompts and supports which promote rich learning and which entice children to explore, create, experiment, consider, theorise and play. Children can move freely throughout all these learning areas and they are taught to tune into and attend to their own physical needs such as food, drinks, exercising and toileting as required throughout the day. This has resulted in children understanding that they are trusted as competent people by teachers.

Children make comments to their teachers about their experience at school, and throughout this chapter some of the children's comments are presented to capture their view on the changes in the school. One of these comments is by Tyson (pseudonym) who is in Year 3. He noted that: 'I like how we get to do projects inside and outside, everywhere in the school. The teachers trust us to learn and to be safe.'

Personalising the curriculum

Personalised learning is tailoring the curriculum and the learning environment to meet the needs of the individual child. Personalised learning at St. James underpins the philosophy and is embedded in everyday teaching and learning. For example, at the beginning of each day children make a plan for their day and develop their own learning goals for the day. Personalised learning at St. James has resulted in children being able to self-regulate, self-select and act independently within the learning environment, without having to have all the materials, resources and equipment provided by the teacher. Children are given a voice in, and ownership of, their learning through making choices and decisions constantly. In this way the staff at St. James have found that children are becoming better decision-makers.

Children assimilate learning into an already existing framework, and so the children at St. James were encouraged to develop their own theories about the world and how it works, through play, projects, contracts (e.g. where a child makes an arrangement with the teacher to complete certain tasks), compulsory and optional workshops (i.e. children enrol themselves within a school workshop on a particular skill, which may be optional – their own interest – or compulsory, where they need to learn skills to meet curriculum requirements), focused teaching (i.e. the teacher gives information to the class), skill development, personal reflection and personal investigations which engage and motivate them. Children with limited skills and knowledge bases are able to join in with the collective through meeting, mixing with and being influenced by more capable peers and adults with whom they make connections to their lives and their world. At St. James, capable adults can be either teachers or members of the community who engage with the school to teach children particular skills (e.g. wood carving). Children become self-directed thinkers and learners. They use initiative, imagination, teamwork, creativity and a broad range of interpersonal skills requiring genuine collaboration. Jenny, in Year 3, notes that: 'I like how we get excited about learning in the passions we like – we do what we are expected to and as we get older we get higher expectations.'

Self-directed thinkers and learners who can collaborate with others are socially connected and independent learners. A research study compared the social connectedness, ability to self-initiate ideas through play, and oral language ability of children attending St. James with a school that maintained a traditional classroom environment. This study by Reynolds et al. (2011) focused on children in their first year of school. They found that children at St. James were significantly more able to self-organise their ideas through play, their play was highly organised and complex, and they were more socially connected than children in the comparison school (Reynolds et al. 2011). The children at St. James were also less socially disruptive to peers and were socially interactive (Reynolds et al. 2011). Interviews with the teachers at each school also confirmed the empirical findings that children at St. James were more self-directed, socially cohesive, and had increased use of language compared with those at the comparison school.

ICT

Today's children live in a world more different from that of past generations than ever before, not least because of technology, which has changed the way in which they are raised and educated. Children are able to interact with and access the world in very different ways than past generations. Effectively using technologies within schools that are available to children out of school should be a key strategy.

Flexible use of contemporary technology as a personalised learning tool enables children to problem solve and engage in relevant learning in this rapidly changing and complex world. Using appropriate hardware and software creatively empowers children to engage with the global society and includes the child as a global citizen, being in and of the world. Technology offers instant, interactive, global and personalised learning in a personalised curriculum. Children are able to flourish through their use of technology in their individual passions, talents and interests. Children are able to self-regulate and self-manage by using meaningful, contemporary and purposeful resources. iPads, iPods, Touch-tables, YouTube, Wikipedia, Weebly, and Skype are just some of the hardware and software that facilitate group interactions where children explore and co-create. Compulsory and optional workshops are run within the school and outside the school by students and adults (i.e. teachers, parents and community members), and these provide opportunities for further capable social peer interaction. Effective use of technology enables children to have a voice which they may not have had without the technology. For example, if only handwriting is allowed to complete a task, then the children with poor motor skills are at risk of not being heard. Creating more personalised and effective use of technologies has the potential to highly stimulate and engage learners as part of a global community.

Voice/empowerment

The children's voices are recognised and listened to, and their leadership skills developed through child-directed and adult-supported student leadership groups named Kaizen groups. Kaizen is a Japanese word meaning 'improvement' or 'change for the better', and staff at St. James have used the concept of Kaizen groups (English and Hill 1994), based on the socially inclusive premise that every child can be a leader and contribute to the overall good in a field that they are sufficiently interested in to take action on. Children in Years 3–6 form teams that are focused on being of service to the school and broader community. Children brainstorm their ideas and discern several areas on which action could be taken. Within the Kaizen groups, a broad range of interests can be catered for, and possible actions could be forthcoming through a focus on social justice, sustainability, construction and maintenance, art and performance, and health and wellbeing.

Parents, staff and children work together to pay attention to what each child is saying, acknowledging that children can indeed help shape and positively influence the world. This empowers children to see themselves as capable of producing positive change and to be included as part of something bigger, the collective. Diversity of thought, talent, skills and understandings can be recognised and celebrated through the collective. The value and importance of interdependent thinking is witnessed in the social interactions of students as they use their diversity of talents to collectively achieve common, worthwhile goals. For example, St. James has an environmental education programme where children work together on environmental issues such as waste minimisation, biodiversity, recycling, animal husbandry and climate change, and children are encouraged to read up and research each of these areas and come up with solutions within the school grounds. Children understand that they have the power for their thoughts to become actions and that they can make a real difference in their world. This is reflected in a comment made by Ella (pseudonym) who is a senior student. She says: 'It's great because we choose areas we're interested in, like sustainability, where we help look after the animals and the veggie gardens.'

Spirituality

Christian beliefs give staff an overarching set of values and understandings which provide them with the foundations upon which they act. Central to student wellbeing is the spiritual/emotional environment, which is based on 'inclusiveness and justice where all children have the right to learn together' (UNESCO 1994).

At St. James, staff recognise that every child has the right to feel whole – to think, to feel, to relate, to act and to make their own meaning. This is at the heart of the school community; it is about the dignity and humanity of each person, so that when a child or a member of staff breaks a bond with someone, they are breaking a bond with their spirit, with their humanity. It is not, therefore, about breaking school rules, it is about breaking relationships. Staff and children work towards repairing and restoring that relationship so that they continue to remain an integral, interconnected part of the collective.

Community and co-responsibility

It takes a village to raise a child.

(African proverb)

At St. James, staff believe that it is the responsibility of the whole community to nurture each child in the school. Parents are their children's first teachers, and a happy healthy home is the best school. St. James staff believe that parents are strong, capable and competent and deeply interested in the welfare and development of their children. Respectful and caring home–school partnerships are key, and are expected and welcomed. Parental involvement in the life of the school is necessary and valued. Parents also contribute their wider community connections to the energy of the school. Grandparents, extended family members and community members in and about the neighbourhood run workshops, mentor children, offer encouragement and stand up for and provide support as the children grow in this very quickly changing world. Teachers and children are out and about a lot more, and are now seen to be an integral part of the local Sebastopol neighbourhood. Increasingly, smaller, more personalised excursions for small groups of children are conducted, making for more meaningful wider community connections for every student. Children and families understand that they belong, and are important, contributing and valued members of the local and wider community.

Teaching staff want their children to be socially aware, appropriately socially connected and know that they have the ability to impact positively on their vision for their world. Staff members are empowering children to create and act upon that vision, teaching the children how to think and how to act on their thinking with actions that lead to making the world better for themselves and for others. The staff have observed that the children are influencing elements of what happens at home and, in some cases, actually teaching their parents how to think. For example, one father came into the school and asked what the teachers were doing. This father continued to explain that when his child Tom (pseudonym) came home from school, Tom insisted on talking to him about school. Tom was so keen about what he was doing at school that when he went home he insisted on including his father in conversations about his interests and school projects. Another example, which many parents comment on with teachers, is that the children talk to their parents about the importance of planning their trips and then, after the trip, reflect on the event with their parents.

Thinking involves language. A second research study, with children in their first year at St. James and children in their first year at a comparison school, explored grammar, vocabulary, and narrative language abilities (Bailey 2010). The study found that, at the beginning of the school year, children at St. James had poorer grammar ability than children at the comparison school. By the end of the school year there was no difference between the grammar skills or vocabulary ability of the children at the two schools, with the children at St. James significantly increasing in their grammar and narrative language ability (Bailey 2010).

Four children from the senior and middle school recently felt that the shelter for the school crossing lady needed a complete renovation. They decided to design a wall painting which showed how the crossing supervisor connected St. James students to different parts of the Sebastopol community. Undaunted by the local council's previous refusal to improve or replace the shelter, the children wrote a letter to Ballarat City Council explaining their concerns about the condition of the shelter and also stating that their gift of enhancing the shelter was their way to thank Heather for her many years of hard work and support. They are still anxiously awaiting council's reply!

Sharing wisdom

Leadership in the St. James school community is based on the 'shared wisdom' philosophy. This means that all members are listened to and their knowledge and wisdom are valued and welcomed. Decentralised and inclusive networks, built on a spirit of collegiality and collaboration, work on short- and long-term projects with people sharing key responsibilities and collective ownership. Children, parents and staff are all included as part of these networks, and each person has the right to be heard and the responsibility to speak. These networks promote the importance of building and maintaining healthy relationships so that the interconnected community is flourishing. This richness of individual community members' unique talents and contributions has enabled the passions and abilities of everyone to shine. This philosophy of shared wisdom creates, in practice, a sense of welcome, belonging and ownership.

Case study

Matthew (pseudonym) was 10 years old when he arrived at St. James. He had been expelled from two previous schools, and when he arrived at St. James he was not happy to be at another school. Matthew was different. He was loud, had quirky ideas, and was dramatic. However, at St. James diversity is valued, and over time Matthew realised that at St. James, his loudness, quirky ideas and dressing up the dramatic were embraced. He was accepted, embraced and valued by the group. After two further years at St. James, Matthew had become a productive, contributing member of his class and the school. He saw himself as valued and as an important contributing member of his community. He was socially connected, happy, and contributed to the larger group.

Conclusion

This chapter has examined the process that brought about this enormous shift from a school where children were not socially connected to a school where children wanted to belong. The hard data from the school reflect this change as well. For example, in 2011, 167 students were enrolled at the school, and of these there were four children with high behavioural needs. During the 5 years from 2007 to 2011, students' sense of wellbeing has risen to approximately the 80th percentile on the Insight SRC data, while student misbehaviour is now around the 20th percentile. In addition to the hard data, other observations of children's behaviour reflect a greater commitment by them to the social community. There is now a respect for each other and each other's tools (e.g. pencils, rulers, scissors), with children looking after their equipment and returning equipment so other children can use it. There is a decrease in truancy, and an increase in engagement through school, with parents coming into the school to talk to teachers. Children now understand and respect social cues and social contexts. For example, when I (first author) first visited the school, I was sitting in a circle with the other authors of this chapter. We were sitting in an empty classroom as the children were having a lesson in the library. The bell rang. Children came to the door, saw us, quietly walked in around us, got their belongings and left. After the children had left, it was pointed out to me that if this situation had occurred the year before (before the changes were implemented) the children would have rushed into the room, walked through our conversation 'circle', talked loudly, and then rushed out. The children now understood that, when you sit in a circle, you are having a conversation, and this needs to be respected. So, you do not walk through the conversation 'circle', you are quiet, you get your belongings and leave. This demonstrated the huge social shifts that had begun in this school and have continued since that first meeting.

Broader implications

There are practical things that schools and teachers can do to increase social inclusion of the children and families within the school community and wider community, but the most important thing required is the paradigm shift in the teachers' thinking. It is a passion for possibilities; what contemporary education can really look like, and the impact this can have for every child and his or her place in the world. Some key shifts that bring about change are summarised in Table 6.2.

Good educational practice has the power to unearth every child's potential, to enable them to find their niche in life so that they see themselves as valuable, thinking, contributing members of a society, and that society can be enhanced through their actions.

Table 6.2 Key shifts required for whole-school change

Adults – teachers

- Whole-staff understanding of and commitment to the school's contemporary learning and teaching philosophy
- Teachers' image of the child as strong, capable and competent, curious and creative. Staff need to recognise and build on children's existing conceptual understandings (constructivism)
- Like-minded teachers who are passionate about children and their learning
- Collaborative teaching teams

Adults – teachers and parents

- Student–parent–teacher connectedness

Children

- Children being self-aware and having the ability to make their own decisions
- Creating a student-focused, empowering learning environment
- An environment that shows that children are valued and respected
- Children sharing their learning through whole-school gatherings and expositions where students organise, prepare and present their projects to the wider school community

Physical environment

- Flexible, purposeful, stimulating learning spaces
- Contemporary and functional learning spaces
- That is, spaces where rows of desks and chairs are no longer suitable for socially interactive learning spaces

Emotional environment

- A place of welcome where diversity is celebrated, and where interdependence is the key to social inclusion
- A school-wide commitment to respectful relationships
- An environment where everyone feels safe to be who they are, to take risks and to learn without intimidation

7 Inclusive service design for young people with learning disabilities who exhibit behaviours of concern

Sophie Goldingay and Karen Stagnitti

Introduction

Service providers across the globe have reported increasingly disturbed behaviour and conduct problems among young people (Hickie et al. 2005; Sainsbury Centre for Mental Health 2009). In the UK, the number of 15–16 year olds with conduct problems at the more severe end of the scale more than doubled between 1974 and 1999 (Collishaw et al. 2004). In many cases, young people are subject to restrictive interventions such as imprisonment or compulsory treatments in order to control what are termed 'behaviours of concern' (DHS 2010b). Such behaviours of concern may include aggression and self-harm (including substance abuse) and crime. This chapter is concerned with considering the needs of children and young people between the ages of 10 and 17 years who have learning disabilities, and who have been identified as having problematic behaviours.

Ongoing incidents of disturbed behaviour and conduct problems among young people are likely to restrict social inclusion for those affected. For example, problematic behaviours in childhood have been strongly associated with unemployment, poor educational outcomes, low earnings, job insecurity, marital problems and criminal activity (Sainsbury Centre for Mental Health 2009). In addition, receipt of restrictive interventions such as imprisonment and compulsory treatment, including hospitalisation and medication, is also likely to impair social inclusion for young people due to stigma, social alienation, impaired access to education, or, in the case of medication, reduced cognitive or adaptive functioning (DHS 2010b: 16).

Causes of problematic behaviours are likely to be complex and multidimensional, and thus this chapter is not advocating a simple cure. Rather the chapter aims to consider one group of children and young people aged 10–17 years, exhibiting behaviours of concern, who may be particularly vulnerable to adverse outcomes, and explore service designs that could be more inclusive of them. The group of young people this chapter considers is those with learning disability. 'Learning disability' is a broad term that can encompass a range of neuropsychological disabilities such as foetal alcohol spectrum disorder (FASD), acquired brain injury (ABI) and autistic spectrum disorders (ASD). ABI can be the result of a traumatic brain injury, chronic use of alcohol or illicit substances, or lack of oxygen to the brain (Jackson et al. 2011), sometimes as a result of suicide attempts (Andover et al. 2011). While intellectual disability may be a factor in having a learning disability, this chapter is concerned with those whose Intelligence Quotient (IQ) is 70 and higher.

The chapter will begin by discussing the impact of learning disabilities on young peoples' ability to receive therapeutic benefit from standard therapies and will estimate the prevalence of these disabilities based on data from adult prison populations. It will then consider the impact of learning disabilities on problematic behaviour and overall functioning. An alternative approach to assessment and treatment will then be discussed based on evidence showing the efficacy of pretend play to improve the ability to solve problems, manage impulsivity, and form and sustain social relationships with others. The chapter aims to be specifically inclusive of the needs of young people with learning disabilities who exhibit behaviours of concern and are in receipt of restrictive interventions as discussed above.

Impact on effectivness of standard treatment programmes

Learning disabilities as a result of ABI, ASD and FASD are likely to impair neuropsychological functioning (Andover et al. 2011) and may be particularly widespread amongst those receiving restrictive interventions such as imprisonment. A study of prisoners in the USA revealed that a large proportion of participants had impairments in neuropsychological functioning. Consequently, prisoners were frequently unable to process and act on the complex cognitive concepts addressed in therapy, and hence interventions which had the aim of behaviour modification tended to be ineffective (Andover et al. 2011). While this study was with adults in custody, people in younger age groups with a learning disability also experience similar difficulties with processing and acting on complex cognitive concepts in therapy, such as the ability to process higher level thinking such as planning, problem solving and working out strategies to solve problems.

A similar prevalence of ABI, ASD and FASD may similarly affect the efficacy of current treatments for young people who display behaviours of concern and are in receipt of restrictive interventions. The number of young people with such disabilities who are in youth justice or mental health facilities is unknown, however, as neuropsychological functioning processes are not routinely assessed. A study with adults conducted by the Department of Justice in the state of Victoria, Australia, identified that 42 per cent of male prisoners and 33 per cent of female prisoners had an ABI, whereas the prevalence in the general population is 2 per cent – demonstrating a substantial overrepresentation of those with ABI in Victorian prisons (Jackson et al. 2011).

Impact of learning disability on problematic behaviour

We will now consider in more detail the functional issues that young people with learning disabilities such ABI, ASD, and FASD experience, which may impact on problematic behaviour.

Young people with acquired brain injury

A wide range of neuropsychological functions can be disrupted as a consequence of an ABI, such as perceptual motor skills, behaviour, attention, working memory, sequencing, problem solving, language, reading comprehension,
auditory processing and learning capacity (Ewing-Cobbs et al. 2003; Catroppa
et al. 2009). ABI with frontal lobe impairment impacts on social communication, including impulsivity, initiation, disinhibition, self-regulation and social
imperceptions. It also impairs the ability to learn from consequences (MacDonald and Wiseman-Hakes 2010: 497–8). As a result of these disruptions to the
normal development of neuropsychological functions, educational performance
(Catroppa et al. 2009; Lewis and Murdoch 2011), building social relationships,
and engaging in appropriate activities with peers, such as play or leisure, can be
difficult for people with ABI (Bedell and Dumas 2004; Galvin et al. 2010).

Young people with autism spectrum disorder

People with ASD are diagnosed on the basis of communication, and social
and imaginative play impairments (Lawson 2006). Explanations of difficulties
within these areas are based on mind theories (Baron-Cohen 1996; Hughes and
Leekam 2004), as well as newer theories such as single attention and associated
cognition in autism (Lawson 2006, 2010). Lawson (2006, 2010) proposes that
people with autism have single attention, which leads to highly focused interests, and as a result they have difficulty with non-literality and find it difficult to
think 'outside the box'. For example, they have difficulty connecting ideas or
concepts, unless they are very interested in the topic. Within a social context,
this makes it difficult to relate without schedules and refocus after being inter-
rupted (Lawson 2006). Thus, people with autism miss the subtle cues of social
interaction, and are poor at social problem solving. Their behaviour can be
misinterpreted as rude and inappropriate in social situations. In addition, people
with autism have difficulties with attention, language and memory, as well as
problems with predictive thinking (Hagland 2009).

Young people with foetal alcohol spectrum disorder

FASD includes a spectrum of conditions including prenatal alcohol exposure.
FASD is associated with neuropsychological issues including language, memory, motor functions, hearing, visual processing, attention, and resulting problematic behaviour (Cone-Wesson 2005; Henry et al. 2007). There are likely to
be problems with longer reaction/decision times, problem solving, attention,
planning, strategy use and working memory (Green et al. 2008). There are
also likely to be problems with social-information processing, which includes
understanding what is happening in a social interaction, such as the meaning
of facial expressions, innuendo, and verbal and non-verbal behaviour (McGee
et al. 2009). Henry et al. (2007: 106) suggest that 'etiologies of challenging

behaviours are rooted in poor executive functioning, cognitive inflexibility, limited social communication, deficits in language processing, and affect dysregulation'. They recommend that the neuropsychological impact of FASD be recognised, and that intervention strategies need to take into account the individual's need for support in learning new skills.

Common links

From this brief discussion of the functional issues experienced by people with ABI, ASD and FASD, common links in neuropsychological disruption associated with these conditions can be identified. These include communication and problem solving, leading to inappropriate or problematic behaviour, and difficulties in attention, memory and social-information processing. Difficulties in these areas have implications for social inclusion due to possible rejection by peers, partners, teachers and employers.

In addition, information processing, problem solving, attention and memory problems caused by these conditions affect young people's ability to process, and act on, concepts used in standard therapies such as cognitive behavioural therapy (CBT). CBT is the treatment of choice across many services in Australia for young people with problematic behaviours (Day et al. 2003). In a similar way (see the prison study with adults by Andover and colleagues discussed earlier in this chapter), CBT is likely to be similarly ineffective in young people with neuropsychological impairments, due to difficulties in attention, problem solving, social-information processing, language and memory (Hagland 2009).

A brief search of the evidence base supporting the efficacy of CBT in young people with mental health problems confirmed that all trials excluded several groups of young people. For example, Gaynor et al. (2003) excluded those who did not complete eight or more sessions of CBT. Westra et al. (2007) similarly excluded those who did not complete CBT self-directed homework tasks or attend all the group sessions. Kennard et al. (2009) excluded those young people with diagnoses of bipolar disorder, autism, eating disorders, substance abuse and females who were pregnant, breast-feeding or not using reliable contraception.

Thus, those young people who have difficulty with planning, attention, problem solving and predictive thinking (i.e. those with neuropsychological disabilities) would be, to a large part, excluded from trials attesting to the efficacy of CBT for young people. Attending courses and completing homework tasks on one's own requires planning, attention, memory, problem solving and consequential thinking skills that neuro-typical people may take for granted. The absence of these may present significant challenges for those with neuropsychological functioning problems, and prevent them from engaging with and benefiting from CBT.

Therefore, alternative approaches that are able to take into account and address the cause of these difficulties can constitute an inclusive approach to service design for those with learning disabilities.

Difficulties in social-information processing, problem solving and language in middle school, adolescence and beyond can be linked to a poor ability to pretend during play in childhood (Peter 2003; Stagnitti 2004). There has been little research in the early play experiences of people with ABI, ASD and FASD, particularly for those with ABI and FASD, as most research in early play experiences has been carried out with children with autism (see, for example, Jarrold et al. 1993). Pretend play during childhood is significant throughout life because, to engage in pretend play, children are required to understand the social context, the roles of other players, the functions of the toys and props, and the meaning within the play (Peter 2003; Stagnitti 2009), as well as use the language associated with that particular play scene (Westby 2000). To pretend in play requires the child to logically sequence and order their play actions (Stagnitti 2009), problem solve and negotiate with peers (Peter 2003), and build on other children's ideas (Whitington and Floyd 2009). All these tasks require flexibility and adaptability in play. A link has been demonstrated between the ability to pretend in play during childhood and the ability to understand the motives and beliefs of others, i.e. social perception (Harris 1994; Baron-Cohen 1996).

Seen in this light, pretend play incorporates many skills that are foundational for social competence, emotional understanding (visceral empathy) and cognitive processes, such a logical sequential thought and predictive thinking. The implications for social competence and flexible and lateral thinking in later life as a result of failure to develop these skills in childhood are often underestimated. As such there is very little literature available at present that acknowledges this connection. The following discussion will therefore include evidence relating to pretend play ability in children and social competence. An example of implications of this for young people will also be discussed in this section of the chapter.

Evidence has linked the ability to pretend in play with positive outcomes in children's development. For example, children who are competent in pretend play have been found to be socially competent with peers (Lindsey and Colwell 2003; Uren and Stagnitti 2009). Pretend play ability has been strongly linked with creative problem solving ability, affect regulation and adaptability (Seja and Russ 1999; Wyver and Spence 1999; Russ 2003), self-regulation (Nicolopoulou et al. 2010) and language (Westby 1991; McCune 1995). Role playing in pretend play develops these competencies as a meaningful context is created to practice negotiation, and explore nuances of social situations. It also engages children in problem solving and negotiation of power relations, including how to obtain help and support from peers and supportive adults.

Göncü and Perone (2005) suggest that pretend play is a life-span activity, and use an example of improvisation (which assumes the adult has developed the ability to 'play out' a situation within a theatre script) to explore affect regulation within adulthood. Göncü and Perone's article is the only article that links skills learnt through engagement in pretend play to skills present in adulthood. This chapter argues that if children have failed to engage in pretend play in childhood, and as a result did not develop skills such as negotiation of power relations, flexible and predictive thinking, problem solving, and understanding of the nuances of social situations, they will not develop them in adolescence or adulthood unless there is targeted intervention. We contend that a more inclusive service design for young people with a learning disability should therefore build skills related to pretend play that these young people have never developed.

Anecdotal evidence with a group of unemployed teenagers aged 16–18 years in a regional Victorian town showed that a trial of activities based on pretend play skills such as role play and thinking of alternative uses for objects, proved too challenging for group participants. This indicates the need to investigate how to unpack the scaffolding required for young people to develop these skills. This raises the issue of whether adolescents can learn skills missed at key developmental stages. Some literature (e.g. Doidge 2010) discusses critical periods in development where learning is maximised and children are most receptive to picking up particular skills (e.g. language, social competence). We recognise that young people aged 10–17 are likely to have passed the critical period for developing social competence, problem solving and flexible and predictive thinking. We therefore cannot overestimate the difficulty young people with learning disabilities such as ASD, FASD and ABI will experience and the degree of scaffolding required during intervention to enable participants to develop in these areas.

An inclusive approach to service design for young people with learning disabilities who have behaviours of concern and are receiving restrictive interventions will therefore address skills that have not have been fully developed in childhood. Both the assessment and intervention programme will be based on the principles of pretend play ability, and its design takes into account neuropsychological difficulties and their impacts on learning and behaviour modification.

Assessment

Assessments will begin by testing associative fluency (Wallach and Kogan 1965). These tests measure a participant's ability in lateral thinking, flexibility and symbolic thinking. In order to determine a young person's ability to quickly understand the perspective of others and how characters interact, they will be asked to set up a movie scene and incorporate characters, roles and a short script (measuring social perception). They will then be given a problem solving task. The assessment itself is straightforward and researchers or clinicians learning to administer the assessment will require only a one-hour training session. The equipment required is simple and includes movie-making equipment, such as cameras and props, and a social skills assessment package which can be purchased online from http://www.pearsonclinical.com.au./productdetails/340. The ease of administration and simplicity of the props means this assessment could be used on a wider scale. The inclusion of these assessments will add to our understanding of the thinking processes of people with learning disabilities. They are a departure from what has traditionally been measured within these population groups, as assessments for ASD, ABI and FASD are typically stand-ardised intelligence testing and tests of working memory, attention and ability to plan and regulate behaviour (executive function).

Intervention

An intervention strategy for the group of young people with low scores in the above assessments can be developed based on the principles of pretend play. The intervention will embed common social problem solving within a playful interactive setting and meaningful context so that, while these skills are required, they are not explicitly focused upon. The purpose of intervention would be to assist young people to address factors contributing to their prob-lematic behaviours, including impulse control and social alienation, through improving predictive and flexible thinking and social competence.

Early evidence for intervention for children with ASD based on building up their ability in pretend play has been found to increase a child's social skills and language (Wolfberg and Schuler 1993; Stagnitti 2004; O'Connor and Stagnitti 2011). Interventions for people with ABI suggest that self-regula-tion, self-awareness and social perception are the problem, rather than social skills knowledge (MacDonald and Wiseman-Hakes 2010). Interventions that were reviewed by MacDonald and Wiseman-Hakes included only five stud-ies for children and adolescents aged 0–19 years. Many of the interventions reviewed had social competencies separated from language or communica-tion interventions. The intervention proposed here includes practice in social understanding, language and communication, and represents a new way of assisting young people with behaviours of concern who may have learning disabilities.

There is no literature looking at the common links in function between ASD, ABI and FASD, and very limited information on the early pretend play of people diagnosed with FASD or ABI. Therefore, a trial and evalu-ation of the effectiveness of the proposed assessment and intervention will add to the current knowledge about these conditions and may help to guide further service design for those receiving restrictive interventions, as well as interventions for young people who are currently exhibiting behaviours of concern who have not yet come to the attention of the youth justice or mental health services.

Thus, our proposed intervention for young people exhibiting behaviours of concern, and who have learning disabilities, is grounded in the understanding that early pretend play ability is important for meta-cognitive development because pretend play involves ability in social competence, language, prob-lem solving and affect regulation (self-regulation). Deficits in these abilities have been shown to be associated with social alienation, poor problem solving and difficulties in self-regulation. These factors contribute to problematic behaviours and, for some, there is a possibility that these will lead to receipt of restrictive interventions.

As mentioned earlier, social competence, social alienation and difficulties in self- regulation are also unlikely to be addressed by standard therapies such as CBT, as these rely on language competencies and the ability to understand, attend to, and remember complex concepts and think predictively and sequentially (Hagland 2009). We contend that by breaking down these skills within a playful interactive setting, young people with ASD, ABI and FASD would be given a safe environment that creates a real-world situation in which to build foundational skills that, we argue, were not fully developed during childhood due to neuropsychological dysfunction such as that created by having an ABI, FASD or ASD. This approach to intervention is in line with the evidence gathered so far on interventions that are most likely to be effective (MacDonald and Wiseman-Hakes 2010).

Wider implications

We suggest that, initially, the programme be trialled with young people who are already receiving restrictive interventions and in whom standard therapies have not been helpful in modifying their problematic behaviours. We anticipate the trial to lead to deeper and more widespread understanding of the thinking processes of young people with learning disabilities. Such understandings could lead to earlier detection of the need for similar interventions based on pretend play, for those who have not yet come to the attention of restrictive intervention services delivered by youth justice or mental health providers. We anticipate that play-based assessments and interventions could be used in a variety of settings for young people with learning disabilities, especially schools, where teachers may be alerted to issues of social alienation.

This chapter has discussed the difficulties young people with learning disabilities may face with language, information processing, attention and memory problems, and has linked this to the difficulty of gaining benefit from standard therapies. We have also discussed the situation for those young people with learning disabilities who exhibit behaviours of concern, the increasing number of young people coming to the attention of mental health and youth justice services, and the negative effect of receipt of restrictive interventions. We have suggested that one way of practising social inclusion for this group is to design treatment programmes based on pretend play, as evidence has shown its efficacy in assisting young people to develop self-regulation, self-awareness and social perception, not just social skills knowledge.

Thus, the proposed programme would address key sources of difficulty in a manner which young people with learning disabilities can engage with, and gain benefit from. A more widespread application of assessments and treatments based on pretend play for those young people with learning disabilities who are not receiving restrictive interventions is possible through schools or other institutions as well. Assessments and treatments based on pretend play could enable those young people exhibiting signs of problems with social competence, language, and problem solving to receive alternative interventions before coming to the attention of restrictive intervention services.

Part IV

Practising inclusion in service delivery

8 Working for connection and inclusion

The role of front-line practitioners in strengthening the relational base of maginalized clients

Mark Furlong

Introduction

Although this chapter is relevant to managers and policy workers, researchers and supervisory staff, it is especially designed for front-line practitioners – for those who are outreach workers and occupational therapists, counsellors and case managers, advocates and community nurses. The premise of what follows is simple: no matter what the role or profession of origin, each person in the service system has some power to assist clients become better connected and less excluded. Although unlikely to be a core demand of the professional's role, this aim can be advanced insofar as the practitioner understands, and then undertakes, everyday practice in ways that recognise, and seek to catalyse, the client's links with their meaningful others.

Alternatively, practitioners can fail to acknowledge the importance of the client's symbolic and practical interdependencies. This positioning has as its inadvertent effect that these linkages are neglected, attenuated or even antagonised. As practitioners we always act in relation to promoting or diminishing the client's prospects for connectedness, regardless of whether we are aware our contact with the client has such an impact. Although it may seem counterintuitive, it is not possible for practitioners to be truly neutral in relation to the client's personal relationships (Furlong 2010).

This chapter summarises, and gives specific examples to illustrate, how those in direct practice roles can advance a social connection agenda. Although this aim is rarely central in how such roles are conceptualised, funded or evaluated it is argued that there is always a degree of discretion in how the practitioner undertakes their everyday tasks. This distinction – between the formal goals of practice and the creativity the professional can utilise in implementing these goals – offers a potential space within which the client can be prompted towards a good-enough quality of social connection.

That a good-enough quality of social connection is fundamental to health and wellbeing is well-established (Berkman and Glass 2000; Wilkinson and Marmot 2003; Cacioppo and Patrick 2008; Wilkinson and Pickett 2009). Similarly, it has been concluded that social exclusion is associated with significant risks to self-image, health and wellbeing (Taket et al. 2009a). The literature on the social determinants of health and social exclusion informs the current exercise, as does the investigation of the 'the process of individualisation' (Bauman 2001, 2003; Howard 2007). This process has multiple dimensions, but fundamentally concerns the delegation of responsibility to the individual for their health and the realisation of their life project, including the demand to calculate unsentimentally the benefits and costs of their personal relationships. These sources are the background to, rather than the focus of, what is put forward.

The material in this chapter has been developed from more than 20 years of clinical practice combined with an extensive background in multidisciplinary consultation and training. Practical ideas will be introduced that can be used by a broad range of practitioners to promote the social connection of those with whom they work. Such people may be formal clients in fields like mental health or substance abuse, homelessness or disability. Alternatively, these people may be deemed vulnerable or at risk, such as those with diverse sexualities in schools, those who are immigrants or refugees, or those who are unemployed. Although it is not formally correct, whether or not the person with whom the professional has contact is officially registered as a 'client', for the current purpose this term will be used in order to simplify the language which is used.

Two specific practices which can be undertaken at the 'locally social' level (Furlong 2009) are described. The first concerns the practice of understanding, and actively relating to, each client as a relational, social being. Addressing the client in this manner involves making it a policy to hail the qualities of interdependence and personal accountability in the client–worker dialogue. A composite case study – Sam – has been constructed from three real-life practice examples and is used to animate this possibility.

The second practice outlined concerns the possibilities of working systemically with individuals with a special focus on how constructive decisions can be made with respect to convening multi-party discussions, for example between a client and an estranged significant other or prospective significant other. Using the same case study introduced earlier, some examination is offered of the process of making complex convening decisions.

Locating the approach

If, as it is often claimed, it takes a whole village to raise a single child, what array of attachments, exchanges and obligations are required to maintain an ordinary adult? Presumably, what is required is an ensemble of reciprocities of a similar complexity and reliability. The nature of adult interdependence may be as fundamental, if not configured in exactly the same way, as that of a child, but an awareness of the importance of adult sociality has been masked, hidden in plain sight, by the iconising of autonomy and choice in popular culture. Leaving theoretical concerns to one side, in practice even one good-quality personal relationship can make a great deal of difference, especially to a person who is unrecognised and alone.

The client's linkages with meaningful others can be considered temporally: those in the present, in the past and/or in the future. That is, the practitioner can make it their business to find out about the quality and number of the client's current relationships. The practitioner may also consider the client's prospective relationships. There may also be the option of keeping an ear out for specific relationships the client has had in the past. Such bonds may appear to be latent but, at times, can be creatively revived. Additionally, sensitive practitioners can be interested in, and find ways to have the client access, timeless relationships – those symbolic departed 'good objects' that nearly everyone has, to some extent, internalised: the aunt who always had a kind word, the teacher who was encouraging or the neighbour (or professional) who maintained their faith.

Insofar as practitioners can 'smell the spring on a smoggy wind' (Mac-Coll 1949) in imaginatively entering the client's relational life-space, we are set up to incite social connection and inclusion. However, unless one is in a community development role, a great deal of professional acculturation and organisational momentum encourages practitioners to have a suspicious attitude towards the clients' associates and relatives. This is not the occasion to tease out this contention, but the reader is asked to reflect how frequently the clients' significant others are framed to appear uncaring and/or exploitative, unsupportive or absent. Of course, the possibility of abuse has to be recognised, but it is not a good pre-condition for relationship building for the practitioner to start with a suspicious mindset towards those who have, or might have, a meaningful role in the client's life. On the contrary, it is more sensible to be primed to recognise the actuality of, and the potential for, loyalty and affection *by and towards* the client. An attitude of respect and optimism towards the possibilities of connectedness positions the practitioner far more effectively than does scepticism.

In summary, the starting point of what follows is simple: even if clients are conferred a full set of benefits and rights, and/or receive the best credentialed, most evidence-based clinical interventions, this will not secure an enduringly positive outcome if the client is not embedded in a good enough mix of relationships. The voice of authority may not traditionally stress the importance of sustainable interdependencies in how practice has been articulated, but practitioners can know better. Third-party funding bodies, peer review conventions and line management may narrowly define preferred methods and measures of outcome, as they must, yet almost every practitioner intuitively knows that being an isolate in your own land is merely to subsist. People may have money, may even have a secure house and have their rights guaranteed but, as Epicurus said approximately 2500 years ago, 'of all the things that wisdom provides to help one live one's life in happiness, the greatest by far is the possession of friendship' (as quoted in Russell 2005).

No professional group has a monopoly on the knowledge or skills that are relevant to strengthening the client's relational base. To think otherwise would be to miss the point.

Addressing the client as a relational being

The presenting problem is rarely loneliness or the desire to relate better with others. More likely, there is a major issue, such as depression or homelessness, a parole condition or the sequelae of an accident. With increasing frequency, there is also the scenario where the client presents with a complex mix of problems which are difficult to disaggregate and prioritise (Keene 2001). Because the practitioner's role is their point of contact with the client, in either case it is inappropriate to launch a different project for which there is neither agreement nor mandate. This made clear, the relationality of the client can be recognised and accentuated in the process and pattern of everyday practice without the matter of personal relationships ever becoming the central, or even a particular, item in the business that is conducted. How might this complementary purpose be achieved?

The simplest way the practitioner can invoke the relationality of the client is to address this person as a relational being. This can be done directly or more implicitly. In its direct iteration the practitioner can voice and bring to attention one or more of the people who make up the client's circle of significant others and to make tangible the client's connection with this named person or persons. Without it overtaking the primary business of the contact, this 'people-ing' of the dialogue with a client enacts an interactional ontology.

In the following vignette 'Sam', who lives alone, is 33 years old and has become unemployed after being made redundant from a telemarketing company 8 weeks ago. Imagine the practitioner is employed in a primary mental health team, a service to which Sam has been referred by a general practitioner, with a provisional diagnosis of depression. As an item, but not a thread, in the initial discussion the practitioner can ask 'interventive questions' (Tomm 1988) such as:

- 'Sam, who is the person you see as most concerned with your depression?'
- 'You have told me you are feeling really alone. Who would you like to be active and caring about you?'
- 'Just about everyone who feels very down gets at least a little preoccupied with themselves. Do you think this might be happening to you in that you are finding you are temporarily less sensitive to, and cooperative towards, those who have been close to you?'

Under some conditions such enquires lead to conversational strings. Such lines of thought – themes – *may* be reintroduced, elaborated and embedded in different ways at different times. Even if there is no apparent continuity, no seeding effect, in this deliberate citing of sociality the client is constructed as a relational, rather than exclusively autonomous, entity. Simply identifying, and then voicing, the names of one or more of those who constitute the client's circle of significant others recognises, and to a degree honours, the primacy of interdependence.

Taking an allied tack, the practitioner can introduce the idea of thoughtfulness towards others. This is a key attribute in effective relating and is endangered when clients experience so much ostracism and injustice that they become defensive and self-preoccupied. For example, a practitioner might say:

Practitioner:	When you get a chance to stop and think, who is it in your mob (circle; ecology; network; group home; extended family, etc.) that you are most worried about?
Sam:	That's such a big question. I get really worried about Mum, but there is also my ex who I kind of dumped who has hit the skids. Yeah, but mostly it's an old friend Zig who I hardly ever see. When I tell you my life is going down the chute, well that's nothing to the on-and-on bad luck that has cursed her.

Depending on the circumstances, it may be reasonable to take this enquiry further:

Practitioner:	If you decided to do something, to go into bat for Zig, what are the options? Might it be best to make a point of calling Zig, or dropping in, and having a friendly word? You know, find a way to show your soft side. Maybe, you could tell Zig how important their life is to you. Or, what about dropping in a little unexpected treat or present? Hey, maybe the simplest thing is to just say soft and clear that "Zig, I have long appreciated you and, right now, am really worried about you." What's your style of showing you are on Zig's side?'

Addressing the client as a relational being entrains dynamic possibilities. This potency can be theorised within several traditions, most obviously symbolic interactionism (Blumer 1986) and narrative theory (White 2007). It is also possible to view the action of addressing the client as an interpersonal being as an 'interpellation.' This idea is taken from the Marxist theoretician Louis Althusser (2006) who contended that when a policeman calls out 'Hey you' as you walk along the street, and you turn around and you pause, in that instant you have been 'made' to be one-down to that symbol of authority and the regime this officer represents. That is, as originally conceived, an interpellation is a verbal command that, if responded to, reconstitutes the status of the person to that of a subservient subject.

In the current work it is understood that the practitioner is also an authority figure, albeit one with a more ambiguous role, who has no choice but to be always summoning particular identities in their exchanges with clients. As such, the practitioner can pick up on, and/or introduce, frames such as reputation and respect, embarrassment and manners, which are inherently concerned with the immanence of being-in-relation. One might talk with a client about, say, the reputation they would prefer to have and, if the preconditions are there, to discuss with the client what they might do to win the reputation they wish to secure. Such a course of action might, for example, include reparation. While apparently abstract, such discussions can quickly become animated in ways where both feeling and behaviour are entwined.

In discussions with Sam, the unemployed person who is being seen because of a diagnosis of depression, *en passant* the practitioner could ask/say:

> For sure, you are seeing things as very stuck at the moment, that nothing can really change – except for the worse. As I say 'depression lies', it warps our vision. But, over some time you'll make up your own mind on that one. What I want to ask you now, and it might sound a bit crazy, is this: down the track, if you do find yourself pulling through this shit-full stage whose respect would you be most likely to win? And, a slightly different question goes along with this too: whose respect would you most want to gain?

Another approach could take the following form:

> People with a mental health issue, like people who are out of work, often feel embarrassed, even shamed. Are there any particular faces that you think are looking down at you, or would look down at you if they knew about your troubles?

There are so many themes that draw out the connectedness of people. Discussion around, even merely mentioning, the importance of appreciating the other can be supportively challenging.

> Maybe it's all too rare, but I bet you have found when, out of the blue, you get a word of thanks or praise, approval or appreciation, your heart swells? Turning this around and looking out and not in, are you aware how powerfully you can have an impact on someone who is, or might be, special to you when you yourself act this way?

If used with timing and taste, 'heavy' concepts – such as reparation and obligation, guilt and remorse – can also be introduced. Seeding the interpersonally literate might only be 2 per cent of the content of a contact, but it can be telling. The two approaches mentioned – the simply direct or the more carefully indirect – should not be confused with 'small talk', that cursory 'How are the kids?' kind of politeness. Rather, there can be a dividend, a more or less immediate pay-off, in raising, having an ear for and then following up examples of the client's connectedness in practitioner–client interactions. Honouring the intimate, and the conflictual, is not to engage in gossip or arid courtesies.

Currently, many practitioners assume it is neutral to privilege autonomy, self-determination, confidentiality, an internal locus of control, choice, and so forth, as if these goals were both self-evident and non-arbitrary. On the contrary, these values, or as discursive theorists say these 'specifications for the self' (Rose 1998), are highly contingent historically, culturally and ideologically. One view is to judge these as 'male-stream' (O'Brien 1981), neoliberal preferences (Furlong 2010). Rather than privileging any one aspect, it seems more healthy that practitioners seek to summon a balance of moments between the autonomous and the relational aspects of selfhood (Paterson 1996).

In talking around themes such as respect and reputation, and in being interested enough to ask clients about their contacts with meaningful others, there is the chance to dynamically construct the client as a relational being (Furlong 2013). This is in contrast to encounters where the client is reproduced as a unitary and amoral agent, as someone whose key business is to be a product of the process of individualisation. It seems natural to those acculturated by this process to believe that 'I must be in charge of my life', that 'I am the boss of me', that 'I must make the most of my opportunities', and so forth (Rose 1989; 1999). Yet, being caught up in this line of thinking can be self-defeating, as the horizon of awareness then becomes bounded by the 'I', Like a dog chasing its tail, the more self-absorbed, the more likely it is that a person becomes, or remains, isolated.

Professional practice is, inadvertently, closely aligned with the above project. In traditional arrangements practitioners function within a language and convention set that positions the client as a solo figure who is separate to, and who acts upon, an inert background. Rather than understand this background as a passive setting, it is possible for the practitioner to animate this background and to co-create it as a spirited environment that is diversely populated and which requires moral responses. To a degree this can be aided if practitioners re-purpose the original meaning of the term 'interpellation' by mindfully interpersonalising the life of the client.

In one sense this is a simple practice, but to do so is contrary to many of the received customs of professional training, organisational practice and the ideology of popular culture. What is characteristic of the 'psy professions' (Rose 1999) – psychology, psychiatry and psychotherapy – is to privilege the neoliberal values of autonomy, self-determination and choice. Similarly, these values hum at the core of professional training in nursing, allied health and social work. Enacted in the formalities and informalities of everyday practice these values construct the client as a sovereign self. Organisational factors, and other institutional patterns, such as the private practitioner's arrangements with third-party funding bodies, reinforce the same bias. 'Cases' are allocated, reviewed, funded, etc., on the basis that the client is an exclusive enclave. Of course, this is entirely consistent with the larger cultural bias. As Elliot and Lemert (2006: 7) conclude, 'individualism is the master idea of modernity.' Relating to the client as a relational entity contests this bias and opposes its problematic legacy.

Systemic work

The second practice that will be introduced concerns the possibilities of working systemically with individuals. Ideally, this includes the option of meeting with one or more of the people who make up the client's interpersonal ecology in order to 'be on everyone's side'. Being able to achieve this kind of engagement – what was originally termed a 'multi-partial alliance' (Boszormenyi-Nagy 1974) – is likely to be a difficult challenge, at least initially, for those who have been acculturated to see themselves as unilateral advocates for their clients.

Even if the professional is positively disposed towards, say, the client's siblings or those who live in the same group home as their client, there is likely to be some discomfort at meeting with the client's others, as these ensembles do not talk with one voice. Things can get noisy or, even worse, deadly quiet when a bunch of people are present. In what follows, brief attention is given to two forms of professional work, starting with systemic work with individuals prior to considering several key principles related to conjoint work.

Talking alone with clients while imaginatively including others

Working systemically with individual clients means being holistic in one's attention and in the purposes of one's actions (Boscolo and Bertrando, 1996; Hedges, 2005). Given the majority of practitioners meet with the single person who is presented to them, this idea can be used as an organising principle around which everyday relationship-building practice can turn.

This work can be conducted 'imaginatively.' That is, the practitioner may only meet with the client but seeks to populate this exchange with named others, key people whose feelings, behaviours and perspectives are elicited and acknowledged, albeit at one remove, as important. Perhaps, the practitioners might also meet serially with one, or even more than one, of those in the client's network without this contact being collectively undertaken. Whatever the configuration, the key point is that there are, or potentially might be, mini-communities of interest within which the client is included. These networks are not ever perfect, but generally are made up of individuals who are doing the best they can.

In the situation with Sam, the practitioner might have the following kind of discussion:

> *Practitioner:* Sam, you say that your Mum has said that emotions are really important and should be given their own space. On the other hand, your ex, Benny, who you still get on well with, knows about you being depressed and has a different view. Can you tell me how Benny understands this depression thing?
>
> *Sam:* Oh I don't know. Benny is unusual and always says 'Let's just move on' when things go wrong.

Practitioner:	How does this view compare with your own? Do you think that Benny, or maybe your Mum, has the most helpful attitude when it comes to your current situation?
Sam:	I don't know, it is hard to say.
Practitioner:	So if you were to tell Benny that you were going to go onto anti-depressants do you think this would be supported or do you think this might endanger your relationship?
Sam:	You know I haven't any mates. Losing Benny's friendship, or my Mum's trust, that is a nasty kind of idea.
Practitioner:	What about we think of them as with us now and get a kind of debate going?

There are many variables, but having multiple points of view present in the practitioner/client dialogue can often be helpful. In relation to different possibilities, one option is for the practitioner to play the role of broker, companion or coach (Carter and McGoldrick, 1999). Task-centred actions to one side (Marsh and Doel, 2005), at the very least seeing, and understanding, the client in their experience of their network illuminates the context and the meaning structure of their lives.

Conjoint work

Conjoint work refers to meeting with more than one participant, and, in itself, is not necessarily helpful. For instance, bringing the client and their significant others together is naïve if the practitioner assumes that 'open communication' will be helpful. Putting people together without structure or an agreement on purpose can be like putting out a fire with gasoline. It is necessary to assume, and often to overtly acknowledge, the good intentions of those involved, but it is not sound to expect that constructive contacts occur organically.

If conjoint meetings are organised there are a number of principles that need to be observed. These can be divided into those that concern both the 'convening' and the 'conducting' of sessions. In relation to the convening of sessions it is important that the people who are key players are sensitively identified. This involves asking the client non-standard questions as to who the key participants are:

> Sam, those who are important to us may not be obvious to outsiders. If we want to get the person, or persons, who might be best able to help you battle against the depression that is pushing you around, who are your possible allies?'

Sam might nominate a sister or a brother, or it might be a non-related neighbour or someone with whom Sam was once friends. It might be a minister or an uncle or aunt. It is simply impossible for a practitioner to guess from the case notes or deduce from convention who is important. What should also be considered is that there are formal connections, and these should not be ignored or discounted. In making a decision about who to involve, there are a round of considerations to be thought through, not least of which is the possibility that the relevant cast may vary over time. Narrative practitioners refer to this aspect as developing 'witnessing circles' (White 2007). Once this level of decision-making is resolved, the practitioner needs to put a substantial amount of time into contacting those who are to be invited. In this contact the practitioner has to introduce himself/herself and his/her purpose, and to elicit, and to closely track, the point of view and sensitivities of each party prior to bringing them together. Engagement begins well before the first meeting.

Those who may be relevant have their own lives and interests and should not be instrumentalised as resources or defined as carers. This is a trap for many practitioners, as their point of reference is 'the client, my client and nothing but the client.' However, each of the client's associates has their own biographies and needs, and the practitioner has to accept that these others do not exist only insofar as they are proxy servers for 'my client'. Often, these people have had negative experiences with professionals and can be primed to feel blamed and shamed. As far as we possibly can, we need to ensure there is not an us-and-them dynamic.

In relation to conducting meetings, several points are crucial. First, the practitioner has a contradictory role. On the one hand, the role is that of a host (Furman and Ahola 1995), and on the other we are visitors, temporary guests in the company of those who have an ongoing, non-artificial bond. As a visitor it is essential to be humble and to ensure that one does no harm to the prospects for relationships in the local ensemble. This is the opposite of being a myth-buster, or any other kind of macho champion. It is not in the client's interest, or anybody else's, to crash about indelicately in the intimacies of others.

In the sense that the practitioner is a host, it is necessary to be welcoming and positive and to take a persistent responsibility for keeping the gathering safe and structured. This can involve being prepared to play the 'traffic cop' and to gate-keep information exchange. There is also the value of being confident, or at least acting confidently, and to feel it is proper to take the floor at the beginning and at the conclusion of the meeting, and, when necessary, during the meeting. Rather than seeing oneself as a facilitator, it is generally better to position oneself as a group leader.

There are other matters that are important to consider, including questions of culture and setting. This noted, what is central is to be appreciative and to recognise that everyone is doing the best they can. Projecting a sense of interest and respect, of being friendly and open, is always a key ingredient. For example, if Sam and you had negotiated that Benny, as ex-partner with whom Sam retains a good relationship, could be a good ally, a first (or last) comment from the practitioner might be:

> It's fantastic you have taken the trouble to join us today. I know Sam recognises how awkward this might be, and so do I. It might feel a bit creepy

me saying this, like I am being a phony or something, but giving your time up for Sam is worth acknowledging in my book.

And then later asking:

> So, Benny what's your view? I know you and Sam busted up some time ago and you don't live in each other's pockets, but what I'd like to ask you about is this: what do you think are some of Sam's values and attitudes that might be good assets, maybe even tools or weapons, that could be used against this depression thing that has so pushed around so much of Sam's get up and go?

There are so many ways to go. One option is to explore one or more of the themes that are inherent to Sam's sociality:

> Benny, do you think Sam might have organised her reputation to be either too hard or too easy with others? What's the go here?

There are, of course, often a variety of contacts that might be activated or reactivated. For example, there might be an estranged significant other or pro-spective significant other, mindful that it only takes one quality relationship to make a great deal of difference. Sam being reminded of Benny's respect might, in itself, be a crucial invigoration.

Discussion

Good-quality relationships cannot be conferred on clients. Unlike a right to a benefit, or any other official entitlement, relationships can only be 'earned and learned', and it is naïve to assert that supportive relationships can be 'accessed' (WHO 2005: 93) as if these are a material good, a resource, that can be deliv-ered on a plate. Practitioners can nevertheless attempt to catalyse attitudes and behaviours that are associated with the attainment of relational competence, but we cannot give those we work with a quantum of connection and inclu-sion. It is possible, of course, to argue that the professional can give the client one relationship – the practitioner–client bond. This option is not developed, as more often it is preferable to consider the professional as a short-term visitor in the life of the client. That is, the working relationship is a means rather than an end. As such, the worker–client relationship should be constructed to be as minimal and as non-mythologised as possible.

To talk of relationships is to engage with a mystery, as we humans can be a perverse lot. For example, in some circumstances identity, strength and pride can be accentuated if I am othered by those who belong to a group that me-and-my-kind look down on. This dynamic acknowledged, more generally if a person senses others are 'dissing' them – the street term for putting down, disrespecting or abusing – this is not merely passingly unpleasant, as a person's longer term health and wellbeing can be compromised if they regularly feel others regard them as disreputable (Wilkinson and Pickett 2009). As inherently social beings we are exquisitely sensitive to the attitudes of those around us: being on alert to, having a radar for, negative signals in one's immediate environment presumably has developed over a million or more years.

Being ostracised from the nomad herd was never a good survival strategy. Similarly, being placed in the stocks in medieval times was an aversive experience, just as many people find being alone in the schoolyard or the workplace disturbing. Nearly everybody has an interest in being popular, respected and cared for, rather than being lonely, disregarded and disliked. Even more pointedly, this is a concern for those who have been officially branded as inferior or transgressive. Being declared by the competent authorities to be mentally unwell, having a marginal citizenship status, being diagnosed as intellectually inferior, being vilified in the popular media, leaving the children's court with your parental status disqualified, is transformative. However inadvert this may be, degradation occurs whenever services are targeted rather than universal. That is, in order to access assistance, what is termed being judged 'eligible for a service', requires the person's identity to be successfully reprocessed (Jones and May 1992). Perhaps, it is more of a problem if someone's significant others think they are a creep, but it is hard to know whether the voices of distant authority figures, such as judges or politicians, or even the encounters that are conducted anonymously on the street, have more symbolic and auto-immunological impact than exchanges with intimates. One hates to be disapproved of by one's mother, or the internalised views of a respected, but now dead, uncle – but it can also be aversive to be deemed a fool by an unknown other. Humiliation can be damning wherever it is occasioned.

A final question merits attention: What is the relationship between social exclusion, as understood in terms of structural factors, such as citizenship status and access to employment, and the matter of interpersonal connection? One position is to view these constructs as hierarchically arranged, for example that a person can have good-quality companionship and peer recognition and still be disenfranchised and excluded (Taket et al. 2009a: 12). The view underlying the current contribution is that the achievement of social inclusion is incomplete unless there is a quantum of good-enough sociality within which there is some giving and taking of affection, respect and recognition.

Reliable attachments within which it is understood a person's worth is recognised and deserved act as an insulation, even perhaps as an inoculation, to the effects of exclusion. Practitioners wishing to encourage such connections require facilitating conditions, such as an affirming professional culture, adequate resourcing and positive forms of supervision and accountability. In terms of their direct contact with clients, the promotion of good-quality sociality can be pursued as an agreed goal with a client or, alternatively, if there is insufficient time to negotiate an agreement, or if the client is so relationship-shy as to baulk at this as an agreed aim, it is possible for the practitioner to work towards the realisation of this aim indirectly. The rationale for such an openly partisan position is that practitioners have no choice but to either act to oppose the atomising process of individualisation or *de facto* to collude with this process. It is impossible for the practitioner to be neutral with respect to social connectedness.

9 Experiments in social inclusion and connection

Cases from Lebanon

Jihad Makhoul, Tamar Kabakian-Khasholian, Michael El-Khoury and Faysal El-Kak

Introduction

The creation of opportunities for social inclusion requires an understanding of the structures and the processes which have brought about conditions of exclusion. Lebanon is a country whose society is characterised by social and communal ties of much benefit to its members, yet the same society has shown exclusionary practices in its laws and values. However, attempts to practice social inclusion for individuals and groups take place. After providing some background on the situation in Lebanon, this chapter will focus on two examples of how inclusion is practiced in service delivery in Lebanon: first, within a psychotherapeutic service in two community-based centres supporting persons struggling with their sexual orientation, and, second, within a research outreach programme on improving childbirth practices.

Lebanon, a small country situated on the eastern side of the Mediterranean, stands out among its Arab neighbours for its democratic reputation, multi-religious co-existence and a refuge for people from the region seeking asylum over the years. Yet, its location in the heart of the Arab world places it also in the midst of the Arab–Israeli conflict and consequent regional political upheavals. The Lebanese civil war of 1975–1990, where the warring factions were supported by regional and foreign interventions, was ended by the Taif Agreement, which made arrangements for the representation of the religious sects in state governance (Haddad 2002). However, social development and the needs of the various sectors of the population were overlooked when the post-war government focused on economic development and the reconstruction of Beirut, the capital of Lebanon (Shammas 1996). The health care sector in Lebanon is currently characterised by ambulatory care provided by the private sector, and, to a small extent, by health centres run by non-governmental organisations (NGOs). Tertiary care is provided by hi-tech private hospitals, which bill the Ministry of Public Health and public insurance schemes. This health care system has resulted in major inefficiencies, and the creation of a culture that is oriented to secondary care and technology (Van Lerberghe et al. 1997).

The Lebanese society, like other Arab societies, is known for establishing social ties and sustaining formal and non-formal affiliations. These communal loyalties provide the Lebanese with a sense of belonging and varied levels of social support, yet also pervade the social as well as the political structure of the country (Khalaf 2001). Similar to the rest of the Arab world, Lebanese civil society, political parties and corporations are dominated by traditions of familial and sectarian loyalty. The country is a mosaic of the 18 officially sanctioned religious faiths, some of which are Muslim Sunni and Shi'ite, Christian Orthodox and Maronite, and Druze. This strong surge of socio-religious conservatism has negatively impacted the health rights of vulnerable groups (Maziak 2009), which includes women and homosexual and transgendered individuals.

Furthermore, Beirut is divided along sectarian lines, where the eastern suburbs are predominantly Christian and the southern and western suburbs Muslim. Poverty, officially connected with income levels, is also unofficially associated with specific groups of people such as Shi'ite Muslims, and the internally displaced (Fawaz and Peillin 2003), who have been historically marginalised and excluded from development benefits.

Case study 1: Psychotherapy within non-governmental organisations for individuals with homosexual orientations and transgender identities

Although it is more tolerant than other Middle Eastern countries, Lebanon, unlike many of its neighbours, has colonial French laws from the 1930s criminalising non-conservative otherness, such as homosexuality (Massad 2002). It is not surprising that this view is internalised by health care providers from this society. A study on physicians' views of clients of different sexual orientations reveals that they perceive homosexuality as a disease that needs medical and psychological counselling, and an overwhelming 93.1 per cent of them have never received any medical training on homosexuality (El Kak 2009).

Information provided here is based on the experiences, understandings and interpretations stemming from 7 years of psychotherapy work within a multidisciplinary team of activists, social workers, counsellors, and founders of two NGOs: HELEM and MARSA. HELEM (Arabic for 'dream') is a community centre founded by volunteers in 2004 to support and protect LGBTQ (lesbian, gay, bisexual, transsexual, and queer) individuals by providing free counselling, awareness, a non-judgmental atmosphere, a 24-hour help-line, and an adequate referral system to relevant services. It was never officially sanctioned by the Lebanese government but, according to Lebanese law, any NGO that does not get an official reply within two months following its proclamation request is considered unofficially official.

MARSA (Arabic for 'dock'), a sexual health centre, was a pragmatic offshoot of HELEM in 2010, mainly due to the labelling of HELEM as supporting homosexuals and queers only, in spite of HELEM's active policy to engage with the general population indiscriminately and provide its sustainable services to the public at large. Thus, MARSA, by proclaiming itself a general sexuality clinic, was able to attain official recognition from the government, improve its visibility, gain community and governmental acceptance, and increase access to care, making it more socially inclusive.

Consumers of both services will be referred to in this chapter as 'therapees', as other wordings may inadvertently contribute to their social exclusion. For example, utilising the term 'non-conforming gender identities or sexual orientations' can imply an exclusion from the hetero-normative majority, while 'gay and lesbian' can imply that this is all that the person is, thus excluding other important parts of their personhood and social-hood. As such, the term 'therapees' will be used to describe the role of these individuals in a specific time (50-minute psychotherapy sessions) and space (social and clinical centres).

Most of the individuals who approach the centres come from low to low-middle socio-economic backgrounds. The majority live with their families but some live on their own, a rare social living arrangement in an Arab country like Lebanon where young people generally remain within their family of origin's home until they get married, irrespective of their age. In their family homes, they commonly have to hide their sexual identity and are under the continuous threat of different degrees of excommunication. Many of their parents are either divorced, have significant familial conflicts, and/or display lack of emotional expression and care. This situation seems to be in sharp contrast to a minority of individuals in Lebanon who usually do not seek out the centres and are more open about their sexuality; they tend to come from families that are generally more tolerant towards their sexual orientation.

Individuals seeking our services seem to be struggling with and suffering from exclusion at many levels, organised here from the general to the specific: global, societal, religious, institutional, familial, interpersonal and intrapersonal. Examples of inclusionary practices at each of these levels are given below.

At the global level, and with the ubiquity of internet use and the world wide web, therapees are well informed about many of the events taking place as they are reported in the global media: gay marriages, sexual reconstructive surgeries, web dating, conferences, training, courses, information on safe sex and sexually transmitted diseases, and so on. They are encouraged by the staff to access sites that provide accurate information (some of which are the official websites of HELEM and MARSA) (HELEM 2013; MARSA 2013), and, for example, are warned to be extra careful during web dating. Some are encouraged to become volunteers and activists, who will participate in local, regional and international training events and conferences that can improve their life skills. These initiatives have helped many individuals engage more with the world, better accept their personhood in general and sexual orientation in particular, and to better appreciate their self-conceptualisation.

At the societal level, it is important to note that Beirut is a 'competitive city' for gay tourism, with the paradoxical co-existence of extreme conservatism and behind-the-scenes 'liberalism'. Depending on the strength of their egos and their resilience (e.g. their ability to withstand other people's derogatory looks, condescending comments and abusive behaviours), therapees are often encouraged by the counsellors and therapists to adapt to these social–contextual differences by revealing various aspects of themselves in different contexts. For example, in contexts where there is a low tolerance of different masculinities, femininities and sexual orientations, therapees can be encouraged to 'pass as normal' by undertaking different ways of dressing, different hair styles, and different body movements and gestures. In other settings that are more tolerant, therapees are encouraged to be more open about their sexuality.

Religion plays a big role in the identity of self, family and community in Lebanon (Joseph 1997). People from all religions have sought help in the centres, and there is no evident dominance of one faith or religion over the other. Most therapees are quite religious and want to hold on to their faith, but find it challenging to integrate their religious beliefs, values, behaviours and expectations with their sexual identity, fantasies, thoughts, emotions, behaviours and relationships. For example, many scholars of Islamic law believe that homosexuality is beyond sin and is a crime (Kligerman 2007). Most, if not all, therapees understand their religion to clearly condemn same-sex behaviours, which places them under severe pressure towards splitting of the self in terms of good/bad, acceptable/unacceptable, sinless/sinful and deserving heaven/hell. Accordingly, the ultimate task of the therapist is in helping them regain the integration of the disparate religious and sexual aspects of their identity (Haldeman 2004).When appropriate, the therapist tries to explore and expand on the belief systems held, and attempts to offer in a questioning format different possible interpretations of the scriptures and God's unconditional acceptance. There have been three main outcomes to this process. First, many therapees have split the two realms of religiosity and sexuality completely from each other. For example, when engaging in sexual behaviour or fantasy, they put their religious selves far into the background, and when praying or participating in a religious ceremony in a church or mosque, they put their sexual identity far into the background. Second, some have become non-religious while at the same time maintaining their belief in a Creator, or have shifted their belief entirely and become atheists. Third, some find relief in maintaining their religious beliefs while not accepting the sinfulness attached to same-sex attraction and sexual behaviour.

At the institutional level, most if not all therapees mention the daily hardships in trying to acknowledge their sexuality at school, university and the workplace. Because many young people start this process during their school years, the educational setting plays a significant role in shaping these individuals, especially when the environment is derogatory and utilises homophobic terminologies (Michaelson 2008). The centres have become a safe space within which to foster normality, acceptance and belonging, where many therapees choose to spend some of their time away from the constant fear of harassment. Also, through the awareness campaigns initiated by the centres and other key individuals in the field, the staff at the centres use the media to increase the current understanding about sexual identities and to challenge stereotypes and misconceptions among the public. Many of the staff use their professional status as, for example, members of prestigious universities, to seek media exposure in raising awareness of tolerance towards LGBTQ individuals (see the short video about key figures in MARSA focusing on inclusion and normalisation (MARSA, 2011)).

There is a saying in Arabic: 'A monkey is a gazelle in its mother's eyes', meaning mothers will view their offspring favourably regardless of any unwanted aspects in their physical appearance or character. Many therapees experience the opposite of this proverb: 'A gazelle is a monkey in its mother's eyes'. The heaviest burden to therapees' mental wellbeing, in addition to that associated with religion mentioned above, is at the familial level, where many therapees have experienced isolation, abandonment and un-belonging. Many also struggle with the prospect of raising a family of their own due to the almost total lack of acceptance within current social norms of raising children by same-sex parents (O'Dell 2000). Depending on the individual, therapy aims at recognising, acknowledging and venting these emotional and relational scars. It moves towards acceptance of both the strengths and weaknesses of each family member, the family dynamics and the different world views each family member may have, salvaging and improving what is still healthy in the family (Saltzburg 1996), and moving away from 'all-or-none' thinking and towards complexity in truths. In a similar vein, the coming out process (revealing one's sexual orientation to another person, family or community) is adapted to each individual in accordance with the strength of his or her ego, the potential risks, and the extent to which this step can improve his or her quality of life. It is important to mention that the therapist does not tell the therapee what to do, but rather explores the pros and cons of the different available options (Haldeman 2004).

With regard to the interpersonal level, a large number of therapees struggle to find and maintain healthy romantic relationships. Many of them do not want to engage in brief relationships limited to physical sex, but due to the low probability and opportunity of finding long-term partners, and the fact that it is relatively easier and quicker way to find sexual companions, temporary therapees often find themselves forced to move in this direction. Depending on their priorities, therapees are encouraged to continue their search for suitable partners, are reminded to expand their intimate relationships to include close friendships, and are taught how to improve their relational dynamics and assertive skills pertaining to initiating and maintaining long-term partnerships. For example, some are coached into taking their time to get to know the other person and to refrain from sex during the early stages of a relationship; others work on improving their negotiation skills and assertive communication; and some work on improving their understanding of what constitutes psychological and physical abuse. The therapists promote safe sexual behaviours and may refer therapees to other members of the team for sexual counselling and skill building.

Finally, social inclusionary practices at the above levels affect the intrapersonal level (psychological self) by enhancing self-esteem, expanding emotional growth and expression, and promoting healthy behaviours and daily functioning. The likelihood of mental distress such as anxiety, depression and suicide may also diminish (Kulkin et al. 2000). The therapeutic process creates an environment free from blame and judgment, where the therapee's feelings of shame and guilt are acknowledged and empathised with, and his or her skills of insight, adaptability and self-healing are developed. This process helps therapees achieve a 'corrective emotional experience' (the term being first coined and defined by Alexander and French (1946) as 're-experiencing the old, unsettled conflict but with a new ending') whereby they re-experience emotions with the therapist in a manner that is different from what has happened to them in the past, and this can eventually help them improve their relatedness to others (in Bridges 2006: 551). Moreover, within these centres the psychotherapeutic effort itself helps therapees to become more inclusive within themselves, mainly through acceptance of their sexual orientation, which helps reduce internalised homophobia. Some quotes from therapees expressing their experiences of social exclusion and inclusion are given in Table 9.1.

Case study 2: Inclusion of women in their maternity care

Women's active involvement in maternity care and the responsiveness of different health care systems to women's needs is a major deficiency encountered in different contexts around the world, in both industrialised and non-industrialised countries (Davis-Floyd et al. 2009). The vast majority of systems providing maternity care around the world seek to avoid mortality by intervening excessively, thus leading to morbidity that could have been prevented (Davis-Floyd et al. 2009). The increase in caesarean births is one substantial example of these approaches (Johanson et al. 2002). These models of maternity care are characterised by their disregard of the scientific evidence indicating improved health outcomes with women-centred approaches, such as the provision of information to women about different obstetric procedures to facilitate women's participation in the process of care by providing informed choices (Davis-Floyd et al. 2009).

More than three-quarters of deliveries in Lebanon occur in private hospitals and are paid for by the Lebanese Ministry of Public Health. Reported hospital caesarean section rates are high at 40.8 per cent (DeJong et al. 2010). A large proportion of maternity care is provided by obstetricians within the private sector (Tutelian et al. 2007). Women are very passive actors and do not take part in the decisions relating to the care they receive. Gender differences, considering that obstetricians are most likely to be male in the Lebanese context, and professional dominance contribute to the exclusion of women from this process. Moreover, organised systems of providing women with information do not exist in Lebanon, and there are differences in access to information according to social class (Kabakian-Khasholian et al. 2000).

In 2001 a group of researchers from four Arab countries established a regional network, the Choices and Challenges in Changing Childbirth research network, and have been actively researching birthing practices and women's experiences

Table 9.1 Quotes from therapees on exclusionary and inclusionary practices (taken from the progress notes of therapy sessions and translated from the Arabic)

Experiences of social exclusion at different levels	Experiences of inclusion in the two centres
'Chatting with men on the net is too much about sex and money. I feel like I'm taking on other people's characteristics to become accepted in society.'	'Here in this therapy session, I want to feel safe and not go through feelings of pain and abandonment as I was feeling with my family.'
'I feel that God is punishing me.'	'Enough is enough from hurting from other people's words and behaviours!'
'I was a severely isolated student at school . . . the teacher used to ask the rest of the students: "Does no one want to be the friend of Jameel?"'	'From now on, I will not allow anyone to destroy me.'
'All my family thinks low of me.'	'It feels good to be listened to and accepted, like pressing the "refresh" button.'
'I don't know you . . . you are not my daughter.' (Parent to child)	'After our last session, I felt like the letters and words [in Arabic to mean 'parts of the self'] are now making sense in full sentences.'
'What did I do so bad that you don't want me?' (Child to parent)	
'It is very difficult for me to accept that my own mother does not love me.'	'I feel now that I exist.'
	'I feel much more comfortable with who I am.'
'I don't want to bring children to this world out of my fear for hurting them like the way I was hurt.'	'Thank you for helping me bring out what has long been caged in my heart.'
'I have no one.'	
'I long to long.'	'I came to realise that it is not my fault that I am gay: I am gay, it's a fact.'
'I love caring emotions but I cannot express emotions.'	'I want to move away from loneliness, confusion, and weakness.'
'I have a lot of caring feeling in me that is going to waste.'	'I feel safe and more in control.'
'I see no light at the other side of the door, only sadness and suffering.'	'This is the first time in my life where I feel like a human being.'
'The only way I can allow myself to feel some emotion is if I imagine the death of a loved one and start crying.'	'Therapy with you was a very difficult journey but I gained a lot of inner strength.'
'Enough waiting, isolation, retreating . . . enough past.'	'I feel now that I belong, if not to anyone at least to myself.'
'I am tripping with myself.'	'Sessions are a place for me to vent and cry.'
	'I am gay but not a criminal.'

in childbirth, with the aim of accumulating evidence and conducting interventions to improve the quality of services and women's experiences. Researchers within the network in Lebanon have attempted to influence women's perspectives and facilitate their inclusion in the maternal health care system through research and practice activities. These activities are aimed at shaping women's demand for a different model of maternity care, through communicating evidence-based information to women and encouraging dialogue on these issues with their health care providers. In this way, mainstream systems of maternity-care or health care systems are, in general, redirected toward adopting inclusive practices that allow women to become major players in these processes. Three different activities will be discussed here: mobilising women to change maternity services, the use of an informational leaflet, and antenatal maternity records.

Mobilising women to take a more active role in the process of maternity care is an act of empowerment that challenges the traditional structures of the health care system and facilitates inclusion of women's voices in this process. In a system where unnecessary, and sometimes even harmful, obstetric practices are used routinely, women are not provided with opportunities to discuss alternative forms of care and to express their needs. Moreover, women are not well informed about best practice, something that explains the lack of demand for alternative forms of care and further deepens women's exclusion from this process. The first example in this regard is derived from an intervention study conducted to test the impact of mobilising women by providing them with information about best practice in maternity care and enhancing their communication skills with providers. This was done with the aim of facilitating their participation in the decision-making process of the care they receive during childbirth.

Following the intervention, women reported being more vocal about demanding specific practices during labour and the postpartum period that were discussed in the intervention sessions. For example, women expressed their preference to not have an enema during labour, and reported being more vocal about demanding not to be separated from their babies during their hospital stay.

This example offers an approach that indicates the possibility of influencing the process through which women receive maternity care, by addressing women's knowledge about evidence-based care and enhancing their skills of communicating their needs to providers. Although this approach does not address all components of this complex system and targets only the consumers' perspective to instigate change, it presents a successful example of an approach that reaches women with information about best practice in obstetrics and builds their self-efficacy in negotiating their care. Women's lack of information about best practice in maternity care, and the intimidation they experience due to the professional dominance of clinicians, is often used for the convenience of health care providers by completely undermining women and ignoring their needs. Women having knowledge of what is beneficial and healthy with regard to childbearing have the potential to mobilise this marginalised group within the system and to shift the power differentials between the different players.

The second example concerns a different approach to facilitating women's inclusion and participation in maternity care by facilitating their access to evidence-based information. The Salamet Hamlik (meaning 'Your safe pregnancy') informational leaflet aims to raise awareness about the various physical, emotional and lifestyle changes, and the possible medical and obstetric problems that can occur during pregnancy, delivery and the postpartum period. It presents information and evidence on different issues that are relevant to the Lebanese context. Nationally, there are no other materials produced in Arabic and distributed free of charge. The newsletter is published quarterly and is distributed to women attending obstetric clinics, both private and public, and primary health care services all over Lebanon. The different editions of the leaflet focus on providing information that is not commonly provided during prenatal visits, including best practice during labour, delivery and the postpartum period. The leaflet also includes messages that encourage women to take a more active role in the care they receive throughout the childbearing process.

Feedback on these leaflets from women and health care providers indicates that there is a high demand for, and use of, the information provided. An important number of women reported applying and using the information given in the leaflet and gaining high satisfaction from its application. Around 86 per cent of women reported that the information they read in the leaflet was new to them, and changed their perception about certain aspects of care and prompted them to inquire about certain obstetric practices during prenatal visits.

The two approaches presented so far have focused on women. They provide women with opportunities to become more vocal about demanding choices and choosing what corresponds to their needs. We acknowledge that these are not enough to change the traditional biomedical approach to delivering maternity care; nevertheless, these attempts denote the importance of the right to know what is best for childbearing women as a first step on the road to including women in the decision-making process.

The third example is an initiative of working with providers to instigate change in the process of delivering maternity care. As a result of the largely private health care system in Lebanon, childbearing women often receive fragmented care, with a lack of continuity from the prenatal to the postpartum period. Many women need to change their health care provider during the course of their pregnancy, for their delivery or for a subsequent pregnancy. These women do not have access to their medical records, which are also not easily transferable from one private facility to the other. This not only creates a situation where health care providers are obliged to compromise on the quality of care offered to women who deliver at a facility different from where they received prenatal care, but also denies women the right to access information related to their reproductive history. The Choices and Challenges in Changing Childbirth group in Lebanon formed an Initiative on Standards of Practice in Childbirth (ISOPIC), which is composed of eminent obstetricians and other health care providers for women and which has developed an antenatal and maternity record in response to this need.

The aim of the antenatal record is to provide a minimum standard package of maternity care, and the maternity record is intended to provide women with access to their own maternity history. The antenatal record is a medical record documenting the pregnant woman's socio-demographic information and medical, obstetric, surgical and family history, and includes a risk assessment and care plan, and details of periodic visits, problems or issues, and any other relevant information pertaining to the course of her pregnancy. The maternity record contains less medical information, and is focused more on educational messages for pregnant women. It is meant to be kept by the woman so that she can keep track of her pregnancy requirements (visit schedule, medication, tests, ultrasound scans), and have the course of her pregnancy documented in case she needs to change her health care provider. The maternity record has been adopted by the Ministry of Public Health in Lebanon, for use by all health care providers taking care of pregnancy and childbirth. The national implementation of the use of maternity record ensures that women from all social classes, receiving care from public or private facilities, will have ownership of the information about their reproductive history. This is another example of inclusionary practice that will provide many women with an important opportunity to participate in the process of their care at some level.

Some quotes expressing women's experiences of exclusionary and inclusionary practices in maternity care are given in Table 9.2.

Table 9.2 Quotes from different studies expressing women's experiences of exclusionary and inclusionary practices in maternity care

Experiences of marginalisation and dissatisfaction with maternity care	*Experiences of inclusion in the process of maternity care*
'They shave you in a hurry, they don't even consider the fact that you are having contractions and you are in such pain. It was one of the most disturbing experiences of my life.'	'I read the information you gave me and I started asking questions about things I did not think about before.'
'The doctor will talk to you about different things but he does not have the time to go into the details.'	'When you go through the process of giving birth you kind of feel like many things that the staff do to you can't be the right thing to do. You kind of adjust because you don't know better. I learned a few things in these two sessions that I will definitely use during my third delivery. Now I know.'
'You don't receive ready-made information just whatever you ask about.'	
'She told me there is no big difference between vaginal and caesarean deliveries and that I can stay awake and see the birth.'	'Two of my patients this week referred to your leaflet when raising questions about labour pain.' (An obstetrician)
'I was in the operating room all alone and not knowing anything about a caesarean.'	

Conclusion

This chapter has attempted to provide examples of how social inclusion can be practiced. This has been done through two case studies focusing on, first, psychotherapy for socially excluded persons and, second, women utilising health care services in Lebanon. The chapter has shown that the inclusionary practices of therapists and the public health practitioners have worked despite the various powerful exclusionary processes that exist within the social and structural levels of the Lebanese context. This was possible because they have used their power to identify and implement ways to improve the situation for the groups in question. The daily and ongoing exclusionary practices at the global, societal, institutional, religious, familial and interpersonal levels can significantly undermine the wellbeing of individuals whose sexual identities, orientations and behaviours are not in line with the *status quo*. The obstacles to inclusionary maternity care, such as professional and gender dominance, overmedicalisation of care and the unavailability of information, reflect the overall culture of the Lebanese health systems and patient–provider, or in this case woman–provider, relationships.

Psychotherapists and public health practitioners who are aware of and committed to social justice are better able to practice social inclusion and, as Barter-Godfrey and Taket (2009) suggest, can reduce the social distance between service users and service providers. Psychotherapists provide a means for therapees to unveil threatened aspects of themselves in an individual-focused, supportive, non-threatening atmosphere. Public health practitioners can make important information related to prenatal and postnatal health care available to women in an appealing way, and this increases women's choices and improves the quality of health care they receive.

There are no straightforward and simple solutions for care providers in dealing with all the challenges and barriers to inclusion at all levels. To be able to practice social inclusion, service providers need to develop an understanding of the people they serve and what is important to them, so that they can offer meaningful interventions and personalised care. Service providers need to capitalise on the team effort and the provision of inclusionary services and interventions at more than one level. They also need to provide opportunities to narrow the distance between them and their service users. Finally, to maximise the benefits of these services, professionals need to advocate for the institutionalisation of inclusionary practices at more than one level.

10 Practising social inclusion

The case of street-based sex workers

Rachel Lennon, Pranee Liamputtong and Elizabeth Hoban

Introduction

It has been widely documented that street-based sex workers experience stigma and discrimination on a daily basis (Jiménez et al. 2011; Sallman 2011). Women who are street-based sex workers are labelled immoral women, drug users, and transmitters of disease, and are generally considered as unworthy members of society (Wolffers and van Beelan 2003; O'Neill et al. 2008). As a result, street-based sex workers often experience stigma and discrimination, affecting their social, physical and psychological wellbeing as well as intensifying feelings of social isolation (Vanwesenbeeck 2001; Pinkham and Malinowska-Sempruch 2008). Fear of experiencing stigma and discrimination also impedes women's access to community-based services and personal support networks, subsequently leading to feelings of immense social isolation and exclusion (Krieger 1999; Kurtz et al. 2005; Pinkham and Malinowska-Sempruch 2008; Strega et al. 2009).

The practice of social inclusion is essential for marginalised groups as it facilitates feelings of safety, wellbeing, reduces mental health issues and provides a sense of belonging (Australian Social Inclusion Board 2010; Smyth et al. 2011). In this chapter, we briefly review the impacts of stigma and discrimination on female street-based sex workers and how this results in social exclusion. The chapter discusses ways to increase social inclusion through exploring the business of St Kilda Gatehouse, a not-for-profit organisation located in Melbourne, Australia, designed to provide services and support for male, female and transgender street-based sex workers and homeless people; male and transgender street-based sex workers are not the focus of this chapter. We will illustrate how a community-based organisation such as the St Kilda Gatehouse can facilitate social inclusiveness for female street-based sex workers and address issues of social inclusion in their service delivery. We will then discuss the impact that the organisation has on female street-based female sex workers in St Kilda who access the Gatehouse.

Sex workers' experiences of stigma and discrimination

The definition of sex work, although it varies slightly within certain contexts, is the provision of sexual services for economic exchange (Harcourt and

Donovan 2005). Women who enter street-based sex work do so for many reasons; however, drug use is the main precursor to entry (Rowe 2003a, 2006; Fick 2005; Kurtz et al. 2005). Street-based sex work is a means to sustain individuals' drug habits and to survive (Dalla 2002; Rowe 2003a; Harris et al. 2010).

The most significant contribution to stigma and discrimination of female sex workers is the assumption that sex workers are vectors of disease, drug users, and immoral, and hence they operate outside the domain in which they should expect public protection (Vanwesenbeeck 2001; Sanders 2004; Fick 2005; Rekart 2005; Pinkham and Malinowska-Sempruch 2008; Jiménez et al. 2011). Sex workers frequently respond to this by internalising these assumptions, subsequently avoiding contact with health care and judicial services providers (Jeal and Salisbury 2004; Kurtz et al. 2005; Hong et al. 2010). Barriers to accessing services and increased mental health problems place sex workers at further risk of social exclusion and violence (Rowe 2003a; Kurtz et al. 2005; Corrigan et al. 2006). Violence, a daily consequence of sex work, is viewed by the public and workers themselves as an 'occupational hazard.' This creates another barrier for accessing support services, as workers are seen as 'deserving' of the assaults and abuse perpetrated against them (Pyett and Warr 1999; Fick 2005; Quadara 2008; Jiménez et al. 2011; Sallman 2011). Street-based sex workers in Australia are not alone in their experiences of stigma-related barriers when accessing services. Studies conducted in the USA (Kurtz et al. 2005), Hong Kong (Wong et al. 2010) and Puerto Rico (Jiménez et al. 2011) found there was a need to implement health programmes, utilising appropriate models of service delivery, that target and reduce stigma for street-based sex workers.

Brief history of sex workers in St Kilda

During 1880–1900, St Kilda became one of the wealthiest suburbs in the state of Victoria, Australia. Subsequently, early in the 20th century, the spread of industry moved the sex-worker population into the suburbs of St Kilda, where the area became known as a 'pleasure centre' for First and Second World War serviceman (Lowman 2000; Rowe 2006; City of Port Phillip 2011). In the 1970s and 1980s, tolerance zones (synonymous with 'red-light districts') were implemented in St Kilda following the decriminalisation of street-based sex work in an attempt to govern and localise street-based sex work in the St Kilda region (Mulligan 2006). In recent years, gentrification of St Kilda and adjoining suburbs resulted in local residents campaigning to rid the area of its long-standing reputation as being a centre for street-based sex work, heroin syndicates and criminal activity. There have been attempts by resident groups, through their local council, to move street-based sex workers out of the area (Lowman 2000). In 1986, the development of The Prostitution Regulation Act was an attempt to decriminalise street-based sex work. Yet the influence of the Victoria Government's Upper Houses of Parliament resulted in the criminalisation of street-based sex work (Arnot 2002; Rowe 2006). In 2002, proposals for tolerance zones re-emerged from the Attorney General's Street Prostitution Advisory Council in response to the growing concerns and complaints about street-based sex workers in the St Kilda. Although recommendations for the introduction of tolerance zones have not been enacted, it remains the only political strategy that has attempted to address issues about street-based sex work in Melbourne (Rowe 2003b). Thus, current regulation is governed through the Prostitution Control Act, (1994), which deems licensed brothels as legal; street-based sex work remains illegal (City of Port Phillip 2011).

St Kilda Gatehouse

The St Kilda Gatehouse (hereafter referred to as 'the Gatehouse') was developed as a not-for-profit organisation in 1992 by the South Melbourne Church of Christ in response to the increasing rate of street-based sex workers, drug usage and homelessness in the area (St Kilda Gatehouse 2013). The Gatehouse partners and sponsors include community groups, local government, churches and charitable trusts. The vision of the organisation is to provide pathways towards life transformation and community connectedness. The organisation operates as a drop-in centre from Monday to Friday that aims to give sex workers a safe and judgement-free space to access support workers who can provide referrals to services, one-to-one support, discuss issues, or simply have a drink and something to eat. The Gatehouse support workers provide referral services, assist women to manage their complex social issues, and support women to develop pathways towards drug rehabilitation, find accommodation and access judicial information. Assistance with child access visits and visits to court, community meals, and celebrations and events are provided. The Gatehouse also celebrates events with women and encourages participation in activities such as joining the local netball team. The organisation is conveniently located in the heart of St Kilda where sex workers work. It has five staff members and two volunteers, and operates under a Board of Governance comprising six members.

The core function of the Gatehouse is to provide street-based sex workers with an environment that is free from stigma and to encourage a sense of belonging and community. As noted on the Gatehouse website:

> St Kilda Gatehouse is based on the Christian principles of inclusiveness, unconditional support, service, and social justice. St Kilda Gatehouse believes every person is worthy of a 'home' environment and a 'way in' to resources and participation in family, community and social life.

The study

This chapter is based on data from a larger study that explores the experiences of stigma and discrimination of female street-based sex workers. Qualitative inquiry was selected as it allows the researcher to develop an in-depth understanding of the participants' experiences and the issues under exploration (Liamputtong 2007). Interview data was collected between October and December 2011. Twelve street-based sex workers participated in face-to-face in-depth interviews which ranged from 30 minutes to 90 minutes in length. As the interviews were semi-structured, participants were asked questions such as 'Tell me about your experiences with the Gatehouse', which prompted more questions and discussion. All participants signed a consent form and agreed to be tape-recorded. In general, few women accessing the Gatehouse are from non-Caucasian backgrounds, and all women interviewed were Caucasian. All but two women did street-based sex work to support their heroin addiction or were on a drug addiction treatment programme at the time of the interviews. Participants were between 22 and 49 years old. For the ten women with children, the age range of their children was 1–29 years. One woman was pregnant and three of the women had mothers who had been sex workers. There was a mother and daughter interviewed who were both street-based sex workers. Seven women were looking for stable housing and three women were homeless at the time of the study.

Ethics clearance for the study was granted by the La Trobe University Human Ethics Committee, and the study was part of a larger study exploring the impact of stigma and discrimination on female street-based sex workers in St Kilda, Victoria, Australia.

Results

Data revealed that street-based sex workers experience low self-esteem and feel unworthy members of the community. On a daily basis, women experienced dirty looks and verbal abuse from onlookers and business owners. While women were working on the streets they were constantly suspicious of other workers, and thereby were reluctant to develop friendships when not working. Furthermore, women lacked the support networks they needed from family and friends to increase levels of self-esteem and their overall wellbeing. Some women were afraid to reveal themselves as sex workers to friends and family, perceiving reactions from others to be negative. Also problematic in the lives of street-based sex workers was stigma and discrimination in the form of violence and abuse. Women not only experienced violence and abuse from onlookers and clients, but also experienced it in their personal lives through interpersonal violence. In discussions about the St Kilda Gatehouse, four main themes emerged: safe and non-judgemental environment; convenience; sense of community; and provision of services. These four themes are discussed below. Pseudonyms have been used throughout this chapter to protect the identities of the women.

Safe and non-judgemental environment

The Gatehouse succeeded in its aims of being socially inclusive of street-based sex workers. For women who lacked support networks, the Gatehouse was a safe and responsive service that harnessed the philosophy of a judgement-free space for all. This had a positive impact on all sex workers interviewed.

Street-based sex workers could access the Gatehouse at any stage of their life and expect acceptance. The organisation assisted women to engage with the local community through fun, social and recreational activities. One-on-one services are available that assist women who wish to exit sex work to transition into other areas of employment. For example, Aimee, who has a steady partner and is the mother of two children, had been a sex worker for 14 years; Aimee did not have a drug habit. Aimee was trying to market her own business and the Gatehouse support workers assisted her to develop her business's website: Aimee could not develop this website on her own:

> Very, very helpful. G [support worker] helped me with my website, L [support worker] has helped socially as a friend and in other ways – anything that I ask, she's there. I love the Gatehouse, this is like my second family, it's good. I love the Gatehouse.

Some of the women took the opportunity to discuss personal issues with the support workers and felt they were supported, regardless of the situation they were in. Despite the sex workers' propensity for suspicion of others, the Gatehouse tended to eliminate this by creating a welcoming and judgement-free environment. Mia felt that the attitudes, non-judgemental philosophies and social inclusiveness of Gatehouse staff and the programmes were examples of the way society in general should be treating sex workers:

> They provide a lot, they do, they really do. They open up their doors. When they're open and as soon as you walk in you see the workers, say it's like, 'Gidday how you going?'. I know the workers that work here at the Gatehouse, but they are a really fine example on how society should be treating us girls.

Corinne, who had been a street-based sex worker for over ten years, has two children and has only recently been introduced to the Gatehouse. When we interviewed Corinne, she was suicidal because she was dealing with recent threats of violence from a group of street-based sex workers. Although Corinne did not seek out 'any support' from the Gatehouse, she experienced the Gatehouse as a stigma-free service where she felt comfortable talking to other workers:

> I come in here [the Gatehouse] and I can literally talk to someone that knows what is going on and they're not going to judge me and they're not going to put me down or whatever else. I honestly I don't know what I'd do without the Gatehouse.

Belinda, who has four children and no longer has custody of them, felt comfortable accessing the Gatehouse knowing that she would not be judged. She appreciated the way in which she could share her concerns with Gatehouse staff. Belinda also admired the way the staff assisted the women to address their personal issues, especially when their lives seemed to be out of control:

> Yeah and it's not just about the food and the drinks and the toilet facilities and stuff like you can come in here and share your . . . what's going on and not be judged you know . . . like last week this woman had the worse time in her life and L [support worker] made everything so much better, got on the phone and did all this for me and did that for me because clearly as if you can be fucked going through half of that stuff by yourself and doing it.

Convenience

Although there were other services in the St Kilda area (specifically close to where the women mainly work, i.e. Greeves Street and Grey Street) that were designed to support sex workers, none compared to the Gatehouse in terms of accessibility, safety, getting provisions (such as hygiene products and food and drinks) and being a non-discriminatory environment for street-based sex workers. The Gatehouse staff provided services to sex workers beyond their position descriptions and appeared to genuinely have an interest in the well-being of the sex workers. For example, support workers often took women to the pharmacy for their methadone treatment, or provided them with transport if they were having trouble getting back to the Gatehouse. The staff developed personal relationships with the sex workers and kept in contact with them even over weekends when the Gatehouse was closed. The Gatehouse was the place where street-based sex workers reported that they came to obtain a sense of belonging and to feel included in a community.

Other organisations within the St Kilda area that also provide outreach and referral services to street-based sex workers include Resourcing Health and Education for the Sex Industry and the Sacred Heart Women's House. However, Nadia felt that other organisations were not as conveniently located, private and quiet as the Gatehouse. Nadia felt that the Gatehouse was a 'God send' because it was located in close proximity to where most street-based workers recruited clients:

> There's the other services all within walking distance but I like this one because it's a quiet street and you don't have to go out on the busy roads for everyone to see and this is the street I work in so I'm not about to take time off work to go all the way up there when I can just come here.

Although Dee, a sex worker who had lost custody of her daughter, had accessed other services in the local area, she felt that the Gatehouse staff had nurtured a relationship with her and treated her less formally than other services. Dee felt that she could 'hang out' at the Gatehouse, whereas she could not do this at other support service facilities in the area. Upon questioning Dee about her involvement in the Gatehouse's regular activities (cooking, helping out with the weekly barbeque), she replied, 'The people know me'. Dee also felt that, if it was not for the Gatehouse and her relationship with the staff, 'There's no way I'd be here'. Dee discussed her experience with other services:

> Before I came here I was hanging around at the women's house, the Saturday night mission and I was always going there. Every day I was hanging out there and starving, then I started to come here and now I don't go to the women's house anymore cause they're a little bit different, the way they treat people and stuff like that . . . Whereas here at the Gatehouse you can do whatever you want, go as you please.

Sense of community

The Gatehouse provided a sense of community for the women. Aimee's experience of the Gatehouse had always been positive, and she believed that it was inclusive for all street-based sex workers. When she visited the Gatehouse, she felt it 'is like my second family'. Despite the lack of support women gave to each other outside of the Gatehouse, women came together at the Gatehouse to chat, play netball in the local netball team and participate in recreational activities such as the weekly barbeque. Aimee believed that, at the Gatehouse, feelings of animosity between workers tended to be overridden. The Gatehouse brought people together, and the women had an opportunity to talk and discuss issues they had with one another. Aimee believed that, if it was not for the Gatehouse, more problems would occur between the workers:

> They look after you well here especially the barbeques. It brings a lot of people together around here as well. It's a lot friendlier and girls . . . there's, if girls aren't getting along it brings them together and they might actually start talking and resolve shit too. I found that. A few girls have done that. They weren't talking and then they have. So this helps. I reckon the Gatehouse is if it wasn't here there'd be a lot more trouble out there. Not just me I'd say a lot of other people as well, I'd say it. There's a lot of good people working in here as well which helps.

Barbara, who had been a sex worker for two years, also viewed the Gatehouse as a place where she could socialise with others, regardless of how frequently she worked on Greeves Street:

> I don't come that often and when I do, I only stay, well, well if I do a lot of socialising because I like coming here and talking to the ladies but honestly when I'm out there I'm only doing a couple and then I go, just do what I need and I have found that the girls down here are all great and everything.

Provision of services

Women who accessed the Gatehouse did so for similar reasons, such as provision of support, referral, to relax, and to eat and drink. Women who went to the Gatehouse were hungry and appreciative of the food that was provided. Every day the tables were set and food, such as biscuits, lollies, fruit, chips, sandwiches and scones, which had been donated, were laid out for women to eat. There was always tea, coffee, cordial and water available for the women. The women that frequented the Gatehouse knew they could come in at any time and help themselves to food and beverages. In addition, the Gatehouse provided women with tampons, sanitary towels, condoms, razors, toothbrushes and other toiletries. A supply of clothes for women to take that had been donated by local businesses, council authorities and members of the public were also available. Women wore the clothes on occasions such as court appearances and job interviews.

Belinda appreciated the small comforts and conveniences the Gatehouse offered street-based sex workers like her:

> But you know little things like that and go get a tampon or a pad or go to the toilet like before you know come like you know half an hour away and my friend we're thirsty, just sit down and have a couple of glasses of cordial just before you have to go out and sit in the sun and try and get work for as long as it's going to take you.

Conclusion

The findings of the study reveal that the Gatehouse creates a safe and non-judgemental environment for female street-based sex workers, thereby promoting social inclusiveness. Most importantly, having a stigma- and discrimination-free environment removes barriers to access for female sex workers (Rowe 2003a; Kurtz et al. 2005; Corrigan et al. 2006), allowing the Gatehouse to actively support these women with their physical and emotional needs. Another barrier to access that the Gatehouse manages to overcome is that women who frequent its services are not seen as deserving of the violence inflicted upon them by clients (Pyett and Warr 1999; Fick 2005; Quadara 2008; Jiménez et al. 2011; Sallman 2011) and can comfortably discuss any personal experiences as street-based sex workers. Women can come and go as they please, and take any necessary personal items, food and provisions. The women are free to engage in casual interactions with other women and the Gatehouse support workers, and access the professional and recreational services provided by them.

One of the limitations of the study was that no female sex workers from ethnically diverse backgrounds were interviewed. Although the Gatehouse serves all women that enter the premises regardless of age and culture, mainly Caucasian women access the Gatehouse. Why this occurs is unknown. Additionally, the Gatehouse provides services to male and transsexual sex workers. However, as this study focuses on female sex workers only, we are unable to make references to male sex workers.

This research suggests that the Gatehouse is an organisation that operates successfully on the ideology of social inclusiveness for street-based sex workers. Sex workers feel they can access the organisation without feeling judged or stigmatised. They experience a sense of community when visiting or simply 'hanging out'. Provisions are available for them and, through the support workers, referrals are made or one-on-one counselling is arranged. There is the opportunity for women to come together and cook or become involved in activities offered by the organisation. Women feel that the Gatehouse is situated conveniently on Greeves Street, St Kilda, where most clients drive by, and it is not as formal as other support services in the vicinity. Another strength of the Gatehouse is that the core values remain integral to the organisation's operation, and they are not influenced or compromised by the businesses and organisations that fund the facility. From the outset, the Gatehouse's mission has been of inclusiveness, unconditional support, service, and social justice for street-based sex workers. This ideology and associated organisational policies and practices have been operational for 14 years. Female sex workers who access the organisation are aware of the socially inclusive culture of the Gatehouse, which, as they have identified, can at times be difficult to find in other support services.

We recommend that the values and mission that underpin the Gatehouse model be considered not only for organisations that support street-based sex workers in Australia, but also for other marginalised populations, such as the homeless and drug-addicted populations. Providing a judgement-free service where these populations can access food, clothes and hygiene provisions, and feel as though they belong to a community would benefit these groups and create a sense of belonging. The Gatehouse has managed over the course of its existence, to practice social inclusiveness and has not deviated from this core value since its inception.

Part V

Practising inclusion in community life

11 Promoting social inclusion of frail older people living in the community

Ann Taket, Sarah Pollock, Lisa Hanna,
Emily Learmonth and Peta Farquhar

Introduction

The increasingly diverse needs and wants of Australia's ageing population, like those in many other societies, are drawing attention to aged care as an increasingly important area of broader health and social policy. Active ageing and a focus on enabling people to remain living in their own homes in the community are two of the key components of this policy shift. The policy shift towards active ageing recognises and aims to support the desires of older people to remain active members of their communities as they age. Active ageing is 'the process of optimising opportunities for physical, social and mental well-being throughout the life-course, in order to extend healthy life expectancy, productivity and quality of life in older age' (AIPC 2008: 26). According to the World Health Organization (WHO), the rights, needs, preferences and capacities of older people should be central to active ageing policies, and these should be framed by a life-course approach to ageing (WHO 2002). The development of age-friendly communities, social inclusion and engagement are emerging as key policy issues in the context of an ageing population (Lui et al. 2009). Recent research demonstrates the importance of a sense of belonging in maintaining a sense of identity and increasing the wellbeing of an individual (Vanclay et al. 2008; Wiles et al. 2009). The sense of belonging that comes about through community engagement also plays a role in successful adjustment to ageing, including prolonging good health and reduced risk of entry into residential aged care (Djernes 2006; Kimberley and Simons 2009; Knapp 2009; Wiles et al. 2009).

Connections between social isolation and lack of community engagement suggest that an absence of community engagement may lead to, or be a consequence of, social isolation. Evidence demonstrates how ageing can increase the risk of social isolation, through reduced social activities due to the death of family members and friends, restricted mobility resulting from ill-health, or changed work and financial circumstances (ABS 1999). Furthermore, as a person ages there is often a reduction in physical and cognitive function, which leads to the loss of independence and an increased need for formal health care, which can increase social isolation (Beswick et al. 2008).

Frail older people living on their own in the community often report isolation, loneliness and social exclusion. This chapter reports on a well-established
volunteer programme run by a community service organisation in Melbourne,
Australia, that has successfully promoted social inclusion for this particularly
vulnerable group, drawing out implications for similar practice elsewhere. The
chapter first gives an overview of the volunteer programme, and introduces a
number of different pieces of research that have examined the programme and
its effects. Following this, the chapter summarises the effects of the volunteer
programme on social inclusion, and then concludes by drawing out implications for policy and practice.

Do Care and social support

Do Care is a social support service provided by Wesley Mission, Victoria, to
address social isolation and assist older people to sustain involvement in or
to become involved with their communities, with the intention of prolonging their independence. Do Care works with each participant to meet their
individual needs. A range of activities are available (see Table 11.1 below),
and participants are able to select those that best meet their needs and interests. The programme includes rigorous assessment of potential volunteers and
participants by the paid coordinators, who also oversee the establishment and
monitoring of matches to ensure that the matches continue to meet the clients'
needs. The programme operates throughout metropolitan Melbourne and surrounding semi-rural municipalities. In 2010, over 890 socially isolated people
and 790 volunteers participated in this service.

Researching the programme

So far there have been four different, linked, small studies that have looked
at various aspects of the volunteer programme. A 2009 quantitative research
study explored mental health in independently living older people and the role
of volunteer befriending in the Do Care programme (Illingworth et al. 2009).

Table 11.1 Do Care activities

Do Care activity	Participant involvement
One-to-one matches	Individual is matched with a volunteer with similar interests, who visits on a regular basis. Social activities are negotiated
Small regular group activities	Activities are run at various locations, including the Do Care offices. Do Care clients have involvement in the selection of activities and groups
Telelink	Provides social support and friendships in small groups over the telephone
Annual functions	A range of one-off functions for special occasions, e.g. outings, Christmas function

This study found that clients' experience of depression was reduced the longer they had been involved with the programme. The findings suggested this was related to the quality of the relationship between the volunteer and client. A second research study (Pennington and Knight 2008) investigated the lived experiences of volunteers and older people in the Do Care programme. This examined the befriending journey and considered the elements that contributed to the volunteer–older person relationship, particularly those elements that led to a deeper sense of connectedness. They found that two different types of beneficial relationships could develop: one where the relationship remained characterised as a volunteer–client relationship, and the other where the relationship became closer and could be described as being like friendship or even family-like. These family-like relationships also resulted in some feelings of emotional obligation, tying the volunteer to the older person. Friendships and family-like relationships resulted in greater levels of enjoyment for both the volunteer and the older person.

Both these studies explored elements of the volunteer–older person relationship as facilitated by the Do Care programme. They give some insight into what comprises a good volunteer–client relationship, and the benefits of this. Reflecting on the findings led the Do Care staff to consider how the projects had been shaped by their own assumptions as professional workers about important aspects of relationships, community and belonging. They wondered how the clients of their programme thought about these broader relationships and what they meant to them. In particular, they were interested in how the older, socially isolated people who formed their client group understood 'community', what they wanted from a community and the role they wanted to take up within in the communities that mattered to them.

This led to two further studies that were carried out at roughly the same time during 2010–11. For both these studies, a qualitative approach located within a social constructivist paradigm (Patton 2002; Brewer 2003) was used, integrating aspects of descriptive phenomenology with aspects of grounded theory (Sandelowski 2000; Annells 2006). While both sample sizes were small, they were both large enough to achieve saturation in analysis because of the richness of the data that in-depth, semi-structured interviewing can yield (Morse 1995; Guest et al. 2006).

The first study looked at the lived experience of wellbeing of people who are socially isolated, frail and in later middle or older age. The project, which involved in-depth interviews with a sample of Do Care clients (eight women and four men), is reported in full in Farquhar and Pollock (2011). It explored how participants understood wellbeing, what it meant to them, what helped their wellbeing, and what made it hard to maintain a sense of wellbeing. The interviews included discussion about their relationship with volunteers, where they had them, although not all the sample had been matched with a volunteer at time of interview. Farquhar and Pollock (2011) summarise the findings from their sample firstly in terms of four elements of wellbeing that participants talked about: connections with others; physical wellbeing and health;

emotional wellbeing and state of mind; and looking after yourself. In terms of what can affect wellbeing, six different factors were identified and explored: control; independence; reciprocity; healthiness; the future; and sense of self. The study demonstrated that the way in which these categories interacted, how they were experienced and how important each of them was, differed for each person. Nonetheless, each of these categories was fundamental to the experience of wellbeing.

The second study (Learmonth 2010) was designed to emphasise the voices of socially isolated older people and to explore their perceptions and experiences of 'community'. In-depth interviews were carried out with a sample of ten female Do Care clients, drawn from a different area to the wellbeing study so there was no overlap in the samples. In this study, one part of the interview explored the participants' views about the role that the Do Care programme played in supporting people to take part in the community. A grounded theory analysis was carried out, entailing data immersion, constant comparison, open and selective coding and thematic analysis. Concept maps were produced to represent findings. Learmonth et al. (2012) discuss the four main factors associated with 'community' that emerged from the data as positively affecting participants' wellbeing: social contact; community dynamics; feelings of support; and positive orientation. Each factor was identified in all or the majority of participants' accounts. There were also three categories of negative lived experiences which inhibited sense of community and impacted negatively on wellbeing: feelings about self; feeling about others; and fragmentation of self. The analysis identified a range of factors implicated in each of these.

In the following sections in this chapter the findings from these two studies that relate specifically to the volunteer programme are discussed. Pseudonyms have been used throughout to ensure the privacy of the people who took part in the studies. The impact of the service received from the Do Care volunteer was to strengthen the older person's positive lived experiences of community and his or her wellbeing, as well as mitigating against or reducing negative experiences of the participants in both studies. The size of the impact varied across the samples in both studies. Both studies reveal that participants relied on their individual Do Care volunteer for a variety of reasons. Figure 11.1 (drawn from the 'community' project but applicable to both) summarises Do Care's impact on participants' interaction and involvement in the community. The four different factors identified in the analysis were: increasing social activity; aiding mobility; friendship; and individuality of service. As these factors are equally present in the findings from the study on wellbeing, they are used to structure the discussion in the following sections.

Increasing social activity

Social contact was something that all participants valued and some participants relied on their Do Care volunteer to provide. Some participants were isolated and had limited communication with the outside world. Do Care volunteers

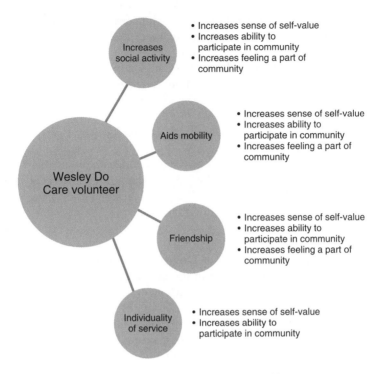

Figure 11.1 The impact of the volunteers on the participants' lives

were acknowledged to provide someone to chat to, a guaranteed visitor in their weekly routine and the company of someone with shared interests.

> Yeah, I go nuts if I don't [talk or see somebody], it's funny you need other contacts you know, that's why it's hard.
>
> (Emma)

> . . . he shows real interest. He doesn't – like a lot of people if you're gabbing on, you can see their eyes go glassy. But there's no movement, no emotion, no nothing. He's really interested.
>
> (Jack)

In discussing Do Care's activities outside of home, participants emphasised their value in terms of something to do, a routine activity to be looked forward to, a chance to participate in a valued activity or hobby, and a chance to get out of the house. There was considerable variation in involvement and feelings of belonging within the community due to these activities, related to participants' individual circumstances and characteristics. The social interaction experienced within Do Care's activities was valued by all participants who attended. Many of these participants discussed how having similarities and shared values with the other service users was important to them and added to their sense of belonging.

The social interaction provided by Do Care volunteers or by the other service users in Do Care activities was often associated with the importance of routine. Emma expresses how much she valued this routine:

> On Monday I usually like to go shopping, on Tuesday I go to the senior cits, on Wednesday, every other Wednesday I go to the [Do Care group] and on Thursday I go to [other group in suburb], on Friday [Do Care volunteer] comes, on Saturday I don't do anything really I do the ironing, on Sunday I am either here or I go with [other group suburb]. I like knowing my week has a routine to it, now I do, yeah.
>
> (Emma)

Additionally Do Care's range of activities were able to give some of the participants an option to take part in something outside of their home while providing them with social interaction. Many of the participants indicated that out-of-home activities were a good outlet and pleasurable way to break up the day. Additionally, the activities gave people something to look forward to, even in the short term. Positive images of the future, however small or near in time, were one of the factors that people identified as having a good impact on their wellbeing:

> I really enjoyed that, getting together with the group of guys [as part of the Do Care activity] . . . that was something I looked forward to.
>
> (Jack)

> I try to keep busy because otherwise I get pipy, as my grandmother used to say and I never knew what pipy was but now I do [laughing] . . . sort of irritable and bit flat, yeah.
>
> (Yasmin)

Aiding mobility

Some of the participants faced considerable mobility issues and discussed their limited access to activities within the community and to transport in general. In many cases these participants relied on their Do Care volunteer to take them to the group activities Do Care offered, and in some instances to complete personal errands such as shopping. Some of the Do Care activities that may have been daunting to some of the participants were made comfortable, as in most circumstances participants said that their Do Care volunteer accompanied them. Gabriella talks about how this improved her experience:

Oh lot of friends, they know me very well, they all hello Gabriella how are you? This and this. I like to be there once a month. I like [Do Care volunteer] there with me . . . I feel more confident with her.

(Gabriella)

Friendship

All participants discussed how friendship was associated with their Do Care volunteer or with the other service users at Do Care activities, and how this impacted on sense of community. Many participants expressed how much they valued their Do Care volunteer and how they had become a close friend or like family, like in Gabriella's case:

We become like two sisters, so yes she's [Do Care volunteer] wonderful and she take me if a day like today [wet and cold] she take me to shop so I can walk around there with a frame, if it's a lovely day we go around outside with a frame.

(Gabriella)

The length of the friendship, having shared values and how this relationship impacted on their life and feelings was also discussed by participants. This is illustrated in how both Jack and Leonie described their friendship with their volunteers:

We got on so well, I mean, the hour's discussion generally went to about three hours and so forth. He had interests same as mine: I liked woodwork and that sort of things . . . So we finished up having a lot in common.

(Jack)

I am happy when I have company . . . he [Do Care volunteer] has always been there to help I was in [name] hospital for 4 months, and he used to come and visit me every second day and his wife would come in sometimes on the other day. So you don't have many friends like that.

(Leonie)

As with Leonie, some participants acknowledged how their Do Care volunteer had provided them with extended relationships, such as becoming friends with their volunteer's families. This was also the case for Jane and Sue:

I went to her place [Do Care volunteer's home] at Easter time, which was nice, she invited me there . . . I know her family yeah. Her husband has been here for dinner, which was nice. They came over here when my son was here for dinner with her, and that was nice for my son to have another male in the house here to talk to.

(Jane)

She's a lovely person [Do Care volunteer]. She has two teenagers they also are happy to sometimes come around.

(Sue)

Other participants appreciated the social contact and company of the other Do Care service users; however, they did not acknowledge these people as 'real' friends. For example:

Well I wouldn't say they [other Do Care service users] are exactly friends because they are in the same boat I am in, they can't drive, they can't come and see you, so you only meet when you go to those functions you know, but still when I have met them outside at [suburb shopping name] or something we have a natter then.

(Emma)

Some participants acknowledged difficulties in fitting in and forming friendships in out-of-home activities, and some felt that they were a stranger to the group when they first joined. Olga and Emma shared their struggles:

I was with them [Do Care activity] oh about six months or so before I got to feel a part of them, because they had been together for a while, cliques had already formed you know and friendships, but now they have accepted me.

(Olga)

Only when you get older I don't think you have that get up and go to do it. I am always open to learning something else, it's not that, it's just friendships are hard to make I think.

(Emma)

The friendships made through the range of Do Care services served to increase participants' sense of self value and therefore their sense both of their wellbeing and of their belonging to a community. The availability of Do Care activities increased their ability to participate in the community and their feelings of being part of the community.

Individuality of service

As can be seen from some of the quotes above, the participants had very different preferences for the types and amounts of social activity that they wanted to incorporate in their lives. All participants valued the individuality of the services provided by Do Care. This included the individual volunteer match up and diversity relating to the range of Do Care activities offered. The majority of the participants talked about how much they valued having similarities and shared values or hobbies with their Do Care volunteer, some crediting Do

Care for having a good individual match-up process. Olga appreciated that she felt no pressure and felt valued knowing she was receiving an individual assessment:

> I have a lady [Do Care volunteer], they [Do Care] asked me if I would like someone to call and see me, for a while I said no, but after a while, they said oh [Olga] I have a lady who would be great for you and you'd get on well with her, she introduced me, and we get on really well . . . And she [Do Care staff member] didn't rush me to have a visitor; she really waited until she found somebody. And I think she realised I am very self-sufficient and there is not much more I would want, you know.
>
> (Olga)

The individuality of Do Care's services led to participants' having an increased sense of self-value and a feeling of being part of the community. Also, participants' had an increased desire to apply self-effort to become a part of the 'community' in that they felt they had the support of a diversity of components of Do Care services.

Conclusion

While the older people had very different views on the type and level of activity they wanted in their life, there were nonetheless strong shared themes about the importance of feeling included in the community. Participants positively valued social contact, including group activities, having something to look forward to, and routine; the level of contact different participants wanted varied considerably. All participants valued the relationship with their matched volunteer, regardless of whether this remained as a volunteer–client relationship, or, became more like a friendship or family relationship. The impact of the Do Care programme is considerable. It gives socially isolated older people the opportunity to reconnect with their local community and form new social networks, and holds a valued and significant role in the lives of participants.

The model of volunteer support in the community, plus, where possible, an associated wider programme of shared activities, is thus one that commends itself for widespread use. A number of aspects of the scheme seem particularly important in bringing about its positive impacts. The first of these is the careful matching of each older person to a suitable volunteer, coupled with careful selection of both the volunteers and the older people. Second is flexibility in the nature and boundaries of the volunteer role, permitting friendships to form where mutually agreeable; and flexibility and choice in the associated programme of shared activities.

In the case considered here, a government-funded programme supporting services for frail older people, younger people with disabilities and their carers (the Home and Community Care Program) provides funds for the paid coordinators who undertake the work of matching volunteers and clients and providing them with ongoing support as and when they need it. This role is vital in ensuring that a quality service can be delivered, often in the clients' homes, in a manner that is safe for both client and volunteer. It is important to recognise that delivering a programme like this need not be of high cost, and for many of the older people, the amount of time involved was small, by their own choice. Perhaps most importantly of all, the older people's involvement at whatever level they chose, was successful in increasing their sense of belonging, arguably the most important facet of social inclusion:

> . . . none of us are independent. I mean we have our freedom and every-thing, but I feel that we are much happier when we feel we belong.
>
> (Olga)

12 Enabling new students to feel that they matter

Promoting social inclusion within the university community

Beth R. Crisp and John Fox

Introduction

Widening participation in higher education has long been proposed as a key strategy for promoting social inclusion in countries including Australia (Gale and Tranter 2011) and the UK (Tett 2004). Consequently, as higher education has been transformed from an elite to a mass education model, universities now attract a much more diverse cohort of students than ever before. However, simply offering places in higher education does not in itself necessarily promote social inclusion unless the institution is prepared to adapt its ways of working to ensure that all students are provided with the means to demonstrate their capacity for learning (Gale and Tranter 2011) and are regarded as full citizens within the university community (Tett 2004). Hence this chapter describes the rationale for, and introduces, an initiative which aimed to enhance the participation of first-year students in the university community.

There is a growing emphasis in Australian universities on the importance of the first-year experience, and in particular on how we might engage with first-year students (Krause et al. 2005). Considerable efforts have been devoted to developing programmes to orient new students to universities along with ongoing provision of support to retain them. However, while such programmes routinely report high degrees of effectiveness, there continues to be a significant minority of first-year students who remain unaware of fundamental university processes and of staff in key roles who could assist them in their transition to becoming part of the university community (Burnett 2009). Such students have typically been depicted as deficient (Lawrence 2002), lacking in the necessary skills (Smith 2002, 2004; Winterson and Russ 2009) or confidence (Burland and Pitts 2007), rather than recognising the complexity of university structures and systems with which they are expected to become familiar in a very short space of time. First-year students, in addition to gaining academic knowledge in their chosen disciplines, are expected to master information about university admissions and enrolment processes, fees, timetables and being allocated to tutorials and assessment processes, including how examinations are organised (Grenfell 2009).

The sheer size of the university results in many students experiencing 'feeling lost' (Christie et al. 2008: 570) or 'feelings of alarm' (Hartmann 2001: 116). At the same time, they may be confronted with greater expectations, than they had previously experienced, that they will be independent learners (Smith and Hopkins 2005). In addition, they are exposed to different methods of learning, particularly those that involve a move away from teacher as expert who imparts knowledge, to teacher as facilitator of student learning experiences. Students who have previously studied on courses where there were right and wrong answers find they are now required to learn processes rather than facts (Griffiths et al. 2005). Hence it is unsurprising that the transition to university has been described in terms of 'shock' (Wilcox et al. 2005: 715; Christie et al. 2008: 570), being 'disoriented' (Ballinger 2003: 100) and a 'struggle' (Leathwood and O'Connell 2003: 607).

Although it has been suggested that students coming straight from secondary school may have greater support needs than other students commencing university (Bartram 2008), a recent Scottish study found that for first-time university students, even those who had attended some other form of post-secondary-school studies, the transition to university was daunting. In particular, the scale of the university campus, being in classes with hundreds of other students and even the enormity of the library were a shock for new students. As a result,

> Students felt that the university was a large, and at times, off-putting environment; the academic demands made of them were higher than they had anticipated; and they found it difficult to manage the competing demands of university study, home and family, and in many instances, paid employment.
>
> (Cree et al. 2009: 891).

Abbott-Chapman and Edward's (1999) claim that diversity is now mainstream is noteworthy here, and suggests that the experience of mature-age students is increasingly becoming the norm of student experience, rather than an exception (Crossan et al. 2003; Clegg et al. 2006). The literature concerning mature-age students reports less engagement with university processes outside of direct learning activities, given other, conflicting demands such as paid work and personal relationships (in particular, caring responsibilities), as well as students' difficulties in accessing student support services, which have typically been designed to service the needs of school leavers (Tones et al. 2009).

The importance of relationships

Although developing a sense of connectedness with others does not necessarily result in students feeling they belong, getting to know others is often crucial in facilitating students to feel that they belong to, and are citizens of, the university community (Crisp 2010a). Hence the significance of interpersonal relationships, including relationships with university staff and with other students, is increasingly becoming recognised as being crucial in the process of becoming a university student as well has having positive effects on learning, retention and course completion (Pascarella and Terenzini 2005). Although 'belonging' (Read et al. 2003; Yorke 2004; Pittman and Richmond 2008) and 'mattering' (Rayle and Chung 2007) are crucial, a study of first-year students in Australian universities found that one-third were not confident that at least one member of the teaching staff knew them by name (Krause et al. 2005). Yet recognition may be particularly important for students who do not conform to traditional notions of who is a university student (Reay et al. 2002; Crossan et al. 2003; Read et al. 2003; Moreau and Leathwood 2006; Christie et al. 2008), who are the first in their family to attend university (Lehmann 2007; Collier and Morgan 2008), parents (Reay et al. 2002) and/or international students (Ramsay et al. 2006; Skyrme 2007; Bartram 2008).

It has been suggested that one key contribution that higher education institutions can make is the provision of appropriate spaces to facilitate the development of and participation in social networks such as accommodation (Wilcox et al. 2005) and 'appropriate social facilities' such as student union bars (Thomas 2002). Notwithstanding the many students who benefit from such initiatives, many others seem to engage with university processes on a selective or strategic basis, with little or no participation in social activities or student services which are offered on campus (Abbott-Chapman and Edwards 1999).

Developments in information technology also have the potential to undervalue the importance of relationships with staff and other students in the university. Many universities are now providing podcasts of lectures and a range of other learning materials online, but assumptions about IT competence may alienate students with limited skills or capacity to engage in online learning communities (Kennedy et al. 2008). Furthermore, being able to use mainstream technologies, such as the internet and mobile phones, does not directly transfer to the use of other forms or uses of specialist technologies in the educational setting, such as bibliographic databases that provide information about 'unstructured' resources such as books and journal articles (Hartmann 2001).

An initiative to promote connectedness among first-year university students

As university teachers, whose responsibilities have included teaching first-year students and the coordination of degree programmes, part of our working lives involves responding to situations associated with the transition to being a university student. Most obviously this includes steering students in the right direction as they attempt to negotiate the myriad of academic, administrative and support systems that are aimed at assisting them realise the goal of graduating with a recognised qualification. We are also required to resource or contribute to university initiatives to orient new students and increase retention rates, some of which seem more effective than others in reaching students on the margins of the university community.

For several years, the first author taught the introductory unit in Deakin University's Bachelor of Social Work degree. A high proportion of students came from socio-economically disadvantaged backgrounds, and many were the first in their family to attend university and arrived at the university knowing no one. Compared to other undergraduate courses, there are high numbers of mature-age students who have family commitments, disabilities and/or physical and mental health issues. As well as having experienced some form of educational disadvantage, many of our students lack critical support structures for their studies outside the university.

In response to these issues, the first author sought to meet with all students enrolled in her first-year unit on an individual basis, twice in their first semester of study to discuss their assignments. Having previously taught in universities in the UK at which all undergraduate students were appointed a personal tutor with whom they were encouraged to meet a few times each semester, she was aware that in Australia large class sizes and the absence of a personal tutor scheme resulted in many first-year students having little or no individual contact with their teachers.

The first semester of studies is recognised as critical, given that this is the most likely period when students will discontinue their studies (Rausch and Hamilton 2006), and consequently staff have explored different ways of teaching students in this unit in an effort to maximise engagement. In 2009, 'Introduction to Social Work' was composed of a weekly one and a half hour interactive workshop for the whole cohort (25 students), which introduced students to the topic of the week, and one-hour small group tutorials (10–15 students per group) in which students discussed the readings of the week and the assignments. In the week before each of their two assignments were due, the group tutorials were replaced by individual meetings with the first author, who was the unit coordinator. All individual interviews took place on the day of the week on which they normally attended both workshops and group tutorials. Students who did not attend group tutorials that week were emailed about the arrangements. A listing of allocations was also placed on the virtual classroom webpage for the unit.

The majority of students (21 of the 25) came to their appointments prior to Assignment 1. This contrasted sharply with the group tutorial attendance, which had a small core of regular attendees and several who attended infrequently. Coincidentally, these meetings were scheduled for the day which was the due date for assignments in two other units which most of these students were enrolled in, and that for some students these were the very first university assignments they had ever submitted. Hence only one student brought with them a draft assignment for discussion, although a number of others had commenced working on the assignment and we discussed where they were at and any issues that had presented themselves. What had not been anticipated was that a number of students would come to an individual tutorial about an assignment that they had not yet started, and in some cases had not even decided which of the four possible topics they were going to tackle. A few students were also not aware of what the first assignment entailed. Conversations with these students tended to be around ensuring they knew how to access the various pieces of information, such as the assignment questions and the library resources. A number of students were more generally confused about university processes and were struggling to make the transition to university studies. These students were provided with information about relevant university processes and services and, if necessary, extensions to the due date for submitting the assignment were also negotiated. In contrast to previous years when a number of assignments were submitted late without having sought an extension, all assignments were accounted for by the due date, either having been submitted on time or an extension sought.

The second individual meetings occurred in the last week of teaching, one week prior to the second assignment being due. A total of 18 students attended on this day, with a further three students offering apologies due to being ill and unable to attend. Of the remaining four who did not attend, three of these were students who had not attended the first round of individual meetings. Although attendance at tutorials and workshops had hovered around ten students for the previous couple of weeks, a number of students who had not been seen in class for several weeks came to this meeting. Again there were a few students who had made sufficient progress on the assignment to talk about specific issues that had arisen for them. As with the first assignment, many of the conversations concerned a range of transitional issues, rather than a narrow focus on the assignment. Many of the conversations were about more general guidance of how to go about the assignment. In a number of instances extension dates were negotiated. By the time the second assignment was due, all but two assignments had either been submitted or the students had been granted an extension. One of these missing assignments was from a student who did not attend the second individual tutorial and had not been seen for several weeks.

Some surprising and promising outcomes followed from these meetings. Scheduling individual meetings with all students not only enabled problems to be identified early but also encouraged contact with students whose studies were going well and who might otherwise not make contact with members of the academic staff. One such student commented at the first meeting that this was the first time she had been in the office of an academic staff member of the university. It seems likely that this student had direct contact with teaching and support staff as part of her secondary studies, but for some reason she had little expectation of contact with teaching staff in the university.

Discussion

Although a sense of social connectedness may be crucial for individuals to sense a place for themselves in a community (Taket et al. 2009a), retaining 'the human element' (Davies 1988) is important in an era in which recipients of information are deemed to be members of a community by virtue of being 'on the list'. In universities a new student's identity can readily become their ID number rather than their name, and students who are unsure of how the organisation functions may not want to identify these concerns in the classroom, particularly if they perceive that other students do understand the university (Davies 1988). By normalising the opportunity to have a discrete conversation with a university staff member, a number of issues that students were experiencing were able to be redressed before they escalated into more serious difficulties (Jacklin and Le Riche 2009).

While individual contact with a staff member may be important in assisting the process of becoming a member of the university community (Tinto 1987), it is necessary to remember that the students participating in this initiative only met with a staff member for 10 minutes on two occasions. But it clearly met a need, given that students who did not normally attend classes and who tended to be more disengaged with the university overall actually participated in these meetings.

As university teachers, it is important for us to acknowledge that universities are very different to the institutions we enrolled in as undergraduates, when many first-year students would have direct contact with and be known to at least some of their teachers. Although universities currently spend considerable amounts of money on orientation and other activities to facilitate transition to university life, in neither of the authors' universities is there a programme for ensuring that all first-year students are able to meet with at least one of their teachers on an individual basis. Rather, within the context of funding constraints and heavy staff workloads, the timely and effective support of the transition of first-year students to higher education is becoming increasingly difficult. The pressure to make savings and efficiencies in transition supports by providing standardised services seems to be increasing at the very time when demands for greater diversity and responsiveness are growing.

However, supporting the first-year transition is not simply a matter of more service provision by universities (Palmer et al. 2009). Without an appreciation of the students' perspective, it is difficult to be confident that any transition support will be successful. Perhaps the most promising approach to considering how students navigate their way into university is the work of a number of authors who have drawn on Bourdieu's (1993) concept of 'habitus'. That is '. . . the norms and practices of particular social classes or groups . . . a set of dispositions created and shaped by the interaction between objective structures and personal histories' (Thomas 2002: 430).

Different social milieus will exhibit different habituses, with that difference reflected in participants' experience of moving between them varying from unconscious and comfortable, to consciously uncomfortable, as Bourdieu put it, a 'fish out of water' (in Thomas 2002: 431). These different habituses can focus on a range of arenas, including peers or friends, family, gender and class or focus on particular institutions, such as secondary schools and universities (Reay et al. 2001). A better recognition of the various spheres in which students are engaged and of the manner in which those habituses do or do not support a successful transition to university is required rather than continuing to view transition difficulties as the necessarily the fault of the student. More particularly, in building socially inclusive university communities, institutions cannot ignore the tensions involved in becoming and remaining a student which arise from the competing demands of students' varied and changing relationships/identities. Supports provided need to recognise these tensions and be able to respond to individual students and not just to identified problem categories for which a student may seek assistance, if they know how to do so.

Conclusion

Although this chapter has focused on promoting social inclusion within a university community, the key recommendations that emerge apply to a much broader range of organisations and communities. Widening participation by encouraging those outside our traditional recruitment strategies to become involved in a community is just the first step. Not only might we need to provide adequate information to new members, but we also need to engage in critical reflection on our habitus or organisational practices with a view to understanding them from the perspective of an outsider. Furthermore, although provision of information may be essential, we also need to ensure there are opportunities for new members to develop relationships with other members of the community. An inclusive community promotes connectedness between its members and also recognises the diversity of community members. These recommendations may seem rather obvious but, as this chapter attests, they are too often overlooked, resulting in communities that foster social exclusion rather than promote social inclusion.

13 Community-driven social inclusion practice

A case study of a multicultural women's friendship group

Lisa Hanna and Jan Moore

Background

The promotion of social inclusion is not restricted to the domain of politicians, policy makers and social, health or welfare professionals. Australian government policy emphasises the importance of a multi-sectoral approach, engaging not just government and business but also community organisations and citizens in order to build community capacity to generate and maintain socially inclusive communities (Australian Government 2010). In this chapter we examine the practice of social inclusion as enacted by community members rather than health professionals or policy makers. We present a case study of how community members themselves can initiate, enact and sustain social inclusion practice. We draw on a programme of participatory research carried out with members of a community-generated, not-for-profit multicultural women's friendship group operating in outer east Melbourne, Australia.

In 2006, the founders of the group, a group of friends who supported the idea of the group, initiated a social gathering to enable older women from diverse cultural backgrounds to meet regularly. The group's president had identified a need for such a group in her community, particularly for those women who had been widowed and were experiencing social isolation as a consequence. The founding committee placed an open invitation in the local newspaper inviting older women to meet once a month to share friendship; 50 women attended the first meeting.

In 2009, committee members of the group approached one of the authors, Jan Moore, requesting research partnership and collaboration. At the time of study (2009–11) the group had attracted over 200 women from 30 nationalities. Members' ages ranged from 46 to 97 years, with many being retired and/or widowed. Meetings were held monthly and varied in content, but typically included educative sessions on life matters appropriate to the group such as legal advice, community services, health issues and welfare assistance. With the growth of the group, some local government funding was secured and recreational activities were introduced such as craft and exercise classes. Three or four times a year members participated in an organised day trip outside of the city to encourage friendship and provide outings for women who may otherwise have few opportunities to travel. Members supported these activities with gold coin donations.

While our participatory research was initially designed to investigate the potential for group membership to enhance social health and wellbeing in older women (Mutisya 2011) and to produce a robust report on the group's functioning and characteristics (Moore et al. 2011), subsequent strands of research have included a further undergraduate project which produced recommendations and guidelines for similar groups (Renton 2011) and a focus on the group's experiences of exclusion and inclusion (data reported in this chapter). Collectively, these case study data offer a rich resource with which to examine community-driven social inclusion practice.

Our data highlight community capacity to develop and apply health promotion principles without formal professional affiliation or theoretical grounding, and provide a rich description of community participation, agency and ownership of the social inclusion agenda. We reflect on the factors contributing to the success and sustainability of the group as a facilitator of social connection, and on the potential formation of similar community-driven groups to enhance social inclusion at a grass-roots level.

Methods

Over the course of the research programme, the research team (including authors Jan Moore and Lisa Hanna, both university academics, and two students) attended and participated in a range of group meetings and events. Documentary material such as group mission statements, committee agendas and minutes was collected to provide background and context to the group's activities and processes. Five focus groups were conducted with group members. Four focus groups facilitated in 2010 by JM and a student researcher aimed to explore group members' perspectives on social health and wellbeing, and analysis of these data suggested that group membership was perceived to be a potent factor in attenuating social exclusion. Therefore, a fifth focus group discussion, facilitated in 2011 by LH, aimed to explore group members' and committee members' perspectives on the group's contribution to the promotion of social inclusion in the community.

Each focus group consisted of 9–10 group members and took place in quiet rooms at the group meeting venue. Forty-three group members participated in total. Focus group discussions comprised participants from diverse cultural backgrounds and included women who identified their heritage as European, Asian, African and third-, fourth- or fifth-generation Australian, and ranging from 46 to 86 years of age. Discussions were between 60 and 90 minutes' duration, and were audio-recorded and transcribed verbatim for analysis. Data were analysed thematically to illuminate our examination of community-driven social inclusion practice as enacted in and by this case study group. Data from the final focus group only (examining the group's practice of social inclusion directly) are presented here, supplemented by our examination of documentary material.

However, all findings and themes are supported by data from the preceding strands of data collection. All participant names used below are pseudonyms.

Overcoming exclusion and promoting inclusion

The Australian Government states that it considers 'a socially inclusive society [to be] one in which all Australians feel valued and have the opportunity to participate fully in the life of our society' (Australian Government 2012). However, our data indicated that older women living in this Melbourne community were susceptible to social exclusion along a number of dimensions, and that the group's community-driven practice involved overcoming the barriers to social inclusion identified by members. Participants' construction of social inclusion encompassed dimensions of sharing, belonging, friendship, acceptance and a reduction in isolation, as shown in the following examples:

> [Social inclusion means] to be friends with anybody you meet and not because of their race or opinions.
>
> (Margaret)

> [Social inclusion means] just not to be alone. Because at times, like, you know what happened in my life, I sort of became very much alone.
>
> (Jane)

Forging an inclusive identity: group vision and leadership

The first step in the group's practice of social inclusion was its formation in 2006 by the president and working group, who had identified a need in their community for a space and place in which older women could connect with each other. The group's vision statement, developed by its initial working group and committee in 2009, is as follows:

> To establish a community group that will assist in bringing together mature women from all nationalities and cultures to help ease isolation and loneliness, promote assimilation and social connection; provide company, support and the exchange of friendship in a safe and trusting environment. A community group such as this has the potential to enhance the social health and wellbeing of its members.

Such an inclusive approach and focus by the group's committee may have contributed to the welcoming ethos permeating the group, as highlighted in the following participant statements:

> I'm only a new member . . . but when I first came in, and I was alone, I found people came up and talked to me.
>
> (Eva)

I feel we should accept people and also we should be the one doing something to mix with people.

(Florence)

Transcending culture and cliques: promoting 'one-ness'

As stated in the group's vision statement, a core component of the group's identity was its multicultural emphasis. A dominant dimension in which group members identified social exclusion as occurring was that of culture, a perception supported by research literature (Women's Health in the North 2006; Maslen 2008; Manderson 2010). Members who were recent or past immigrants to Australia shared their experiences of perceived discrimination and potential exclusion from the local community due to their cultural status or language ability:

Mine has always been, 'Oh you speak very good English' [laughter]. And again so there . . . they have put you in a box, because of how you look or what colour you are you shouldn't be speaking such good English . . . They just tend to size you up and again, see, I may be wrong in coming out so strongly but people say that racism does not exist, I beg to differ.

(Linda)

However, another participant identified that the group contributed to the breaking down of language barriers due to its diverse ethnic and linguistic membership and its pervasive ethos of altruism and willingness to help those in need:

Sometimes I feel that especially among the [ethnic] community, a lot of them fear to speak up in English . . . they think that it's the language barrier, and they say 'Oh, I can't speak good English, I don't think I could join'. And I often told them, I said 'Forget about this, we can help each other. I am sure among us there are people that can speak your language'. Like last time, when I left here, one of the ladies from [country], she asked me to help her ring up a taxi and I did help her. And then she said 'Oh, stay with me because I'm scared to talk to taxi driver'. I said 'Of course I will'. So we are sort of helping each other and she said to me she didn't feel like coming, you know, in the beginning because she found that it is hard for her to speak the language. I said 'You shouldn't worry about this, any time you know we will help you'. So she seems to be really happy after that, yeah. And besides the taxi driver didn't turn up and at last one of our members, whose husband did go and take her, and I asked help from them and they immediately was willing to take her to [suburb] and the couple lives in [a different suburb], but they said 'Oh, it doesn't matter'. So we really are helping each other, so I was ever so happy to see that.

(Florence)

The group's strong emphasis on multicultural acceptance and inclusivity – its 'levelling' ethos – was perceived to be very important to its success in promoting and practising social inclusion within the wider community:

> Well, any race, any kind of person, it doesn't matter what age you are, it's all included, you know?
>
> (Jane)

> We don't see differences . . . no religion or any religion, all accepted. It's not discussed. And colour, race. In fact it's quite exciting really, with the different races it's very exciting in fact . . . it's the best part of it actually [others agree]. My best outing I say in this year was an outing with a Croatian, a Spaniard, an Irish woman [laughs, others laughing], what was the fourth, we were all different nationalities . . . We had the most wonderful day . . . it was so exciting, it was a beautiful day, it was good to be alive, actually [laughs].
>
> (Patricia)

However, while remaining a central facet of the group's identity, the group's name did not include the term 'multicultural', focusing instead on 'friendship'. The group president explained that this was to ensure that women from all cultural and ethnic backgrounds, including third-, fourth- and fifth-generation Australians, would feel welcome:

> *Margaret*: I think when we started it was called multicultural group, that's what attracted me, then we had to drop that, hadn't we, Anne?
>
> *Anne*: No, I wouldn't say we dropped it, it wasn't the most predominant. Because I think Aussie people sort of thought, oh if it's a multicultural group it's not for us . . . I still sort of say to people, or I always mention that there are thirty nationalities involved. I think that's the big thing, but, we're all one. We've always said that . . . When I [went to] the council, I've spoken up there, they have the Macedonian group, they have the Greeks, they have the Chinese, they have their specific days. And I said, where do I fit in? You know you're saying we don't need another group in the community, but we've got Fijian, we've got a woman from Libya, we've got a woman from Kenya, you know, there's nothing for them unless you're the big, you know, groups. So that's what I think is so great about it, and then we're all one.

While acknowledging that monocultural community groups or social practices may provide security and comfort to migrant groups, many participants also identified that cultural insularity could be a source of exclusion to those outside a particular cultural community and lead to a lack of social cohesion in the community as a whole:

One thing I've noticed is that the [ethnic] community, they sort of hang around each other, and then [nationality] people, they mix with their own selves, and then you get like, you know, whatever . . . if I went into that group, would I be included? And often the answer is no, because they are cliquey groups . . . and I think that would be very difficult.

(Margaret)

Members strongly emphasised the inclusive nature of the group, and described active steps taken by the committee and the group's president to avoid insularity, and in doing so purposefully encouraged active engagement of all members with each other:

And there are no cliques in our organisation. Nobody feels excluded because we are all encouraged to mix, and [Anne, the president] makes a point, at least once a year we have to sit at a table with other [women] than our friends. So no cliques are formed, but friendships are formed.

(Patricia)

Creating space for women: emphasising friendship and togetherness

Group members also felt that the women-only nature of the group and its emphasis on friendship were strongly appealing, and friendship has been shown to be an important contributor to older women's wellbeing (Martina and Stevens 2006; Stevens et al. 2006; Eshbaugh 2009; Pinquart and Duberstein 2010). Some participants felt able to connect more easily with other women due to shared life experiences that transcended cultural background or offered a sanctuary from the demands of daily life:

So that's what I think is so great about it, and then we're all one. We all come together, like [member] said at the luncheon the other day, cooking – women love cooking, women love talking about food, we all enjoy food . . . we all come together with a cup of tea, a cup of coffee, doesn't matter what you have, a biscuit, but you all come together as one. And you've all got sort of the same interests, you're family people, you know . . .

(Anne, group president)

My sister joined the [nationality] club . . . and there's all these men there, and they always play cards, play whatever and they just carry on, and all the men stick together and all the ladies stick together. And I thought, I don't want to go into a group like that, I prefer to go to a group that's only ladies and we all share the same interests, and we can understand because we're mothers, grandmothers, cooking, sorrow – we can talk so much. Men haven't got the time for things like that . . . That's what attracted me, it's all ladies. I quite like the word friendship actually. Women's friendship . . .

that's why I joined up because I needed a day . . . because it was friendship, because it was only ladies, and I just wanted a day to myself in the sense like . . . I can just talk, I can just be among women . . . It's my day . . . it's away from my daughter, it's away from my husband, it's my day. It's my time. That's why I like it. This is the first time I've done something for myself. To be among other people in a different way.

(Eva)

Women together: overcoming isolation and social stigma

Gender was also identified as an important facet of social exclusion by participants. Women (particularly older women) were perceived by participants to be vulnerable to isolation and social exclusion:

Well a lot of women are at home, aren't they? So you get excluded from the community.

(Jane)

There was that other thing you said to us one day about the lady who hadn't spoken to anybody for days, she was home alone – there's a lot of people out there like that, I'm afraid.

(Margaret)

These perceptions are corroborated by research evidence; older women have been shown to be at risk of social isolation, loneliness, social disconnectedness and stress (Beal 2006; Rice et al. 2007; Cornwell and Waite 2009; Durey 2009). The consequences of the group's community-generated practice was the alleviation or attenuation of these forms of stress and exclusion:

Being alone is another exclusion, I think . . . it's just so good to be in a group where you're accepted. To come out to a friendship group like this at least once a month you get to socialise in one form or another, whether it's a speaker or whether you go out somewhere or whatever, and then if you join up on Wednesday mornings you're doing your exercises . . . and it's really fun.

(Jane)

Group members' narratives acknowledged that puncturing the emotional isolation inherent in many older women's lives was important to promote social inclusion. For example, group sharing of members' life experiences, whether celebratory or sorrowful, was practiced:

We share the joy and sometimes maybe the sorrow with each other – I suppose like one day we have a person's birthday – we celebrate with them and then we sing happy birthday. And unfortunately sometimes we may have our members pass away and we remember them too. So we share.

(Florence)

In addition, many participants identified that their status as bereaved women contributed to potential social exclusion, a finding also supported by existing literature (Aday et al. 2006; Eshbaugh 2009). However, the gendered nature of the group promoted social inclusion by creating a safe space for widowed or single older women to attend without discomfort:

> I've been a widow 15 years this year . . . you go through a bad time, because before you have friends, you know husbands and wife, and first you get invited to things [other participants agreeing 'that's right' 'exactly' etc.], you go and feel out of place, they ask you and you say I'm not coming so then they don't ask you any more . . . your life completely changes. So coming to [the group] was the best thing, I made so many friends, [Anne, the president] said 'turn around and make friends with somebody else', that's helped me a lot.

(Maria)

Group members also reported that the group facilitated social inclusion of women who may have experienced multiple contributors to exclusion, such as gender, age and ethnicity. For example:

> I saw [an Indian woman] standing all by herself and she looked so . . . miserable, and I said, 'Are you by yourself, love?' and she said yes, and I said, well there's six of us, come and join us, and then I gave her [Anne's] phone number and she joined . . . she said, 'Oh, this is the best thing that's ever happened.' She told me . . . 'I've only been a widow for three years, I got to the door of this place with all the people, and . . . thought, I can't stop here, but I said to myself, you've got to' . . . so that's what she did. But now, right now, she's . . . part of the group.

(Margaret)

> We've included women, we've included all sorts of things, all nationalities, we've included all races, we've included [all] ages.

(Patricia)

Consolidating social inclusion: strengthening social networks

The group's emphasis on openness and inclusivity did not preclude the establishment of smaller groups of friends among group members, further consolidating social connections and support between these members and supporting social inclusion outside the group's meeting times:

I think it's happened here . . . a lot of the women now are meeting in little groups together and go and do things. Like they've met here so they'll go to the movies or they'll go to [shopping centre] or they'll go for lunch.

(Anne)

However, members were keen to emphasise that these smaller groups of friends encompassed women from a range of different cultural groups and/or nationalities:

In the women's friendship group, when we were forming the committee, I said to a [nationality] girl, 'You'd be good, come on in' so we got her in, I didn't even know her name, and she was absolutely brilliant, she did all the finances for a couple of years, two or three years and everything . . . [we] became great friends and I meet all her friends and we all laugh and talk together . . . and I meet all her friends on Sunday, and the Indians are in it too . . . And you know I'm part . . . I could go off with them and have coffee and be happy as anything.

(Patricia)

Encouraging inclusion: minimising resource demands

The fact that the group was not a profit-making organisation and therefore its cost did not prohibit membership was important to these older women:

It's not profitable, there's no money in it, that's why it will always be an interest for all of us because none of us gain financially anything out of that. All we gain is friendship.

(Eva)

The group does [bring people together], in a simplistic way. You don't have to have grandeur and I believe you don't have to have money.

(Anne, group president)

The low cost of group membership was important in promoting social inclusion as it is known that older women are at risk of socio-economic disadvantage (Kimberley and Simons 2009). Participants identified feeling excluded from other groups or activities that they were unable to afford due to their limited financial resources:

They say to you, as they've said to me, why don't you join [organisation]. Well to join [organisation] you're up for money. And if you're a pensioner, there's no way you'd be able to keep up with trips [interstate] . . . then you feel isolated . . . then you feel different if you can't go. And left out.

(Patricia)

Extending social inclusion: the practice of group expansion

The group recruited new members largely by word of mouth and the enthusiasm of existing members:

> And it was through some other people that told me that there was this friendship group. And so I contacted [Anne, the group president] and that's how I came into it, and it's really good.
>
> (Jane)

> I pick them up everywhere! We'll be having coffee and someone says can I sit here, well by the time they've gone they've got the card, they come and see . . . [laughs] Then they'll tell someone else, you know. It's like a chain. If we keep working I think we'll grow.
>
> (Margaret)

This was a deliberate strategy, as the committee considered the marketing of the group detracted from the purpose and values of the group. Thus, such a process of organic, community-generated group expansion and growth reflected the centrality of informal social networking and the importance of friendship to the group's identity:

> We don't advertise – you don't advertise for friends.
>
> (Anne, group president)

The consequences of social inclusion: empowerment and capacity building

As illustrated above, the group's practice of social inclusion enhanced members' sense of social and interpersonal belonging, provided a source of valued companionship and facilitated societal involvement. Another critical consequence of the group's activities was its contribution to building further capacity for social inclusion among its members by increasing confidence and life skills:

> Once you start building up your confidence you can start branching out to other groups.
>
> (Jane)

> You've got to develop confidence and friendliness and it's terrific.
>
> (Patricia)

Further to this, participation in group activities, with their strong altruistic dimension, augmented these older women's sense of social contribution and value to wider society, and hence their sense of empowerment – congruent with previous research findings that women's empowerment is maximised by activities with a relational and community emphasis (Peterson and Hughey 2004; Echeverría et al. 2008; Maidment and Macfarlane 2011). The group's organised efforts to help other people (both within and outside the group) enhanced members' self-esteem and promoted social inclusion more broadly:

> We're a great bunch of ladies and work cooperatively for the greater good of the group. It's also confidence-building for a number of us who would otherwise not be aware how we could contribute to society.
>
> (Patricia)

> Well you won't come if you don't want to give something back.
>
> (Margaret)

In addition, the group president, who played a critical role in the initiation of the group, in its ongoing administration and generation of further momentum, encapsulated her personal vision for the group in the following way:

> I always think that if you can enhance someone's life, you've done something in your life. And our motto is 'A friend is a gift you give yourself'. So you got to feel good . . . to give joy to other people less fortunate. It's not just you're taking . . . I think that's the big thing, it's like with the council, you know, we're so pleased, we get money from the council . . . but with that we can generate and give things back and that's why the council have supported us and are behind us.
>
> (Anne, group president)

Conclusion

This chapter has presented a case study of community-generated social inclusion practice. Our programme of participatory research has illustrated that a community-generated and maintained friendship group for older women from diverse cultural backgrounds has successfully promoted social inclusion and increased members' capacity for social citizenship (Buckmaster and Thomas 2009). Over the five years of its growth to date, this group has demonstrated increasing strength and the likelihood of its sustainability. The emphasis on friendship by the women is critical to the group's success. The effects of empowering women's social health and wellbeing through the community action of like-minded women cannot be underestimated. Our data show that the group has created a safe and nurturing space for its members, has promoted friendship and acceptance, and has contributed to social inclusion by 'providing people with the fundamentals of a decent life: opportunities to engage in the economic and social life of the community with dignity; increasing their capabilities and functioning; connecting people to the networks of local community' (Cappo 2009: 5). The group illustrates the potential for community capacity to develop and apply health-promotion principles without professional affiliation or theoretical grounding, and demonstrates the potency of community participation, agency and ownership of the social inclusion agenda. Given the case study group's success at facilitating social connection and inclusion, this chapter demonstrates the potential for similar community-driven groups to enhance social inclusion at a grass-roots level.

Acknowledgements

The authors acknowledge the contribution of Deakin University students Teresia Mutisya (supervised by JM and LH) and Tracey Renton (supervised by JM) to the programme of research. We also extend our sincerest thanks and appreciation to the president, committee and members of the case study group for their enthusiasm in participating in the research and the warmth of their welcome.

14 Practicing social inclusion

Comfort Zone – a social support group for teenagers with high-functioning autism

Jessica Gill, Pranee Liamputtong and Elizabeth Hoban

Individuals with a disability are often excluded from society because of their differences either physically, mentally or socially (Kitchin 1998). In order to tackle this issue of exclusion, social networks must be built with the aim of including these individuals into society. The notion of building social inclusion is described by Pierre Bourdieu (1977) as 'social capital' where resources are embedded within social structures and networks rather than in individuals. By encouraging social inclusion, individuals' quality of life is enhanced by allowing more access to support, resources and relationships.

Individuals with high-functioning autism spectrum disorder (ASD) have deficits in their social and communication skills. These issues hinder their development of friendships and intimate relationships, which can lead to feelings of isolation (Freeman 2008). It has been recognised that the adolescent years are a particularly difficult period for the individuals on the autism spectrum and their families (Kunz 2009).

This chapter focuses on a community-based social support programme for teenagers with high-functioning ASD, called Comfort Zone, which aimed to increase social support. The authors argue that the foundations and aims of the Comfort Zone group have allowed the group to promote social inclusion of individuals with high-functioning ASD into the community. Despite some limitations, this group can be used as a model for promoting social inclusion for other groups within the community.

Introduction

ASD is best described as a group of disorders with a similar pattern of behaviour in three key areas – social interaction, communication and imaginative thought (Autism Victoria 2009). Those individuals diagnosed with high-functioning ASD are the most physically and socially active individuals along the spectrum, and display odd 'autistic' features (Eisenmajer 2006).

Individuals with high-functioning ASD have many social issues, but they must make their way through the social world without many of the protections available to those with more intensive autistic traits (Gray 2002). Due to their average to above-average IQ, many high-functioning ASD children are placed in mainstream schools instead of schools for children with special needs (Gray 2002). Gray (2002: 735) contends 'they are people with a disability who must deal with the social world as if they were not disabled'. Not only are these issues concerning for the autistic person themselves, but can also be an anxiety for parents, who may feel the need to advocate for their child throughout their schooling life, ensuring they are receiving adequate education that accommodates their special needs, and assisting with interactions with community members (Gill and Liamputtong 2013). Often, those individuals with high-functioning ASD experience stigmatisation due to their anti-social behaviour, in a world where they are expected to be 'normal' (Gill and Liamputtong 2011).

Those individuals diagnosed with high-functioning ASD are at their most vulnerable between the ages of 13 and 18 years. This particular period is difficult for the individual and family, as during this time a child undergoes many psychosocial transitions such as starting secondary school and shifting from family to more peer-based social situations (Klin et al. 2000). The combination of these events is described by Kunz (2009: 8) as 'the perfect storm'. Individuals on the autism spectrum aged 13–18 years deal with many social issues that hinder their development of friendships and intimate relationships, such as a fear of unknown situations, unfamiliar experiences and social judgement; this can lead them to feel isolated (Freeman 2008). While individuals on the lower end of the autism spectrum appear socially aloof, individuals with high-functioning ASD are interested in pursuing friendships but, due to difficulties with understanding social interactions and gestures, these friendships are usually quite unstable (Freeman 2008).

Many individuals with high-functioning ASD are well aware of their social limitations, and often become frustrated with their inability to understand the world around them (Howard et al. 2006; Freeman 2008). This frustration can often lead to anxiety, depression and a low self-worth (Howard et al. 2006; Freeman 2008). Adolescents with high-functioning ASD present with high levels of anxiety equivalent in intensity to those diagnosed with an anxiety disorder (Farrugia and Hudson 2006). This highlights the need to embed these individuals in an organised social group at an early stage, as well as educate these individuals about not only obtaining friendships and relationships, but maintaining them in an appropriate manner.

Disability and the need for social inclusion in a community

In most societies individuals living with a disability tend to be excluded (Kitchin 1998). Social exclusion of these individuals is based on society's assumptions of deviance either in the disabled person's behaviour (anti-social actions) or biological conditions (physical ailments) (Martin 2004; Liamputtong and Kitisriworapan 2012). What seems to propel this exclusion is that these groups of individuals are labelled as 'marginalised' 'vulnerable' or 'disadvantaged' (Liamputtong 2007). With this sort of labelling, it has been shown that people with a disability are stigmatised or discriminated against by others in society (Bedini 2000). This has led to their exclusion from 'mainstream' social groups (Bedini 2000). Often, individuals experiencing stigmatisation would avoid certain social situations, leading to 'self-regulated exclusion' (Taket et al. 2009a: 39).

It is important for individuals who have been labelled as being in marginalised groups to feel supported within their community. This is particularly relevant for people living with a disability or impairment, where community ties and community participation have been associated with an improved quality of life, enhanced independence and self-determination (Wehmeyer and Bolding 2001; Carmien et al. 2005; Schalock et al. 2008). Furthermore, it has been suggested that individuals living with disabilities who feel supported in their community develop better ways of coping with their impairments (Scotch and Schriner 1997; Scotch 2000; Schriner and Scotch 2001; DePoy and Gilson 2010).

This can be seen in the case of a teenager living with high-functioning ASD, who has recently joined a social support group run through the local community. This teenager previously felt anxious, depressed and isolated due to their anti-social behaviour and difficulty communicating with others. However, once belonging to a group of other teenagers struggling with similar issues, their communication and social impairments would not be as apparent as they might be at school or in other social areas. Such a support group could also provide this teenager with an opportunity to practice social and communication skills in a comfortable environment so as to cope better in other social arenas.

The idea of building social groups or networks within a community was first developed by Bourdieu (1977). His theory of 'social capital' outlined the need to include people with a disability into social networks in order to better embrace them into our society. Social capital can be conceptualised as one of the building blocks that bond together individuals with disabilities and communities (Taket et al. 2009a: 36). Boateng (2009) and McMichael and Manderson (2004) both contend that social capital enables information sharing, provision of support networks and friendships, builds a sense of belonging to a place, and improves physical and mental health, both preventive and recuperative. Social capital is not only about providing individuals with access to resources such as social networks. Bourdieu also suggests that there must be quality invested in the production of these resources to ensure social connection between individual and community (Taket et al. 2009a: 67).

There are many ways in which a person with a disability can feel connected in the community (Leiter 2011). There are geographic communities (i.e. connections with people who live locally or are involved with the same activities), disability-based communities, (i.e. connections with other individuals living with a disability, through specific activities involving the disabled, such as wheelchair basketball, or a multiple sclerosis social support group), religious communities (involving connections with people in church) and virtual communities (connections with people via chat rooms or other virtual communication facilities) (Leiter 2011). It is important, when developing social networks, to improve the social inclusion of people with a disability that these communities intertwine, so that these individuals might feel socially included in all aspects of their life (Leiter 2011). It is also important to develop networks for children and adolescents, as social participation and inclusion among youth with disabilities may be considered a means for them to improve their social capital and health into adulthood (Leiter 2011).

It is paramount that, when building these social networks for disabled individuals, their family is involved wherever possible (Moxley et al. 1989). This is particularly relevant for children and adolescents, where parents play an important role in the care-giving and development of social opportunities for their disabled child (Gill and Liamputtong 2013). Because of their large role in their child's life, parents of children with disabilities suffer from high levels of stress and depression (Gray 2002), and are often not adequately supported or included within their community. It is therefore relevant to include these families in social networks so as to not only assist their child in developing social opportunities with others living with a disability, but so they too can feel supported.

As mentioned earlier, it is well recognised that people living with disabilities and their families are labelled as marginalised within the community. Despite this, many government and health care agencies have fallen short of their aims of socially including these groups in the community. Advocacy, for themselves and their children, is then left up to the care-giver(s) (Gill and Liamputtong 2013). The following sections provide an example of how these gaps may be overcome.

Method

This chapter is based on a larger study concerning the lived experience of a group of individuals diagnosed with a higher functioning form of ASD. As there is little in-depth understanding about the life of these individuals, qualitative inquiry was adopted in the study (Liamputtong 2013). The data reported in this chapter were obtained through one-on-one interviews with the founders of the Comfort Zone group and their daughter who is an active member of the group, volunteers and parents involved in the group, the coordinator of the community centre where the group is currently running, as well as the Development Project Worker of a not-for-profit organisation funded by the Department of Human Services (Victoria, Australia) who had an affiliation with the group. In each interview, participants were asked what they thought were the benefits of the Comfort Zone group, as well as what they thought were the limitations, necessary improvements required and perceived future outcomes of the group. The data were analysed thematically (Liamputtong 2013). All names used in this chapter have been changed to protect the privacy of the participants.

Comfort Zone and its benefits

An example of local community members advocating to make change was a Melbourne (Victoria, Australia) family with a high-functioning ASD teenage girl, Laura, who took on the challenge to develop a social network for those with high-functioning ASD. The idea was developed when this family went to Sweden for a 6-month period when Laura was in Year 7. While attending a local Swedish school, Laura joined a youth group, connected to the school, for children with high-functioning ASD. The purpose was solely to get together with minimal interaction from teachers. The group ran every Friday and was a free service.

Upon returning to Australia, the family began researching whether a similar group was run for autistic youth in their local area. They discovered no such group existed. As a result, Janet, the mother, contacted her local community centre, where she met Sharon, the coordinator. This community centre was supported by the Baptist Church, through the organisation Baptcare, which is a not-for-profit organisation that supports children, families, people with a disability, the financially disadvantaged, older people and asylum seekers. This organisation addresses the needs of community members, particularly those who are marginalised or disadvantaged (Baptcare 2011). The community centre, with the assistance of Janet, Richard and Laura, set up the group, with Richard taking on the role of coordinator. Laura named the group 'Comfort Zone', which originates from the saying 'getting out of your comfort zone':

> Because people with autism need to stay in that comfort zone or they will probably get pretty distressed, but they aren't used to stepping out of it, so I wanted to create something where everyone would feel comfortable.

The overall aim of Comfort Zone was to create a safe place for teenagers with high-functioning ASD to go and interact with others who have a greater understanding of their difficulties, strengths and shared interests. This is particularly important for teenagers with high-functioning ASD, who often feel isolated or different from their typically developing peers, leaving them feeling socially excluded from the community. According to Laura, in the beginning the group was quite small, about four to five members. Although the community centre advertised through its community newsletter, the group seemed to grow by word of mouth.

When discussing the beginning of the group with Laura, she said that 'More often than not the sessions would just be run at the community centre and we would just hang out together, making up games from the top of our heads like drama activities or octopus – to release some energy!' The family then decided to set up a network with the local girls' grammar school, from where Year 9 volunteers were sourced. Richard, the father, explains that the reason the family decided to have volunteers of a similar age to the group members is that these volunteers 'model ideal social behaviour'. Given the gender imbalance within the group (predominately boys), it was seen as a good idea to involve a girls' school to assist the few female members of the group.

Richard also set up a virtual chat facility for members and their families to communicate with each other outside of Comfort Zone hours. This programme had a similar set up to Facebook, but Richard had control over who could access the site, thereby ensuring the privacy and safety of all members and their families. This facility was an innovative way for members to stay in touch throughout the week, developing true friendships within the group. For a time, it was also used as a way of notifying families of the upcoming weekend activity, before a term programme was introduced. Unfortunately, over time this virtual chat facility was not maintained, as Richard eventually stepped down as Comfort Zone coordinator. In addition, members wanted to access mainstream virtual chat facilities, such as Facebook.

Initially, the group was financed by the families involved, and Comfort Zone activities were organised by the founding family. Parents would pay five dollars per person per week to hire the community centre or pay for an outdoor activity, for example bowling, go-carting, or horse riding. Parents would usually stay around the community centre while their child interacted. Parents supervised their children, but also witnessed the benefits of building 'social bonds' between families who were dealing with similar issues. These families shared information and resources as well as provided each other with emotional and social support. According to Aimee, mother of Luke, a previous Comfort Zone member:

> The parents were lovely, that's where I got a lot of knowledge of different services for things that could help us, and different information about high-functioning ASD. I can remember one day a mother came to the group very upset having a bad day with their child. And we could all understand and relate to this, which I'm sure made her feel comfortable and supported, something that other parents of mainstream children cannot understand.

Another benefit for parents is the relief they felt when they saw their child socialising outside of the school environment and having their child 'nurtured' through the social connection process. This was described by Kate, a Development Project Worker at a not-for-profit organization funded by the Department of Human Services, who built a network with Comfort Zone during late 2010. Kate remembers when she first dropped her son off on his first day of school:

> I came home and I cried all day, and I cried because I was just hoping and praying that he would find a friend. As a parent, I just want my child . . . I don't care if he is a huge academic, I just want him to have social connection and to be happy, and I think that's what parents, whether they have a child with a disability of not, that's what they want. So that's what programmes like Comfort Zone provide . . . it's not about the child becoming a star cricket player, or scoring the most goals at basketball, it's about them belonging.

The Comfort Zone group provided an arena for parents to create social connections for their children. It is important for group models such as Comfort Zone to be a family-based social support group, so that all family members are involved in creating a comfortable and supportive environment for their high-functioning ASD child to socialise, learn and belong.

In late 2009, funding for the group was obtained from the Banyule City Council and Watsonia Returned Services League (RSL), which enabled a coordinator to be sourced to organise activities. The money was also used to fund some activities, which took the strain off families to pay for their child's participation in the group. However, once a coordinator was sought, most parents decided to use this time as respite, rather than stay and assist the group with supervision and continue the social network that had been developed. With the lack of parental supervision, increasing group numbers and school-aged untrained volunteers, the coordinator decided that there was a real need to access volunteers with experience in the field. The volunteers who were sourced were mainly university students requiring volunteer hours for their degree programmes. One of the volunteers, named Louise, who had worked and conducted research with individuals on the ASD spectrum and their families for several years, found that volunteering for Comfort Zone provided her with an avenue to be more involved with, and supportive of, the community in a fun and active way. Through her volunteering experience at Comfort Zone:

> I not only gained opportunities to participate and interact in new ways with adolescents on the autism spectrum and their families, but I was also able to identify areas I could address better in my own practice through a new understanding of the needs adolescents on the spectrum face in this stage of their development.

From 2009 until now, it has been evident that Comfort Zone has successfully provided social support for teenagers with high-functioning ASD. The group has met its overall aims of creating a safe place for its members to go, where they can interact with each other in a non-threatening environment. By providing this social avenue, these members began to feel included in their local community. From a member's perspective:

> The group lets us do what a normal teenager would do without having to be like a normal teenager. It lets us have a non-judgemental group if you will . . . .it just makes you feel a whole lot more comfortable knowing that you are with someone who probably won't care if you are a bit weird.
>
> (Laura, member)

Laura's mother, Janet, added:

> I think it's also an instant place that they can go to without having to do all of those things that are difficult for people with autism, like arrange things,

ringing people up and asking whether they want to do this or that, that executive function that isn't often present. They also get a chance to do things, like bowling, that they perhaps aren't usually invited to by other people, or they might not be invited to birthday parties or things like that, so they might not have much to do on the weekend.

Aimee, mother of Luke, suggested that:

> It was within Comfort Zone that Luke realised he had high-functioning ASD. That's when it actually came through to him . . . the group made Luke realise that it was OK to be different and that there were other kids like him.

Comfort Zone and the future

The key issue hindering the sustainability of this group is funding. Unfortunately, the organisations that awarded grants to Comfort Zone could not provide continual funding for the group. Inevitably these one-off grants were spent, and once again the group was without financial support, resulting in ongoing grant applications and fundraising efforts in order for the group to stay afloat.

Furthermore, the community centre that hosts the Comfort Zone group has not previously run a teenage group, nor has it run a group for individuals on the autism spectrum. Due to funding shortfalls, those providing administration and managerial support to the programme lacked the experience and time to devote to the tasks required in this area. As a consequence important tasks were not completed.

The general consensus among those who were involved in Comfort Zone is that the group had marked potential to expand; however, they also acknowledged that expansion is not possible at this stage until the group works on quality and safety. Change must occur in the areas of volunteer training, new family assessments before entry into the group, an improved enrolment procedure that ensures all medical and behavioural information is indicated prior to a member starting, and providing better care when taking members to activities outside of the centre (such as first aid kit and at least one volunteer who is first aid qualified). There must also be more appropriate activities developed to suit all ages and promote social development, to better integrate members into society.

The authors think it is important for the group to remain at the current community centre so that its members can continue to be supported through Baptcare funding. However, if the group remains at this centre there are some administrative and managerial changes that must be made to ensure a quality programme that is safe for all those who attend. Perhaps in order to successfully make changes, Comfort Zone should build a network with the Department of Human Services organisation mentioned earlier. This organisation offered to assist Comfort Zone in late 2010; however, it has proven too difficult to bring a Department of Human Services organisation into a community centre. Being such a high-level organisation, it is possible they could assist in certain tasks such as family assessments or volunteer training. Kate, Development Project Worker at the Department of Human Services organisation observed:

> I believe more organisations need to come together and help each other, we all need to link hands, share and go forward.

According to Aimee, parent of Luke, who was a past member, it is important to reintroduce the parents into the group. 'When parents stepped aside, the group lost its "grass roots" family based feel.' The authors recommend that the group considers a parents committee be established to work on grant applications and fundraising, which should take the burden away from the coordinator, as well as reintroduce the social-support aspect of the group for these parents. The group should continue to ask parents for their financial support in the form of a term membership, as external funding to cover all the administration costs of Comfort Zone is not feasible. It is therefore important that parents contribute if they can. In order for the group to remain inclusive, there could be a fee reduction or instalment system for those families who cannot afford the term fee.

The authors also recommend the reintroduction of the virtual chat facility for members to ensure the social inclusion of the Comfort Zone members. By re-establishing this website the group will provide a bridge between the virtual community and the disability community. This could potentially contribute to the establishment of connections between group members and ensuring that true friendships are built and maintained.

The authors posit that these recommendations will ensure a high-quality and sustainable group for high-functioning ASD teenagers and their families. The Comfort Zone model can be used to develop other social groups for individuals on the autism spectrum, as well as others living with a disability in the community.

Finally, Comfort Zone could share their model with other councils, community centres and health care agencies, so that the expansion of this idea can become possible. This may lead to the social inclusion of many other disability groups in a community.

Conclusion

In this chapter, the authors have argued that the foundations and aims of the Comfort Zone group have allowed the group to promote social inclusion in community life for individuals with high-functioning ASD. Despite some limitations, the authors contend that the 'Comfort Zone' model should be adapted into other community centres, councils and health care organisations so that teenagers on the autism spectrum, and those living with other disabilities, can be included in the community. This will assist them with social development, reduce isolation and provide them with a better quality of life. Inevitably, these individuals will feel a greater sense of social inclusion in the wider Australian society.

Part VI

Practising inclusion in research

15 Preventing HIV through social inclusion using community-based participatory research

Suzanne M. Dolwick Grieb, Ndidiamaka Amutah, Jason Stowers, Horace Smith, Kimberli Hammonds and Scott D. Rhodes

The HIV epidemic is one of the most severe health crises of our time, and the United Nations Development Programme (UNDP) cites HIV as being responsible for the greatest reversal in human development (UNDP 2005). In areas most affected by HIV, life expectancy has been reduced greatly, economic growth has waned, and household poverty has deepened. Although declines in new infections are being witnessed in some countries, an estimated 2.6 million new infections occurred globally in 2009 (UNAIDS 2011). Currently an estimated 33.3 million people globally are living with HIV, and each year almost two million people die from AIDS (UNAIDS 2011). Increasingly, it is the poorest and/or most marginalised segments of societies that are affected by HIV/AIDS (Parker 2002).

The HIV epidemic is complex and necessitates social and political solutions in addition to biomedical solutions. Increasingly, researchers have realised the need for a comprehensive approach that includes the participation of impacted community members as active researchers and advocates for change to address behavioural, biological and structural vulnerability to infection.

Promoting sexual health and HIV prevention requires a comprehensive understanding of the social and cultural fabric of a community, and the acknowledgement and inclusion of diverse perspectives, norms, values and behaviours (Reece and Dodge 2004). Community-based participatory research (CBPR) therefore provides an important option for community and academic partners to effectively address local HIV/AIDS epidemics. CBPR provides a partnership approach to research that includes community members and academic researchers in every aspect of the research process.

This chapter aims to explore how HIV is being confronted in the USA through social inclusion using the principles of CBPR. After a brief overview of CBPR, we provide examples of how community–academic partnerships use CBPR to facilitate social inclusion and better understand and prevent HIV in their communities for three particularly vulnerable groups within the USA: African Americans, youth, and sexual minorities.

Commmunity-based participatory research

Increasingly, academic researchers, health care providers, and community members are becoming frustrated by the disconnect between research, research translation and policies to improve health (Israel et al. 1998; Green and Mercer 2001). CBPR provides a bridge between academic researchers and communities through shared knowledge, capacity building, co-learning, and commitment to action around issues of priority in the community (Israel et al. 2005).

CBPR has been characterised as:

> [A] collaborative process that equitably involves all partners in the research process and recognises the unique strengths that each brings. CBPR begins with a research topic of importance to the community with the aim of combining knowledge and action for social change to improve community health and eliminate health disparities.
>
> (Community Health Scholars Program 2002: 2)

Thus CBPR is a partnership approach to research that involves community members and academic researchers in all stages of the research process; all partners share their expertise, mutually make decisions, and claim ownership of the research. The aim is to improve understanding of an issue, and then integrate the resulting knowledge into interventions, including social change and policy solutions (Israel et al. 2005).

CBPR diverges from traditional research approaches by including the people most affected by the issue of concern in the development of the research question, the design and implementation of the study, the analysis and interpretation of results, and the development of the solutions. Explicit in CBPR is the democratisation of knowledge (Ansley and Gaventa 1997); the knowledge community members have gained through experience is valued and incorporated in the research process, and knowledge previously contained within the 'ivory tower' of academia is physically and intellectually accessible to community partners (Minkler 2004).

Harnessing CBPR to blend the lived experiences of community members, the experiences of organisational representatives based in ongoing public health practice and service provision, and rigorous scientific methods has the potential to develop deeper and more informed understandings of health-related phenomena and produce interventions that are more relevant and culturally congruent, and more likely to be adopted and maintained over protracted periods of time. Consequently, these interventions are more likely to be successful (Cashman et al. 2008; Wallerstein et al. 2008). Similarly, study designs, including those used to evaluate interventions, that are informed by multiple perspectives may be more authentic to the community and its members' natural ways of doing things.

CBPR is therefore not a method, but an orientation to guide the research process (Shalowitz et al. 2009). Nine principles guide CBPR:

(1) CBPR acknowledges community as a unit of identity; (2) CBPR builds on strengths and resources within the community; (3) CBPR facilitates a collaborative, equitable partnership in all phases of the research, involving an empowering and power-sharing process that attends to social inequalities; (4) CBPR fosters co-learning and capacity building among all partners; (5) CBPR integrates and achieves a balance between knowledge generation and intervention for the mutual benefit of all partners; (6) CBPR focuses on the local relevance of public health problems and on ecological perspectives that attend to the multiple determinates of health; (7) CBPR involves systems development using a cyclical and iterative process; (8) CBPR disseminates results to all partners and involves them in the wider dissemination of results; and (9) CBPR involves a long-term process and requires a commitment to partnership sustainability (Israel et al. 2005).

Israel et al. (2005) caution, however, that no one set of principles is applicable to all community–academic partnerships. The values and principles guiding partnerships should instead be a reflection of the collective vision of the partnerships. Indeed, these principles are applied in various ways within community–academic partnerships, demonstrating multiple approaches to CBPR.

Addressing HIV prevention through community-based participatory research

We present examples of CBPR being undertaken in the USA to address HIV prevention through social inclusion within three vulnerable groups: African Americans, youth, and sexual minorities. We use these examples to highlight various parts of the CBPR process, explore the various approaches taken, and demonstrate how the CBPR principles are operationalised in practice.

The Life Changing (TLC) group: Addressing HIV among African Americans through individual and structural intervention

Almost half of all new infections in the USA occur among non-Hispanic blacks (CDC 2011a). The Greater Rosemont community of west Baltimore, Maryland, is a predominately African American community that has been severely affected by HIV/AIDS, with three of the four zip codes reporting a higher incidence of HIV compared with the city (Maryland Department of Health and Mental Hygiene 2009). Additionally, the community is severely affected by unemployment, poverty, drug use and crime, all of which affect and are affected by the HIV epidemic (Adimora and Schoenbach 2005). This community, once a thriving centre of African American culture, sees itself as a community with identity. There are numerous grassroots organisations working within Greater Rosemont; however, the challenges are daunting at times.

To address the issues and challenges facing Greater Rosemount, a partnership was formed between two community resources: GROUP Ministries Baltimore (GMB), a non-profit community-based organisation providing transitional housing and job training services to ex-offenders and former sub-stance users, and the Johns Hopkins Medical Institutions (JHMI), including the Johns Hopkins School of Medicine, the Johns Hopkins Bloomberg School of Public Health (JHSPH), and the JHSPH Center for Communication Programs. This community–academic partnership is working with residents in Greater Rosemont to address structural risks for HIV in the community. Multi-level interventions focus on African American males between the ages of 21 and 50 years who have been released from prison or jail within the past 2 years.

Greater Rosemont is one of the most common re-entry points for citizens leaving prison, the majority of whom report a history of drug use (Visher et al. 2004). The project aims to promote positive changes in individual and struc-tural risks in order to decrease the prevalence of substance abuse and HIV risk behaviours among this population. Through an ecological lens, which is important in the CBPR framework, the connection between employment, housing and health is realised and addressed.

GROUP Ministries' CEO/President and Deputy Director began collabo-rating with the JHMI partners initially through the organisation's participa-tion in JHMI- and Baltimore City Health Department-based projects; these projects served as an initial foundation for co-learning and capacity building. Subsequently, a JHMI partner joined the GMB Board of Directors, co-wrote a grant with GROUP Ministries, and served as a project evaluator for several GROUP Ministries projects. These interactions, occurring for over 5 years, facilitated the development of a mutual history, trust and mutual respect, as well as a clear understanding of the framework through which the issues of concern were viewed by all involved: community members themselves, organisational representatives and academic partners.

In 2006, the Abell Foundation approved a grant that allowed GROUP Min-istries to purchase a new house and provide job training in the home con-struction trade to ex-offenders. This undertaking builds on the strengths of the community by using local talent and businesses to train ex-offenders in housing construction, a vital service needed by the ex-offenders as well as the community at large. This project provided a catalyst for the expansion of GROUP Ministries' services. The continued collaboration and joint interest in GROUP Ministries' services and expansion plans led to an expansion of the GROUP Ministries–JHMI partnership and development of the research project incorporating these ideas.

This partnership and project, called The Life Changing (TLC) Group, grew to include the initial GROUP Ministries and Johns Hopkins partners, as well as others in the community, city and university who joined the efforts to address the structural impediments to successful re-entry and recovery among ex-offending substance-using African American men. The community–academic partners developed a memorandum of understanding for the TLC partnership, and by signing the memorandum partners acknowledge the community iden-tity and targeted issues of local concern, provide a commitment to participate in the co-learning processes, develop and implement action plans to facilitate structural change, practice social inclusion, and contribute to the sustainability of the partnership.

In 2009, the TLC partnership was awarded a grant by the US Department of Health and Human Services' Substance Abuse and Mental Health Services Administration (SAHMSA) to conduct a multi-level intervention based on GROUP Ministries' existing services and to increase HIV testing in the community. As before, the TLC Group seeks to provide members of the local community with stability through addressing employment and housing needs immediately upon release. This is provided through job training in construction and transitional housing. These programmes strengthen the potential for success after re-entry among African American males, and allow them to join a supportive environment.

While in the housing or job training programme, the men receive two evidence-based interventions: motivational interviewing (Carroll et al. 2006) and *Modelo de Intervención Psicomédica* (Pemberton et al. 2009). The interventions, designed to reduce drug use and high-risk sexual behaviours, are delivered individually by a trained peer educator from the community, and are supervised by GMB's Deputy Director. The peer educator is a community resource that, through careful training, can be harnessed; being a member of the community he or she understands what is meaningful to those who are similar. The peer educator also builds his or her capacity that can be key for communities as they address other issues within communities.

The community–academic partnership developed an expanded programme that combined GROUP Ministries' service components and the Connect to Protect coalition building model (Ziff et al. 2006), and addressed SAMHSA's goals of increasing HIV testing among vulnerable groups. The TLC Group partnered with the Baltimore City Health Department to conduct HIV testing in the Greater Rosemont community in mobile HIV testing vans and through HIV testing at the GROUP Ministries offices.

Using the funding from the Abell Foundation, SAMHSA, and from an additional grant received from the Open Source Institute, the TLC Group programme expanded GROUP Ministries' service efforts to ex-offenders and former substance users, improved the stability and wellbeing of the community, and redeveloped its neighbourhood through employing local community members in housing renovation projects. Through the SAMHSA grant, GROUP Ministries was able to expand its services by utilising local strengths and resources, hire additional staff members from the local community, and train four housing members as community outreach workers and educators (including ex-offenders and former substance users). The outcomes of these activities will be evaluated to demonstrate the role of individual and structural intervention in reducing substance use and HIV risk behaviours.

The evaluation will provide the partners with the necessary detail to guide group decision-making; it will focus both on the outcomes for ex-offenders and former substance users and the application of CBPR. This commitment to evaluation aligns itself with CBPR principles, including co-learning, capacity building and knowledge generation. Through evaluation, partners can discover what works and what does not work, and this information can be used to improve both programming and the CBPR processes.

The community–academic partners developed the survey to evaluate whether the HIV testing and evidenced-based interventions were reaching the target population, to identify additional needs and resources of the population, and determine if the interventions were successful in meeting their goals. The community and academic partners created two versions of the surveys used to evaluate the programme. These were developed over 11 months through discussions and negotiations about the question material and wording. Some questions were required by funders; however, the additional questions were discussed, debated and tested until all partner members were comfortable with the content and wording. The survey development was an iterative and co-learning process, and partners had equal participation throughout, blending sound behavioural theory with the lived experiences of community members.

These direct services activities complement the structural change focus of the community coalition, whose members are working to produce an environment where employment and housing are available. Through this, it is believed that the community's reliance on drug use and related high HIV risk behaviours will be reduced. By applying to the state for Community Development Corporation status, the TLC Group works with a community coalition of community leaders, advocates and city representatives to acquire houses for renovation by local community members who have been, or are to be, trained in construction.

The TLC Group partners understand that broad community-level change is a long-term process. Committed to sustainability, partners are working to develop a business plan that will allow this work to continue without dependence on external funding. An important component of CBPR is the commitment to sustainability, and by developing this business plan it is hoped that the TLC Group can continue its work without reliance on external grant funding.

YOUR blessed health: A faith–based intervention to holistically address HIV prevention for youth

Young people are another subgroup at persistent risk of HIV and other sexually transmitted infections (STIs), for a number of behavioural, biological and cultural reasons (CDC 2011b). Although young people make up only 25% of the sexually active population in the USA, they acquire approximately half of all new STIs (CDC 2011b). Youth of minority races and ethnicities are particularly affected (CDC 2010a).

YOUR Blessed Health provides an example of a programme aimed at increasing the capacity of faith-based institutions and faith leaders to address HIV/AIDS and other STIs among 11 to 19 year old African Americans. YOUR Blessed Health was developed in collaboration between the YOUR Center,

Flint Odyssey House Health Awareness Center, Faith Access to Community Economic Development, Pastors' Spouses of Genesee County, and the University of Michigan School of Public Health (Robinson et al. 2010). The primary partner was the YOUR Center, which was established by a social worker in the Flint, Michigan community in response to a community-wide survey that identified gaps and barriers affecting community health and wellbeing.

A crucial component of CBPR is the translation of research into action strategies that address local issues of concern. In Flint, Michigan, HIV and other STI infections were plaguing youth (Michigan Department of Community Health 2007). The YOUR Center, which had become an established local authority in HIV/AIDS prevention and outreach, was approached by a group of pastors' wives who were concerned about the increasing rates of STIs and teenage pregnancies among African American youth. The pastors' spouses desired guidance in increasing their role in providing HIV/AIDS and STI education and outreach in their churches (Robinson et al. 2010).

Faith-based organisations are considered to be the cornerstone of African American communities and have historically served as an entryway to the community. In response to the pastors' spouses request for guidance, the YOUR Center director asked the faith-based institutions about the possibility of developing an HIV-prevention intervention to be conducted within the churches.

In studies examining the obstacles precluding African American churches from taking a more active role in HIV prevention, the negative religious and moral attitudes about behaviours associated with HIV have been noted. These attitudes include perceptions about sexual behaviour outside of marriage, homosexuality, and intravenous drug use as routes of transmission for HIV (Francis and Liverpool 2009). Partners therefore felt it was important to frame HIV/AIDS as a health issue, not as a sexual or moral issue. The goal for the YOUR Blessed Health was to provide HIV-prevention information to youth in the Flint area by improving the capacity building of churches to discuss sexual health and HIV prevention with their congregation in a non-judgmental manner.

From continued meetings with the pastors' spouses, the YOUR Center director began developing an intervention that respected and built upon the faith-based institution's capacity to address HIV prevention. The director approached the intervention development with the viewpoint of the churches as autonomous units whose dignity and self-worth were to be respected (Griffith et al. 2010b). These concepts are fundamental aspects of a CBPR framework (Israel et al. 1998). The director then reached out to academic researchers and staff from the University of Michigan School of Public Health for further assistance.

Based on the partner's knowledge of the community, the YOUR Center director's history of work in the community and discussions with the pastors' spouses, the partners developed the multi-level intervention YOUR Blessed Health. This intervention was respectful of church doctrine and built capacity around HIV prevention within the faith-based organisations. Although training young people was the primary goal of the YOUR Blessed Health programme, changing the norms of faith-based institutions as well as communities was a secondary goal. Through continued engagement, the YOUR Center staff cultivated support for the intervention concept with local faith-based organisations.

YOUR Blessed Health is a unique programme for addressing HIV among youth because it educates and trains both youth and adults to address HIV/AIDS, utilising a culturally congruent curriculum for the church setting. Its development was informed by inclusion of the pastors' spouses, participation of the YOUR Center and University of Michigan School of Public Health staff in the churches, and iterative discussion with the church members. The YOUR Blessed Health intervention has five components: (1) a 10-hour, five-session youth training programme using the HIV Outreach, Prevention, and Education curriculum (HOPE), which focuses on the basics of HIV/AIDS, STIs, sexual knowledge, communication skills and helping young people to create individualised risk-reduction plans; (2) a 10-hour, five-session training programme for adults in the church and community based on the HOPE curriculum, which provides basic STI and HIV/AIDS knowledge; (3) initial (16-hour) and ongoing training and support for pastors, pastors' spouses and other church leaders who will conduct the youth and adult training sessions to provide them with the basic knowledge, skills and resources to lead the YOUR Blessed Health sessions and conduct other church HIV/AIDS educational activities; (4) church-wide activities, including sermons and presentations during the primary weekly service to raise awareness and reduce stigma of HIV/AIDS; and (5) community-wide activities such as health fairs that educate and raise awareness about HIV/AIDS and promote collaboration among different faith-based institutions on HIV prevention (Griffith et al. 2010a).

In response to the expressed needs of the pastors' spouses, and through continued discussion with them, the YOUR Blessed Health intervention was developed to allow church leaders and members, including the youth, to select from a menu the activities that they desired. Activities included in-reach activities by the church leadership (i.e. 'Boys Nite In'), participation in community events (i.e. AIDS Walk Flint), HOPE parties, and pastor-led education in their churches and within the larger community (Griffith et al. 2010b).

YOUR Blessed Health was piloted in 2006 and 2007 in 12 churches using evaluation materials developed collaboratively by partners through an iterative and co-learning process. Following the pilot, the partners received funding to expand the intervention and evaluation to 30 more churches who were interested in the programme.

YOUR Blessed Health utilised the strengths of faith-based organisations and ensured that intervention messages and components were consistent with the teachings of faith leaders, demonstrating respect for the denominational doctrines and visions of the pastors and their spouses. Working with faith leaders, the partners were able to accommodate the individuality of faith-based organisations and their congregations to improve the acceptability of the curriculum and the comfort of the faith leaders and their congregations. For example, several of the churches did not incorporate all components of the YOUR Blessed Health curriculum (e.g. non-abstinence forms of safer sex) until support from the congregation increased, and some churches began distributing condoms and providing condom-use skills building activities off church grounds to improve the comfort level of congregational members. While the core materials and goals were consistent throughout church settings, churches were able to determine the frequency and timing of sessions that the outreach activities required. This allowed the church leaders and congregants to adhere to their institutional beliefs, doctrines and cultures.

Through the process of developing and piloting the faith-based HIV-prevention intervention, the partners demonstrated that interventions must consider how HIV/AIDS and its routes of transmission can be discussed and acknowledged in ways that are respectful to the churches' culture. Working with the pastors' spouses, the YOUR Center and academic partners were able to create an intervention that allows organisations to maintain their individuality and that respects the doctrine and vision of the pastor. Building on strengths in the faith-based organisations, an important principle in CBPR, the YOUR Blessed Health curriculum was aimed at producing a sustainable and systemic change in the way that faith leaders and members of congregations address the HIV epidemic in the African American community, and they accomplished this goal through practicing social inclusion in research.

CyBER/testing: An online intervention to increase HIV testing among men who have sex with men

Men who have sex with men (MSM) are a behaviourally defined subpopulation that is severely affected by HIV/AIDS in the USA, representing more than half of new HIV infections each year (CDC 2010b). For many MSM, the internet has emerged as an important tool for social networking and support, meeting friends and sexual partners, and building community (Rhodes et al. 2008). However, seeking sex on the internet has been found to be a risk factor for HIV and STIs among MSM (Rhodes et al. 2002). Thus, many community-based organisations, AIDS service organisations, and public health departments and clinics provide HIV education within internet spaces such as chat rooms that facilitate social and sexual networking among MSM (Noar et al. 2009).

Cyber-Based Education and Referral/Men for Men (CyBER/M4M), an internet-based intervention designed to reduce HIV exposure and transmission among gay men and MSM who use geographically defined chat rooms, was developed through a community–academic partnership in North Carolina that has existed for more than 10 years and has over 50 current members. The evolving partnership reflects demographic trends and the ongoing impact of the HIV epidemic. Partners include representatives from public health departments (local and state level); six AIDS service organisations; community-based organisations, including Latino soccer leagues and teams, the North

Carolina lesbian, gay, bisexual, and transgender (LGBT) pride organisation, a local LGBT foundation, local businesses, including media organisations, Internet companies, bars and clubs, a video production company, and *tiendas* (Latino grocers); the US Centers for Disease Control and Prevention; and five universities. Partnership members may be involved with and committed to different projects; however, the partnership is not study specific. Members may join and leave, but despite transitions the partnership remains. Moreover, partners are not merely tied to a single study or funding source; rather, within the CBPR partnership, members are passionate about HIV prevention and committed to one another – with or without funding. CyBER/M4M developed through this partnership as a result of a request for assistance from a local AIDS service organisation to develop and evaluate an online intervention.

In developing the intervention, however, the partners also looked outwards and took intervention ideas and materials to groups of MSM in the community to get their feedback. Often these MSM were less involved and had perspectives that were not affected by ongoing participation in a partnership. Partners understand that the members of their partnership differ at least slightly from those who are not as involved, and the interventions are designed for those who are not involved. Partners, however, valued all perspectives and believed that an intervention for internet-using MSM could benefit from the perspective of someone who is not a gay man or MSM. Thus, the dialogue that partners engaged in as ideas and perspectives are shared contributed to creativity in intervention development. Not only did the partners want to have diversity of sexual orientation, for example, but they valued diversity of geographic location; it is known that chat-room use differs by geographic community. Partners also recognised the differences in perspectives that socio–economic status influences. Thus, the partnership goes beyond race/ethnicity and orientation and sexual behaviour, and worked to ensure diversity in other proxies of privilege.

Based on piloting the resulting intervention, CyBER/M4M, and the promising results regarding improving HIV testing (Rhodes et al. 2011), the partners refined the intervention to focus solely on the promotion of HIV testing. The refined intervention was known as CyBER/testing. This intervention was based on natural helping (Eng et al. 2009), and was implemented by an interventionist from the local gay community who had an intimate understanding of the online and geographic MSM communities and who was employed by a community-based organisation partner. The interventionist was trained in HIV transmission, disease progression, and local testing options and processes, as well as in social cognitive theory (Bandura 1994), empowerment education (Freire 1973), effective communication, and the ask–advise–assist model (Whitlock et al. 2002). Collaboratively, the partners developed the training manual used.

The interventionist entered chat rooms designed for social and sexual networking among MSM in the catchment area at preselected times of the day and posted standardised triggers about HIV testing and his availability to provide information. Once contacted by a chatter, the interventionist could provide information about HIV and HIV testing, as well as answer questions.

To be respectful of the cultural context of the chat room, the interventionist did not send unsolicited instant messages to other chatters. These details
are good examples of how social inclusion can positively impact implementation. By working closely with community members, the intervention meets
community expectations; at no time was the interventionist removed from a
chat room. After all, the intervention takes place in internet rooms designed
for social and sexual networking. It was important that the community was
involved in the development of the intervention and its protocol to ensure that
the intervention met its potential.

Over a 6-month period in 2009, the interventionist recruited the chatters
to complete a brief online assessment by posting instant messages in the chat
rooms advertising a quick and anonymous survey using a different alias. The
seven-item survey used binary or drop-down lists to expedite completion and
reduce respondent burden. The survey asked about demographics, HIV testing,
and knowledge of and interaction with the interventionist. For those who had
interacted with the interventionist, an additional question asked if the chatter
viewed a video recommended by the interventionist. Preliminary evaluation
data of this pilot intervention, based on this quasi-experimental, pre-test–post-
test design, suggested this intervention had promise to reach MSM and increase
HIV testing rates. However, the partners wanted to confirm this through the
use of a longer and more rigorous design.

To develop the more rigorous evaluation study, all partners fully engaged
one another in intensive decision-making about all aspects of this study, including research and evaluation methods, intervention strategies, and implementation and dissemination plans. A repeated cross-sectional matched-pair community randomised design with intervention and delayed-intervention arms
(Murray 1998) was selected to evaluate the effectiveness of the CyBER/testing
intervention. Randomisation of individual participants was not practical due
to the communication structure of chat rooms (e.g. all those in the chat room
can see public instant messages), and thus one community within each matched
pair was randomised to the intervention or delayed-intervention group. As a
result of concerns about the ethics of withholding a potentially valuable
intervention from some members of an already vulnerable community, a
delayed-intervention design was utilised. Evaluation is ongoing.

The partnership was successful in using a stepwise approach, moving slowly
from formative research and pilot studies to more rigorous designs. During this
process, community members learned about the power and usefulness of evidence, and non-community members learned what is both feasible and meaningful within communities.

Conclusion

The projects discussed above utilise the nine CBPR principles to include
community in the research, intervention and evaluation process to reduce
HIV/AIDS disparities in the USA. No one set of principles is applicable to all

community–academic partnerships (Israel et al. 2005), and these examples demonstrate the diverse ways in which partnerships and projects use CBPR as a form of social inclusion. The principles guiding partnerships are instead a reflection of the collective vision of the partnerships. These principles, therefore, are applied in various ways within community–academic partnerships, demonstrating multiple approaches to CBPR.

As documented through these examples, CBPR can address the immediate risks to HIV infection through the development of community-relevant research and interventions to address individual behaviours and structural vulnerabilities. As other research has demonstrated, CBPR can also address the deep-seated causes of disparities through social inclusion and building community capacity to address social determinants of health (Schulz et al. 2002). Throughout this chapter, we have provided detailed examples of how CBPR is being used in the USA to include affected communities in research to prevent HIV/AIDS through community–academic partnerships. The partnerships that develop are unique, as are the projects chosen to address local HIV prevention, and thus we have provided a snapshot of a diverse field by describing these projects at various stages in the research process. However, guided by the principles of CBPR, these partnerships and projects are united in their belief that, through social inclusion in research, community–academic partners can develop a more comprehensive approach to prevent HIV among our vulnerable populations, and address the inequities in health.

16 Inclusive research with people with intellectual disability

Recognising the value of social relationships as a process of inclusive research

Erin Wilson and Robert Campain

People with disabilities have repeatedly called for increased inclusion in disability research. The involvement of people with intellectual disability is complex, and has been explored in an emerging research model known as 'inclusive research'. This chapter outlines an inclusive research project with people with intellectual disability. In particular, we present the model of inclusive research used, critique its capacity to achieve emancipatory and participatory outcomes, and argue for an acknowledgement of the social process as the aspect most valued by the people with intellectual disability involved. It is intended that this will inform others who may wish to engage in inclusive research with people with intellectual disability.

Defining inclusive research

Historically, research in defining and exploring the experience of people with disabilities has largely been conducted without their involvement. Barnes argues that the emerging 'socio-political interpretation of disability' in the 1970s and 1980s, led to both the 'theorisation of disability as social oppression' as well as a new emancipatory approach to disability research (Barnes 2003: 5). In line with other definitions of emancipatory research, Barnes (2003) defines it as an individual and collective empowerment process of the oppressed group via transforming social and power relations, and processes of knowledge production. Within this approach, people with disabilities are researchers and experts of their experience in contrast to 'the power of the researcher-expert . . . [with] control over the design, implementation, analysis and dissemination of research findings' (Barnes and Mercer 1997: 6–7). Similarly, participatory research emphasises people with intellectual disability as involved in varied aspects of the research beyond that of just research subjects or respondents; however, the political elements of the approach are less prescribed (Walmsley 2001) as the participatory paradigm incorporates a broad array of approaches (Reason 1994).

However, concern about the relevance of such approaches for people with intellectual disability, whose cognitive impairments limit the level of owner-ship, direction setting and participation in research available to them, has led to the establishment of an 'inclusive research' model. This model draws heav-ily on practices and goals from both emancipatory and participatory research, while adapting these to the context of research by and with people with intel-lectual disability. Inclusive research is described as 'research in which people with learning difficulties [known also as people with intellectual disabilities] are involved as more than just research subjects or respondents' (Walmsley 2001: 188). Walmsley and Johnson expand this definition to explain that this involve-ment includes people with intellectual disability taking on roles as 'initiators, doers, writers and disseminators' (Walmsley and Johnson 2003: 9). To achieve this, because of people's cognitive disability, researchers without disability are required to support and work collaboratively with people with intellectual dis-ability who adopt roles as researchers.

To date, the complexities of enacting this model have not been well explored. As Bigby and Frawley state, 'seldom . . . does research that claims to be inclusive give detailed descriptions of the involvement of people with intel-lectual disability, their roles, contribution, the challenges encountered, or the support provided' (Bigby and Frawley 2010: 54). This echoes a critique pro-vided by McClimens, who suggested that this absence of published discussion of the 'grittier and messier aspects of collaboration' may be due to a publishing bias towards 'successful' projects (McClimens 2008: 273). Another explanation may be that inclusive research for people with intellectual disability, at least in Australia, has not become firmly established (Bigby and Frawley, 2010), and remains not only underpinned but overshadowed by the expectations and ide-als of emancipatory and participatory paradigms. These expectations potentially silence more detailed and nuanced accounts of the process.

We undertook an inclusive research project with a group of people with intellectual disability in the western suburbs of Melbourne, Victoria. While including some innovative elements, of more importance than the model is the analysis of the complex reality of enacting it, and what this tells us about the key ingredients and practices of inclusive research when it is allowed to stand somewhat apart from, though informed by, its antecedents.

Food Court Friends: An inclusive research project

Between 2006 and 2008, Scope, a disability service provider in Victoria, Aus-tralia, undertook the Food Court Friends project (Campain and Wilson 2010). Central to the project were the members of a Scope community group who worked as co-researchers in the project. The community group comprised indi-viduals with a range of intellectual disability. Some were more independent than others and required relatively low levels of support, while others needed more intensive support on a daily basis. All of the group members had the capacity to communicate thoughts and feelings verbally, though for some this was limited.

Prior to the commencement of the project, people with intellectual disability involved in this project had been increasingly accessing local indoor shopping facilities. In doing so, they were experiencing a range of issues that were impacting their experience. The project aim was to identify these issues largely through the interviewing of shopkeepers and security personnel with regard to their experiences with people with disabilities as shoppers. The project implemented a range of strategies to address the issues identified (see Campain and Wilson 2010).

Our inclusive research model

From the inception of the project it was envisioned that an inclusive research process would be adopted. The project offered three researcher roles. People with intellectual disability worked as co-researchers (to varying degrees at different stages of the research), secondary school students acted as student partners to support the activity of data collection, and both groups worked together with the formally trained lead researchers (the two authors of this chapter). The following outlines the model that we adopted but, as we subsequently discovered, the reality was both more and less than this.

Lead researcher role

The Food Court Friends project incorporated an explicit role for us as the two lead researchers who had previous research training and experience. The feminist researcher, Patty Lather, describes this role as a 'catalyst' (Lather 1986), while within an emancipatory methodology, it has been described as a 'challenger' (Freire 1972) or 'critical friend' (Carr and Kemmis 1986) to the participating group. Stone and Priestly (1996) argue that the formally trained 'non-disabled' researcher must not be detached, but work closely with people with disabilities and be guided by an ethic of improving the lives of the people the researcher works with. In this sense, the researcher's skills should be at the disposal of people with disabilities. Within inclusive research approaches, the role of the formally trained researcher, usually a researcher without disability, has also been labelled a 'research supporter' acting in a variety of roles including facilitator, advisor, trainer (Williams and Simons 2005: 10) and mentor (Bigby and Frawley 2010). In the Food Court Friends project, the lead researchers adopted these roles as well as designing the research, analysing the data, and authoring documents about the project.

While the lead researcher role was dominated by the management of traditional research tasks and responsibilities, it also involved significant contact and relationships with the co-researchers. Lead researchers participated in social events related to the research which were in keeping with a process of building relationships between colleagues. This process of relationship building and engagement in the social world of co-researchers is a feature of participatory research whereby relationship building enables an understanding of the social and cultural context of participants' views (Freire 1972; Bishop 1996). The emphasis on relationships is part of recognising that working together as a group is always more than a technical activity, involving a myriad of roles and responsibilities to members and the group as a whole (Bishop 1996).

Co-researchers

In keeping with aspects of an inclusive research methodology, the project aimed to engage people with intellectual disability (up to 12 Scope community group members) as co-researchers in the planning of the project, the collection of data, and implementation of the project over its three-year life span. Co-researchers engaged in a range of socially valued roles (Walmsley 2001) including:

- Training (along with the student partners) over several weeks each year relating to: the skills of interviewing; data documentation; dealing with negative feedback or difficult situations during interviews; and the associated issues of ethics and confidentiality.
- Collection of data via interviews to identify the main issues affecting shopkeepers and security staff in dealing with people with disabilities. Co-researchers worked with teams of student partners to do interviews with shopping centre personnel inside the nominated shopping centres.
- Meetings with shopping centre management to discuss findings and propose suitable interventions to address issues raised by shopping centre personnel.
- Implementing some of the planned interventions in shopping centres, such as delivering a communication guide to shopkeepers.
- Group discussions at the completion of the project about the findings, recommendations and limitations of the project. In addition, co-researchers reflected on their experiences, motivations and feelings about involvement in the project.
- Concluding events such as social time with all members of the research team.

Finally, part of the co-researcher role involved dissemination of the findings at conferences.

Student partners

An innovative element and strength of the research design was the involvement of senior secondary students as partners in the project. In each of the three years of the project successive groups of students (around 15 each year) worked as student partners to support co-researchers in the collection of data in the shopping centres. This occurred once a fortnight across eight to ten weeks each year. This involved participating in training, and working collaboratively to collect data with co-researchers to interview shopping centre personnel. Teams of co-researchers and student partners adopted the roles of interviewer and note-taker according to preference. They were assisted by Scope disability support staff who were present – if needed – to address any issues arising. This approach is a considerable expansion of an inclusive method in that it aligned two groups of non-formally trained researchers as partners. However, its most significant value (to be discussed later) was seen to be its potential to foster relationships and to change attitudes as research team members interacted during both research activities and social events.

The disorderly reality: Findings/critique

The adopted inclusive research model was an ideal to guide the research, although the reality was much more complex given the agency of individuals and a changing, unpredictable social environment. We, as lead researchers, discovered that our concerns over the project and our role in the collaborative endeavour led to ongoing reflection and doubts as to whether we were meeting the requirements of inclusive research, including its emancipatory ideals. Owens argues that what is required by social researchers is a degree of reflexivity 'because it draws attention to the researcher as a part of the world being studied and the ways in which the research process represents, and is part of, that study' (Owens 2007: 302). As lead researchers, we engaged in continuous reflection on the process and sought out the views of co-researchers, both formally and informally.

The following explores two areas of reflection: the complexities of inclusive research, including consideration of the issues surrounding emancipatory and participatory paradigms; and the need to value the multiple dimensions of the research experience.

The emancipatory and participatory ideals of inclusive research

Through adopting a reflexive approach, we frequently considered whether the research project was emancipatory and truly participative. Emancipatory and participatory ideas are powerful drivers for the design of inclusive research. However, it is important that whenever formally trained researchers argue for the merits of people with intellectual disability undertaking roles as researchers, with all the expectant benefits, that the ideal does not obscure the more nuanced reality. Issues of participation and emancipation are not straightforward in this context, nor are they the only criteria by which to judge the value of inclusive research.

A commonly identified issue of involving people with intellectual disability is that of 'tokenism' (see for example Walmsley and Johnson 2003) and we considered the extent to which our approach was limited to this. A 'tokenistic' research process is one 'in which the disadvantaged person is isolated from decisions about research commissioning, from setting the research agenda, from formulating appropriate research designs or from influencing the nature and content of research dissemination' (Ramcharan and Grant 1994: 228). In our case, constant feedback was sought from co-researchers, and their input was considered seriously and became part of the ongoing research process. However, while the research arose from the concerns of people with disabilities, it was the lead researchers who sought the funding, designed the research method, and organised participants and resources. It is fair to say that the ultimate authority resided with the formally trained researchers who made decisions while striving to ensure the input of people with intellectual disability. Whether this went beyond tokenism is open to question.

Of course, in striving to meet the ideals of inclusive research it is important that people with intellectual disability are not coerced, with consideration given to their desire to be involved. As Cameron and Murphy note, 'A significant tension exists between ensuring that people with learning disability understand the nature and implications of their involvement in research and at the same time avoiding any coercion' (Cameron and Murphy 2007: 113). In our research, the co-researcher role was initiated and designed by the lead researchers, with people with intellectual disability free to consider their level of involvement in the research. Co-researchers were encouraged and supported to choose the types of ways in which they wished to participate. A small number were interested in the processes and tasks of the research, most appeared more interested in involvement as a social activity. A couple of the co-researchers were keen to be involved with meetings with shopping centre management to discuss the research and their possible involvement, while others were content to take part in the activities that were of a group nature with their fellow co-researchers. This suggests that the lead researchers, in their aim to meet inclusive research criteria, cannot exclude the fact that people with intellectual disability may be willing to cede control and the doing of tasks.

In considering issues of participation and tokenism, we were also mindful of needing to ensure that people who had originally given consent to participate in the project could opt out if they wished to do so. Throughout the project, particularly at the junctures where an activity was soon to commence, we sought to again discuss the project and co-researchers' choice to be involved or not. We were mindful that potential participants may feel obliged or wish to be agreeable to us whom they had come to know and feel comfortable with. We sought to address this by making clear that whether the person chose to take part was entirely up to them and would have no bearing on their relationship with us. Co-researchers chose both to opt in and out throughout the research process. They indicated that the choice was sometimes based on the value they gave to the positive relationships they had with us and others involved in the research, more so than the valuing of their own research roles. As Cameron and Murphy note, it is paramount that 'non-disabled' researchers be 'skilled at establishing rapport and social closeness with participants' (Cameron and Murphy 2007: 117) and that 'an ongoing relationship between researcher and participant which uses accessible methods of communication . . . is critical'

(Cameron and Murphy 2007: 118). In this way, relationships between lead researchers and co-researchers can act both as a reason to participate in research as well as the foundation to comfortably decide to withdraw.

An area of participation in inclusive research that requires more attention is the impact of cognitive ability on the level of understanding about the research aims and processes, which may determine the variety of ways people with intellectual disability could be involved. It was often difficult to ascertain the extent to which the co-researchers understood various aspects of the project and their role as researchers at all times. Some were enthusiastic and understood the aims of the project and were able to provide suggestions and insights, while others participated in activities and seemed less able or willing to grasp the intricacies of the research. This needs to be recognised as an inherent tension of inclusive research with people with intellectual disability. While the provision of appropriate support has been identified as a key strategy to increase involvement of people with intellectual disability in research (Bigby and Frawley 2010), in our case people could also be present in research and social activities without expectations of involvement that may exceed cognitive capacity.

These issues speak to differences in participation, roles, and responsibilities held within the research team. Where there are obvious inequalities between lead researchers and co-researchers this must be acknowledged, and there is little to be gained in pretending otherwise. As the main authors of the project, we were guiding and controlling the process overall, including leading discussions, assisting the co-researchers, initiating contacts with others, arranging timetables and co-ordinating activities. Equally significant was the use of our academic research skills and experiences, including the initiating and writing of reports and publications. As the Burton Street Research Group discovered, one of the areas of inequality they experienced was based on differences in the technical skills of research, where professional researchers were necessary to produce publishable research:

> While we aim for all researchers in the group to be equal, the academic structure around researching is far more easily accessed by professionals. We hope this will change but it is the reality for us at the moment.
>
> (Abell et al. 2007: 123)

Bigby and Frawley (2010) also note the importance of acknowledging inequalities of skills and knowledge in the area of research, asserting that collaboration should not require the pretence of equality with regard to this technical expertise.

Inequality of research roles is also evident in the area of payment for people with intellectual disability as co-researchers. In considering issues of equality and the valuing of people with intellectual disability as co-researchers, it has been argued elsewhere that disability research must address the issue of payment given that the formally trained, professional researchers are paid for their work (Walmsley and Johnson 2003). The co-researchers stated that the issue of payment for their involvement was important. As well as a financial incentive, it is likely that financial payment legitimised their efforts and was significant to the way in which they regarded themselves as important contributors to the project. Co-researchers were paid $20 for the work they undertook in the shopping centres, which took approximately one and a half hours. They were not paid for the training sessions which they attended (totalling between two and six hours each year). This does raise questions of fairness. In hindsight, there were times they could, and should, have been paid – such as for the training sessions, conference presentations and meetings with shopping centre management. In determining levels of payment, there is also the issue of how to fairly evaluate the various contributions of the co-researchers. Due to motivations and cognitive abilities, the input of some people was much greater than others. It is fair to say that the involvement of some did not go beyond their attendance. Does this matter? These are difficult issues to resolve and it is questionable whether we got the issue of payment right.

This discussion requires us to consider to what extent we empowered people with intellectual disability, or to what extent we maintained their marginalisation. On the one hand, members of the research team held unequal positions, exemplified by levels of payment. Lead researchers exercised considerable control of the research, and their level of professional expertise in research, as well as their non-disabled status, risked marginalising or silencing the voices of people with intellectual disability (Woodill 1994). This was a likely reality of this project despite our efforts, and was not altogether avoidable given the differing interest levels and cognitive abilities of the co-researchers. On the other hand, the involvement of people with intellectual disability as co-researchers was a strong element of the project. Overall, the use of co-researchers in this project served as a progressive step toward empowerment by offering socially valued roles as co-researchers and providing people with intellectual disability input into the project. It meant that the co-researchers could have a 'voice' and be involved in the research in a manner that was significant to them. Working with people with intellectual disability served as an ongoing reminder for lead researchers that disability research must be guided by an ethic of ultimately assisting people with disabilities in a manner that is both life-enhancing and empowering.

Overall, the approach could be described as a collaborative one where people with intellectual disability were 'allies' with formally trained researchers (Walmsley 2001), although they did not lead and direct the research. However, despite not fully achieving inclusive research goals, it would be wrong to discount the emancipatory outcomes altogether. Rather than a finite state of emancipation, there were emancipatory moments. These included people with intellectual disability seeking out new roles and exerting their agency in the project; new relationships being formed across groups (between co-researchers, the student partners and the lead researchers); and fostering individual self worth and the collective status of people with intellectual disability via occupying valued roles, either as researchers or as people in valued social relationships.

Valuing the multiple dimensions of the research experience

The above discussion begins to suggest that inclusive research may be valued in a range of ways including, but not limited to, elements identified by emancipatory and participatory paradigms. This leads to the consideration of the need for recognising multiple dimensions of inclusive research beyond those related to knowledge production. In broad terms, the project highlighted the value of inclusive research as a process, perhaps more so than its value in producing a substantive product that might later contribute to localised (possibly emancipatory) change. While process, in particular via the participation of people with intellectual disability, is an area of discussion in the literature of inclusive research, the tenor of this discussion does not capture our experience. In this project we found that, for people with intellectual disability, the social value of the research process was of prime importance. In addition, this social process generated valued outcomes in terms of unanticipated social changes. These are discussed below.

Inclusive research has been shown above to be an inherently collaborative process. It was clear that the social process of being together was a key motivator and benefit for people with intellectual disability, in some cases, more so than the research itself. Abell and colleagues reported that a desire for a 'sense of belonging . . . and to continue to spend time with other people in a group and feel part of something' were prime motivators to forming an inclusive research group (Abell et al. 2007: 121). In our case, the social nature of the work meant that people with intellectual disability were engaged in activities that not only fitted the paradigm of research, but also incorporated other socially valued roles. Co-researchers often remarked how much they enjoyed being with the student partners and being involved together in the key tasks of the project. Throughout the training process there was time for various social activities, while the project tasks were also somewhat social in that people worked together in interviewing the shopping centre personnel. Meetings with the research team conducted throughout the research enabled people to get together and socialise before and after. Concluding events at the completion of the data collection included playing computer games, followed by the awarding of certificates to all those involved. Each year, co-researchers attended the Scope researchers' Christmas lunch function along with other Scope researchers and associates. While not explicitly a part of an emancipatory or even an inclusive research agenda, the social interaction had significant value for all those involved.

This social process of the research contributed in an unforeseen and significant way to achieving the research aim. A stated aim of the research was to build relationships and break down barriers to social inclusion. It was originally envisaged, as with most research, that this aim would be achieved by the implementation of actions to address the key findings of the research. It was not anticipated the extent to which the process of the research, rather than the expected product (i.e. findings), would achieve the stated research aim. Social interaction between parties to the research was a fundamental aspect of the research process for the Food Court Friends project. Even where contact between parties was limited (for example, a short interview between shopkeepers, co-researchers and student partners), there was a chance for those without disabilities (shopkeepers and student partners) to learn something about people with disabilities. This led to unanticipated consequences, such as significant attitude change on the part of the student partners, and the manner in which they related to people with disabilities, which changed throughout the duration of their time working together. There also appeared to be a degree of confidence building for the co-researchers in their interactions with others, as evidenced in both our observation and as expressed by them (Campain and Wilson 2010).

Similarly, people with intellectual disability, in their roles as co-researchers, engaged with people in the wider community, particularly shopping centre personnel. This, somewhat innovative, aspect of the research design required co-researchers (along with the student partners) to interview shopkeepers, meet with shopping centre management, and return to retailers to distribute information and resources designed to address key issues identified through data collection. This role is somewhat at odds with most published inclusive research examples, where the emphasis is on people with intellectual disability collecting data 'about them[selves] and their lives' (McClimens 2008: 271). This draws on a fundamental principle of inclusive (and participatory and emancipatory) research, that disadvantaged groups are 'experts by experience'. While there is some critique of this notion, for example Bigby and Frawley (2010) and Barnes (2003), there appears to have been little involvement of people with intellectual disability as researchers of topics where information is gathered primarily from people without disability. While the social change outcomes of this broader engagement are difficult to gauge, this aspect of the project opened up – albeit in an unanticipated way – opportunities for social change outcomes in the form of increased awareness and understanding of people with disabilities and their needs.

Finally, the value of the research was also in its contribution to an academic knowledge base, where new understandings were generated about the research topic as well as about its unexpected outcomes discussed above. However, in our case, the inclusive research approach, while producing new knowledge in new ways, posed some difficulties in terms of meeting the standards of academic rigour. This was largely the result of a significant part of the data collection being done by people with intellectual disability and the student partners who were not academically trained researchers. Overall, the data were lacking in the detail that we hoped to gather. This is not a criticism of the co-researchers and the student partners, but an observation that utilising others to do the data collection means that formally trained researchers have to relinquish control – and even expectations – and accept the limitations this may involve. Additionally, the unexpected 'findings' from the project posed another problem regarding academic rigour. As discussed above, one of the significant outcomes of the project involved the relationship building between the team members and the attitude change indicated by the student partners, which were only belatedly recorded using anecdotal and observational information. As unplanned and *ad hoc* activities these are unlikely to meet academic criteria. Further consideration needs to be given to how to value and validate such findings. Inclusive research must ultimately have value to people with disabilities and this may compete with meeting academic standards. As Walmsley and Johnson state:

> Many researchers struggle to resolve the tension that exists between research which is academically rigorous, acceptable to funding organizations and publishable, and research which is of use to the people who are subject to it, which is relevant to their needs and can inform and promote needed subject change.
>
> (Walmsley and Johnson 2003: 9)

Overall, the social relationship and social change outcomes of the inclusive research approach were highly valued and perhaps of greater significance than those resulting from the anticipated product of the research. However, parameters of research paradigms, ethics applications, and research questions, can often narrowly define the research and constrain what gets valued or accepted as 'legitimate' findings and outcomes (Ramcharan and Grant 1994). These unexpected social and social change outcomes are at risk of being discounted if we adhere too closely to dominant academic traditions, which are confined to a particular system of research conduct and accountability.

Conclusion

Inclusive research is inherently a social process. If inclusive research is about 'researching together' (Williams and Simons 2005; Abell et al. 2007), then it is necessarily premised on fostering relationships between all team members. Therefore, it is important to explicitly foster this social element as both a legitimate process as well as outcome of this approach. Our experience is that this social element is valued in its own right by people with intellectual disability. Recognising the importance of the social aspect of inclusive research is an example of the need for sensitivity to the needs and priorities of the people with intellectual disability involved in it, who may value this element beyond any value they place on the research itself.

Our experience suggests that it is possible that the social process of the research contributes to a diverse range of research outcomes. As has been discussed, social interaction provides an opportunity for emancipatory moments as people with intellectual disability further experience valued roles and relationships. Social interaction also fosters the possibility of positive social change for a range of research stakeholders, including people without disabilities, who interact with the project and its research team. Our approach has identified a potential value in building researcher roles for people with intellectual disability that go beyond researching the experiences of peers with a disability (as is often the case with inclusive research), and instead provide the opportunity to undertake inquiry in and about society at large.

While the paradigms that guide and shape research are important, a more fluid interpretation of the emancipatory and participatory approaches that underpin inclusive research is needed. These paradigms are important in providing guidelines and focus for the work, but need to be seen as guides rather than 'strait-jacket[s]' (Walmsley 2001: 189) for inclusive research. Rather than an emphasis on achieving full or 'true' participation or emancipation, what may be more helpful is a focus on fostering emancipatory moments through a diverse range of strategies. Researchers who collaborate with people with intellectual disability need to be reflexive throughout the research and be critical of their role, accompanying actions, and the research process and aims. It is also important to equally reflect on the specific and contextualised needs and interests of people with intellectual disability involved in the project. Without this, there is the risk that research paradigms can be applied dogmatically, and may then run counter to the needs and valued outcomes of people with disabilities.

Inclusive research appears to have a complex set of benefits and outcomes that are far more than a research product. It is not an easy or straightforward task, and involves wrestling with a range of tensions, as discussed here and in other literature. This understanding of the complexity of inclusive research is important. Without it we risk devaluing inclusive research and the benefits that arise from it.

17 Examining the notion of informed consent and lessons learned for increasing inclusion among marginalised research groups

Nena Foster and Emily Freeman

Introduction

This chapter examines some of the barriers to obtaining informed consent from those who are deemed vulnerable, disadvantaged, marginalised and underrepresented in research to participate in research studies. First, the chapter examines the underlying principles of informed consent, before examining the challenges that formalised and regulated informed consent procedures present for context-dependent data collection processes and the differing needs of potential research participants. Next, the chapter examines the notions of trust and researcher responsibility, and their significance for negotiating and maintaining a mutually accepted form of consent that can enhance, rather than diminish, participant autonomy.

In order to illustrate the challenges and solutions of obtaining informed consent, we present research carried out with a group of predominantly African migrants aged 50 years and older, and living with HIV in a socio-economically disadvantaged area of East London, UK. We examine the challenges presented by utilising standardised, informed consent procedures, by which respondents to an anonymous questionnaire and participants in a series of focus group discussions were required to give written and signed consent. The case study illustrates how underlying assumptions about the nature and acceptability of approaches to verifying consent for research participation can exclude or include participation from populations who are typically excluded from research. Here, adults with uncertain immigration status, poor literacy, poor English language, poor mental and physical health, felt stigmatised or suspicious of the consenting requirements.

Furthermore, this chapter will argue that, while it is important to have an initial discussion to obtain consent, the use of formalised consenting procedures acted as a hurdle to building and maintaining potential participant trust, and that the insistence of ethical committees on formalised processes hinders the inclusion of marginalised groups for a number of reasons. One of these reasons is the underlying assumption that verbal consent is not often sufficient evidence of informed consent. For those with uncertain immigration status, poor literacy, poor mental and physical health and who may also feel stigmatised, obtaining written consent can raise suspicion and can act as a barrier to research inclusion. Drawing on our experiences, we argue that the model of written informed consent, in some cases can, and where possible, should, be exchanged for other forms of informed consent, such as implied consent, in order to include groups that we often know the least about, such as marginalised groups.

The underlying principles and process of obtaining informed consent

Social science research typically involves collecting data from the population of interest. There is a wealth of technical literature regarding methods for recruiting and retaining these research participants (e.g. Gledhill et al. 2008; Breland-Noble et al. 2012; Kubitskey et al. 2012). This literature recognises that recruitment strategies must vary according to the unique characteristics of the sampled population.

Although research studies using participant observation methods, both covert and overt, are a hotly debated exception, it is generally accepted that, in most studies, researchers must inform potential participants about their participation, what that participation entails, that they have the right to decline to participate in the study, and that refusal to participate will have no personal consequences for the participant. Researchers must also adopt a stance of 'non-interference' in the potential respondent's decision-making (Stoljar 2011). Non-interference is emphasised as important for research ethics as it helps to provide some of the necessary and sufficient evidence that participation has not been coerced or forced in any way. It is only under these conditions that research participants can be regarded as having given informed consent to participate (Beauchamp 2011).

As noted, the process of obtaining informed consent in research therefore emphasises individual human rights, individual autonomy and choice. It should also take into account a potential participant's wellbeing (Wiles et al. 2005; Miller and Boulton 2007). Researchers working across all disciplines hold regard for these principles, but many question the extent to which these conditions can be fully ensured (McCrady and Bux 1999; Hoeyer et al. 2005; Miller and Boulton 2007; Lloyd et al. 2008; Stoljar 2011).

Like research ethics more generally, informed consent is as much about abiding by inherent researcher values or morals and professional guidelines, as it is about enforced or enforceable regulation. Many of the guidelines that underpin ethical codes of conduct for researchers, e.g. the Universal Declaration of Human Rights (UN 1948) and the Declaration of Helsinki (World Medical Association 1964), prioritise protecting research participants from harm and exploitation and were drafted in response to past atrocities that very few researchers condone, e.g. research carried out by Nazi physicians on prisoners at Auschwitz, and who were later tried before the Nuremberg Military Tribunals (Pellegrino and Thomasma 2000), and the Tuskegee syphilis study, a longitudinal study conducted in Alabama from 1932 to 1972 in which 399 Black men were denied treatment for syphilis in order to document disease progression (Jones 1981).

These guidelines have been incorporated in the codes of practice produced by numerous professional associations and localised research ethics committees (RECs). However, rather than being used purely to guide researchers in making good ethical judgements, these bodies have increasingly become involved in the regulation and enforcement of the codes. For example, submission of research proposals to a body that reviews them based on these guidelines has become enshrined in government and research funding regulations in many settings (Wiles et al. 2005; Miller and Boulton 2007).

The increased influence and popularity of RECs has been criticised in recent years. Some researchers have commented that the level of scrutiny from RECs is too bureaucratic, unnecessary given researchers' own abilities to make ethically sound professional judgements, and may discourage researchers from engaging with ethical problems that arise once REC approval has been awarded (Guillemin and Gillam 2004). Others have argued that the guidelines are too influenced by natural science research models and are not appropriate for social science research in general, and qualitative research in particular (Lincoln and Tierney 2004). With regard to health and health-related research, non-invasive studies are very unlikely to involve risk of the type of harm to participants that the guidelines were intended to avoid, and so should not be assessed using the same criteria (Rhodes 2005; Wiles et al. 2005; Burgess 2007; Walls et al. 2010). Many researchers argue that introducing a formalised approach assumes a universalism in which ethical guidelines become dictats that should never be deviated from. Assuming such a position is neither desirable nor achievable (Reissman 2005), and raises a number of theoretical and practical issues for eliciting informed consent from potential participants (Miller and Boulton 2007; Tekola et al. 2009a).

The problem of formalising consenting procedures and the conceptual mismatch

Increased regulation in the process of obtaining research participants' consent by governing bodies has been mirrored by increased formalisation of these processes. In many cases, and across disciplines, informed consent is obtained and demonstrated using a participant information document and requesting participants sign a form to acknowledge their consent to participate. Some researchers have argued that this formalisation has not only increased the bureaucratisation of research, but has served to remove the researcher's ability to make situationally or contextually appropriate decisions about consenting procedures based on what best suits individual participants (Punch 1998; Small 2001; Tekola et al. 2009a). For example, consenting procedures used in medical or other forms of more invasive research may not be appropriate for use in qualitative social science research.

According to Miller and Boulton (2007), the notion that social research is governed by the same regulations as medical research is worrying. Members of RECs, especially within health research, are typically recruited from natural and medical sciences. As a result, they are often uninformed about social or qualitative research and the social context in which this research is carried out. Furthermore, RECs have been accused of emphasising aspects of informed consent that prioritise emic – and typically Western – understandings of informed consent, research and participation, that may not be appropriate for all research participants (Miller and Bell 2002). These aspects are often incompatible with socially complex research realities and the needs of particular populations, for example, children, the elderly, those with specific health or dependency issues, and those who are poor or illiterate (McCrady and Bux 1999; Arnot et al. 2000; Barbour 2009; Nordentoft and Kappel 2011). RECs may also be accused of reproducing unequal power dynamics between the researchers and researched by using regulations and guidelines that dictate what is best for potential participants, thereby limiting participant choice and autonomy rather than promoting it as intended (McCrady and Bux 1999; Stoljar 2011).

Researchers have argued that rules-based approaches to ethics strip away the researcher's power to utilise their contextual expertise to make judgements about ethical issues or elicit informed consent that reflects participants' values and understandings. As a result, the experiences of potential participants who cannot or choose not to adhere to formalised consenting procedures, such as written consent, go undocumented in research (Hong 1998; Coomber 2002; Kiltzman 2006; Miller and Boulton 2007; Lloyd et al. 2008; Huang and Coker 2010). Burgess (2007) and Murphy and Dingwall (2007) further argue that such regulation and the systematic bias of governance bodies for formalised consenting processes can influence the data eventually collected to the extent that it becomes very difficult or impossible to carry out certain types of research, such as ethnographic research. Indeed, Miller and Boulton (2007) argue that, since 'informed consent' is a socially constructed notion, the meanings attributed to it and the procedures used to attain it, shift and change according to societal and contextual influences. In practice, this may mean deviating from or altering planned consenting procedures during the course of data collection to suit research interactions with a heterogeneous group of participants.

Social science and qualitative researchers are not alone in their critique of REC ideals and the formalisation of procedures for eliciting informed consent. Other health, medical and clinical researchers have also expressed concern that such procedures alter the dynamic between researcher and participant and can stifle participant recruitment (Arnot et al. 2000; Apfelbacher et al. 2009; Yates et al. 2009; Wilson et al. 2010). Corrigan (2003) and Stone (2004) have noted that medical research participants are more likely to participate in studies in which the researcher, the research institution and the purpose of the study are deemed to be trustworthy, but that such trust can be difficult to establish and is undermined by the blanketed application of consenting procedures.

The importance of trust and researcher responsibility to the research interaction

Trust is implicit to the process of obtaining informed consent, but is more difficult to build or maintain with groups who are fearful, vulnerable, feel stigmatised or for whom research and researchers represent an institution or set of institutions that they believe to be untrustworthy (Tekola et al. 2009a, 2009b; Huang and Coker 2010). For example, Huang and Coker (2010) experienced difficulty recruiting African American participants due to deep-seated, historical mistrust of research and researchers that was further fuelled by the technical language used in consent forms. Other researchers working with African American populations have noted that, despite attempts to use 'lay' language, the very concept of informed consent appears elusive and raises further suspicion (Corbie-Smith et al. 1999; Mason 2005). Additionally, those who are fearful or distrusting of research and researchers question the motives of researchers and view them as profiting from, rather than trying to assist, researched communities (Thompson et al. 1996; Corbie-Smith et al. 1999). Researchers must be mindful of these issues in order to establish participant trust.

It is for one or a combination of these reasons that many minority or socially excluded groups are underrepresented in Western research. While trust-building can foster research participation, trust is often particularly important for those on the margins of research and society. For many of these groups trust is in short supply. Uniformly or insensitively applying a rules-based approach to eliciting informed consent can potentially jeopardise, rather than develop and protect, trust relations, raising potential participants' suspicions about research institutions and researchers (Wiles et al. 2005; Huang and Coker 2010). Trust can be breached or questioned when forms are produced and signatures are required, and thus formalised ethical processes can be counterproductive to their aims (Burgess 2007; Miller and Boulton 2007). In research with professional researchers, Wiles et al. (2005) noted that, even among this informed population, familiar with research processes, producing and requiring a signed consent form for participation was seen as damaging to the trust relationship that had been established between the researcher and the participant, and caused some to reconsider or refuse to participate.

Building trust with participants can take time and effort which dedicated researchers often invest not just for the sake of recruiting another study participant, but due to a sense of responsibility and commitment that they might feel to their research and research participants. Miller and Boutlon (2007) note that building relationships is an important aspect of obtaining consent, as is establishing rapport with potential participants. Establishing 'genuine' rapport often helps to diminish the power imbalance between the participant and researcher and puts the researcher in a trusted position, one which facilitates better research (Oakley 1981; Finch 1984). As a result, researchers often feel a great deal of responsibility towards representing their participants' accounts accurately, ensuring their safety and wellbeing, and taking care to manage and meet the participants' expectations of the research.

Therefore, it is important for both researchers and those who regulate and enforce consenting procedures to be mindful of the social, cultural and historical contexts of the prospective participant groups, and of the challenges that these differences present for research participation and obtaining consent (Wheeler 2003). Undoubtedly, it is the job of researchers to make ethical governing bodies aware of these challenges, but this requires educating both ethics committees and researchers about these challenges and the effectiveness of alternative forms of obtaining consent for participation (Miller and Boulton 2007). As these groups are often those researchers know least about, we may not know what consent procedures are appropriate until data collection has begun. Recruitment and consent processes must therefore be flexible in order to respond to the needs of the group as those needs are identified, either through recruitment or data collected. This will also require a shift in the thinking of ethics committees in terms of values and the emphasis placed on uniform and inflexible regulations, and the timing of applications to committees within research projects.

Barriers to obtaining consent: a case study

In the ideal world envisioned by ethics committees, health-related research would involve participants who do not just report, but who fully understand the aims and nature of the research being carried out. These participants would also be clear on their involvement, not confusing their research participation with part of their standard treatment (Huntington and Robinson 2007) or the receipt of any additional care. They would also understand the research process and the role and function of ethical governance bodies when explained. However, researchers know that these participants are a rarity and research is never quite this straightforward. In many research realities, no matter how well notions of anonymity or confidentiality are explained or how brief the study information sheet is, there may be some participants who do not, cannot, or perhaps care not, to take these notions on board. Potential participants may see research as something they should undertake as part of their civic duty, or be willing to participate in because of a relationship/understanding they perceive has been established with the researcher or the institution carrying out the research (Oakley 1981; Miller and Boulton 2007; Huang and Coker 2010).

Additionally, the potential participant may be pressed for time, feeling unwell, or just impatient and want to 'get it over with' (Walls et al. 2010). Or they may even indicate that they are willing to participate and provide consent, but provide a false name or signature. Many researchers also encounter participants for whom English is not their first language or who have problems with literacy and comprehension (Bhutta 2004; Newton and Appiah-Poku 2007; Lloyd et al. 2008). Finally, poverty may be an issue and may be one of the many factors complicating the potential participant's ability to take part in the research. Many researchers utilise cash or financial incentives to incentivise research participation, which can cloud or influence the judgement of those with financial difficulties (McCrady and Bux 1999). The challenges detailed above have been well documented in the literature by researchers working with vulnerable or marginalised groups as presenting barriers and challenges to securing genuine 'free' participation in research studies.

Many of these challenges were faced in a study conducted with HIV-positive people aged 50 years and older living in a socially disadvantaged part of east London. Below, we will explore these challenges and the problems posed for recruiting participants into this pilot study. We detail the lessons learned by challenging the governing REC's requirement for obtaining written informed consent.

In 2010–2011 the authors and other members of the study team conducted a small-scale pilot study in the east London borough of Newham, a socially disadvantaged area of London with the second highest rate of HIV infection in the UK (Health Protection Agency 2010). In East London, HIV clinics treat a greater proportion of black African and heterosexual patients than clinics elsewhere London, meaning the epidemic in East London is very different compared to the national UK picture (Health Protection Agency 2012). This research aimed to explore the needs and experiences of those living in or accessing health services in the borough, aged 50 years and older, as ethnic minority populations were underrepresented in previous research among the substantial proportion of HIV-positive older adults in the UK (Magalhaes 2007; Health Protection Agency 2010; Power et al. 2010). Data were collected using a 44-item health and demographic questionnaire as well as from a set of focus groups. Participants were able to participate in one or both parts of the research, or, of course, refuse to take part.

Ethical approval for this study was obtained from both a National Health Service (NHS) REC, the lead researcher's university, as well as by the research and development office of the hospital where the majority of the study's participant recruitment would take place. In order to obtain ethical approval to begin recruitment, applications had to be submitted to all three of these bodies. The most intensive and demanding of the applications was that to the NHS REC. Along with the application, final drafts of information sheets for participants and consent forms were required. These specified that, to satisfy the conditions for informed consent, participants must initial each statement of a six-point list to indicate their understanding and agreement, as well as sign and print their full names. This form had to be countersigned by the recruiting researcher who discussed the study with the participant. Participants were provided with a copy of the counter-signed consent form and a copy was retained for the study records. It was also required that participants retain a sheet of printed information about the study, referred to as a Participant Information Sheet (PIS).

In the clinical recruitment setting, potential participants were introduced to the research team by their clinician following their routine appointments. The consenting discussions began with an explanation of the purpose of the study using the PIS, written in simple English. This explained the details of the study, and what study participation would involve in brief. The PIS also contained information about ethical approval for the research as well as the lead researcher's contact details, all of which was required by the REC. After the PIS was explained, participants were given the consent forms and offered additional reading time. However, many participants indicated that they preferred to have the information explained verbally. Copies of the PIS were also made available in the clinic's reception area for anyone interested in reading about the study while waiting to be seen for their appointment, and during the consent discussion potential participants were asked questions to ascertain their comprehension.

By REC regulation, participants should be given a reasonable amount of time to decide whether or not to take part in the research. The research team had therefore received permission from the REC to obtain potential participants' consent to contact them in due course to gauge their interest in participating. This consent was ascertained using a similar form to those outlined, requiring initialled statements, signature, printed name and a telephone number. If, when contacted, potential participants agreed to participate, arrangements were made to meet at the clinic where they could sign the participation consent form and complete the questionnaire, or attend a focus group where a participation consent form would be completed before the discussion began. If potential participants did not want to participate, they were not contacted again by the research team.

Several of those who agreed to take part in the research chose to complete the consent form and questionnaire in the clinic without waiting for the offered 'thinking time'. This was allowed, although no provisions had been made for this in the ethical proposals. It was felt that not allowing participants not to take up the 'thinking time' only undermined their choice, and served to exclude these individuals from the taking part.

This consenting approach posed a greater challenge for potential participants who spoke very little or no English. In these cases, translation assistance was required. In some cases these participants had attended their appointment with a professional interpreter provided by the hospital or a family member or friend. While friends and family were able to help translate the research, professional interpreters were unable to stay with their client after their clinic appointment to interpret for the researcher unless the researcher had booked (and paid for) their services in advance. In these cases, or where follow-up was needed, hospital or agency interpreters were booked for both subsequent phone calls and consent form and questionnaire completion. Although this required additional time and resources, these potential participants were included to avoid excluding the large portion of patients attending the clinic who were non-native English speakers and who have traditionally been left out of HIV research. Not only did language present an additional challenge for obtaining consent, but the actual forms posed a number of problems. As the forms were not translated into potential participants' languages (due to resource constraints and the vast number of languages spoken in the recruitment site), willing participants were required to add their initials, names and signatures next to text they could not read themselves, but had to trust had been translated correctly.

As noted above, producing and requesting that the consent form be signed before the questionnaire could be completed caused issues with a number of potential participants, mostly those from African communities. It is well noted that HIV is highly stigmatised within African communities in the UK, despite the high prevalence and a large proportion of the community being affected by HIV (Owuor 2009). Despite assurances that the consent form would be kept confidential, stored securely, and would not be seen outside the study team (or at the request of the REC), many did not feel comfortable having their name and signature recorded. Some wanted to know who the members of this REC were and why they had a right to this information. After discussions with the research team it was posited that this reluctance could be attributed to a number of reasons: the title of the study was on the consent form, participants may have been concerned that by signing they were disclosing their HIV infection to anyone with access to the form. Others may have been residing in the country without legal documents or with falsified passports, and penning their name raised anxieties about being handed over to the immigration authorities.

Likewise, the requirement for written consent also raised additional suspicion among migrant and non-migrant potential participants about the researchers' motives and why signatures were needed, rather than just verbal consent. It was clear to these potential participants that the information collected in the questionnaire would be anonymous, and therefore it seemed contradictory to then require a signature. Perhaps these participants were also concerned about the leaking of these consent forms to external sources, but also that the questionnaire and consent forms might be paired up, lost or possibly accessed by someone else. Despite providing lengthy explanations about anonymity, confidentiality, data storage and protection, many of these individuals were still unconvinced.

Further discussions with the research team based on a comment made by one participant in particular who wanted to know why providing verbal agreement was not 'good enough' sparked discussion about trust and trust-building. We suggest that the consent form was potentially seen as a breach of trust for these potential participants who felt their verbal consent was being devalued and, therefore, negating established trust and rapport with the researcher. Other concerned potential participants commented that being asked to sign the cumbersome form and the length of the PIS raised suspicion that participation must include more than 'just' a questionnaire. These potential participants associated such intensive consenting procedures with intrusive medical research, making them worry that they had misunderstood – or were being misinformed by the recruiting researcher – about the research and were consenting for something other, and more sinister, than a questionnaire. Lastly, some felt that completing this additional form was unnecessary and they wanted to get on with completing the questionnaire. These potential participants seemed to value the research and understand the process, but viewed the consent form, and therefore the researchers, as wasting their time.

As a result of the numerous hurdles raised by the use of the consent from, it was deemed important to make a case to the approving REC and ethical bodies to change the consenting procedures for the remaining period of data collection. The process of changing required the submission of a 'substantial amendment' form for review by the REC. This form required the changes be outlined, and revised consent and PIS forms to be included. The research team felt that removing the consent form for the completion of the question-naire would increase participation, particularly among African communities, and that removing the consent form provided a more inclusive approach to undertaking this research. We proposed in our amendment that the PIS and consenting discussion remain; however, the notion of 'implied consent' would be applied if a potential participant chose to complete the questionnaire, thus a completed and returned questionnaire would indicate consent (Veatch 2007). This would mean that signatures were not needed and this detail would not be kept for those completing questionnaires only; however, the consent form would remain for the focus groups for which the same problems had not been encountered (probably due to self-selection).

After several weeks of amendment preparation, submission, additional cor-respondence and committee deliberation, the amendment to apply implied consent for the completion of the questionnaire portion of the research was granted. Due to the length and complications of this process there was not sufficient time remaining in the data-collection phase of the study to note a real or noticeable difference in participation. However this ruling helped to set a precedent in consenting procedures with vulnerable research groups for RECs. As noted earlier in the chapter, presenting these challenges to the REC helped to elucidate some of the contextually specific issues that arise during the consenting process that require deviating from the standard model of written informed consent, thus helping to pave the way for future research of this nature.

The importance of exploring alternative methods of obtaining informed consent

As noted throughout this chapter, researchers have provided, and continue to provide, evidence to highlight the challenges posed by obtaining informed consent, a concept rooted in theory, but flawed and not entirely fit for research practice. As explored in the discussion above and highlighted by the case study, reconceptualising informed consent is not only an interesting and worthwhile academic exercise, but impacts upon research participation; formalised consent procedures can make the experiences of some visible while pushing others fur-ther into the margins. In the long term, this process serves to perpetuate social exclusion by eliminating these groups from the data on which health and social policies should be based.

It is for these reasons that it is important for researchers to pursue alternative methods of obtaining consent in order to engage potential research participants, particularly those underrepresented in research. Equally, it is important for RECs to support the use of these measures. Alternative methods for addressing these challenges involves enhancing participant understanding of the consenting process, which can be done using visual aids, decision-making aids or audio-recorded PIS alongside verbal consent (Lloyd et al. 2008; Brehaut et al. 2010). Researchers also argue that it is worth rethinking about which form of consent is most appropriate for the research; implied, presumed, simple or waived consent, and the form of consent used should correspond to the invasiveness or intrusiveness of the research (McCullough et al. 2007; Veatch 2007). Other researchers likewise argue for a more tailored approach to consenting procedures based on the unique research context and population (Tekola et al. 2009a), and allowing for more flexibility in applying the consenting procedures based on the individual research interaction (Miller and Boulton 2007).

Whatever measures are used, Stoljar (2011) argues that the means of obtaining consent should maximise individual autonomy and give voice and choice to participants rather than RECs. In order to ensure that alternative consenting procedures are possible and become more widely accepted, it is important for researchers to challenge RECs to consider the plurality of issues that can arise when researching those with complex health, social and cultural realities (Rhodes 2005). This challenge involves a change in the Westernised and often medicalised view of consent held by RECs, which does not accommodate researching those who do not utilise the same framework for understanding or attach the same meaning to the concept of informed consent.

In summary, this chapter does not advocate doing away with obtaining consent or the consenting discussion for research participation. Such discussion can be crucial to building rapport, allying fears and establishing trust. Instead, this chapter argues for a revision of now standardised procedures for confirming participants' consensual participation, taking into account alternative and more flexible methods. The professional judgement, responsibility of researchers to participants, and intimate knowledge of their research populations should hold sufficient weight for justifying deviations and fostering research practices that promote inclusion in research.

18 The invisibility of childlessness in research

A more inclusive approach

Melissa Graham

Childlessness is increasing in Australia (ABS 2007, 2008) and other westernised nations (Berrington 2004; Abma and Martinez 2006; Biddlecom and Martin 2006; Dyer 2008; Frejka and Sobotka 2008; Boddingtom and Didham 2009). Despite substantial increases in the prevalence of childlessness in the past two decades (ABS 2007), Australia is still predominantly a pronatalist society (Dever 2005; Heard 2006); even with greater choice and equality for women, mother-hood is still the prevailing position. Under a pronatalist discourse, motherhood is the presumed life path for all women, and it is presumed that the act and desire to mother is central to women's roles and identity (Gillespie 1999, 2003). As such, womanhood has become synonymous with motherhood (Arendall 2000). A consequence of this has been the exclusion of childless women from life-course discourse.

Alongside this, a typology of childlessness has emerged which defines women without children as voluntarily, involuntarily or circumstantially childless. Voluntarily childless women are defined as those who are not childless due to infertility or external circumstances, rather they are firm in their commitment to avoiding motherhood, have freely chosen not to have children, and would still choose to remain childless even if circumstances permitted them the opportunity to have children (Cannold 2004, 2005). Involuntarily childless women are those who desire to have children, but due to infertility (the inability to achieve a viable pregnancy after one year of regular and unprotected sexual intercourse) are unable to have biologically related children (Letherby 1999; Daniluk 2001). Circumstantially childless women are those who desire to have children, but have had childlessness imposed upon them by external circumstances such as having no partner, having a partner who is voluntarily childless, or an inability to negotiate paid work with the demands of motherhood (Cannold 2005).

This chapter will highlight the health research evidence where childlessness is visible, and provide examples of health research which has included childlessness, demonstrating that it is possible and that such an approach can contribute to more rigorous life-course research. Methodological implications of including childlessness as a variable in research will then be considered. The chapter will conclude with recommendations for the inclusion of childlessness in health research that does not focus solely on (nulli)parity as the indicator of childlessness.

Childless women in research

Fertility trends demonstrate that the proportion of a woman's reproductive lifespan she spends as a mother is decreasing and the prevalence of childlessness is increasing. For example, the median age of mothers at first birth in Australia increased in 2007 to 28 years (Australian Institute of Health and Welfare National Perinatal Statistics Unit 2009), with 42% of all first births attributed to women aged 30 years or more in 2008 (ABS 2010), and about 32% of women are childless (ABS 2007). Taken together, it is clear that more and more women are spending a greater proportion of their reproductive life without children. One consequence of being a woman who does not identify as a mother is exclusion from life-course discussions, including exclusion or invisibility in health and wellbeing research.

Childlessness affects a woman's daily life and its determinants across her life-course. It is not just about having or not having a child; it is about living in a specific state of childlessness which intersects with other aspects of one's life. This is an important consideration when examining the physical, mental and social health of the population. Research across the life-course can be conceptualised in two ways: firstly the childless-centric research that focuses on childless individuals and populations, and the comparison of women with and without children; and secondly non-childless-centric health research. Childless-centric research is briefly considered here to demonstrate that differences exist between women with and without children with regard to demographic profiles and health and wellbeing outcomes.

Childless-centric research

The body of literature that has examined the implications of childlessness for demographic characteristics and health and wellbeing has shown that, in comparison to women with children, childless women are more likely to attain higher levels of education and socio-economic status (see, for example, Hoem et al. 2006; Hardy et al. 2007; Miranti et al. 2009), which are factors known to be associated with better health and wellbeing outcomes (see, for example, Wilkinson and Marmot 2003). As a result, childless women's higher socio-economic position has often led to assumptions that this population group experience better health and wellbeing.

Indeed a number of positive health outcomes have been identified for childless women when compared to women with children, including lower levels of obesity (Lawlor et al. 2003; Bastian et al. 2005; Hardy et al. 2007; Blaudeau et al. 2008), decreased risk of metabolic syndrome (Gunderson et al. 2009), higher levels of physical activity (Włodarczyk and Ziółkowski 2009), superior sexual satisfaction (Botros et al. 2006), higher bone mineral density (Allali et al. 2007), and increased high-density lipoprotein (HDL) cholesterol (Gunderson et al. 2004).

However, childlessness has also been associated with negative health outcomes. Childless women, in comparison to women with children, have been found to have higher levels of loneliness and depression (Beckman and Houser 1982; Koropeckyj-Cox 1998; Chou and Chi 2004), poorer mental health (Holton et al. 2010; Graham et al. 2011), an increased risk for all-cause mortality (Grundy and Tomassini 2005; Grundy and Kravdal 2008, 2010; Tamakoshi et al. 2011), increased rates of health-risk behaviours such as cigarette smoking and alcohol consumption (Galanti et al. 2002; Kendig et al. 2007; Włodarczyk and Ziółkowski 2009) and poorer nutrition (Włodarczyk and Ziółkowski 2009).

As highlighted here, childless women's apparent higher socio-economic status has not led to better health and wellbeing outcomes in all areas, indicating that health determinants for this population group extend beyond socio-economic status. This also implies that socio-economic status is not a sufficient proxy to account for childlessness in population samples of adult women, but instead requires its own visibility and measurement.

Childless-centric research has been important in understanding the health and wellbeing consequences of childlessness. While much of this research has been conducted with older women, it can provide useful insights into the health and wellbeing of childless women across their life-course. Childless-centric research has demonstrated difference between all women and stratum-specific associations, suggesting that effect modification and confounding may be present in non-childless-centric health research.

Stratification, the approach predominantly used in the childless-centric research, while an accepted method to control for confounding, is limited in its ability to include multiple factors while maintaining an adequate sample size for analysis. For example, if we were to examine prevalence of heart disease, simultaneous stratification by mother/childlessness status (two categories: women with and women without children), age (seven categories: 25–29, 30–34, 35–39, 40–44, 45–49, 50–54, 55+) and physical activity levels (three categories: low, moderate, high) will result in 42 strata. Even with large sample sizes, an artefact of this level of stratification is diminished cell size, making meaningful associations difficult to determine. Multivariate statistical modelling is required to estimate the strength of an association while simultaneously controlling for a number of confounding factors – which is not possible via stratification alone. A confounder is a variable that distorts the association between a study factor and the outcome factor of interest as a result of a strong association with both of these variables. To be a confounding variable, the variable must be associated with the study factor, be an independent risk factor for the outcome of interest and must not be an intermediate variable. Essentially, a confounder confuses the observed association between the study and outcome factors. Given that we often do not know what factors are likely to confound an observed association, all suspected or known risk factors for the outcome of interest (particularly those known to be associated with the study factor) should be considered as potential confounders (Oleckno 2002; Buettner and Muller 2011). Similar to a confounding variable, an effect modifier is a factor that modifies the effect of an association between a study and outcome factor, but it does so differently to confounding. While confounding is apparent when crude measures differ from strata-specific associations, effect modification (interaction) occurs when strata-specific differences are also observed (Gordis 2009; Buettner and Muller 2011).

As evidenced by the examples provided, many studies that compare women with and without children demonstrate differences in outcomes for those two groups. However, outside of the childless-centric research, childlessness status is rarely considered either during the data-collection stage or during the analysis stage to control for the potential effects of childlessness on health outcomes. It is an area of research that has the potential to increase the visibility of childlessness within health and wellbeing research, and may also increase the sophistication and thoroughness of emerging models of women's health determinants, and will now be discussed.

Inclusion of the childless in health research

Childlessness status is not routinely considered or accounted for in health research. Despite the relationship between childlessness and health, few studies on health across the life-course consider childlessness as a variable and, as such, there tends to be an invisibility of childlessness in the non-childless-centric research. While childlessness becomes more visible in research on (in)fertility or specific women's health concerns, for example, menstruation, hysterectomy (Cooper et al. 2008), breast cancer (Adami et al. 1980; Anderson et al. 2007; Grundy and Kravdal 2010) and cancers of the female reproductive organs (Grundy and Kravdal 2010), it is less visible when the research outcome of interest is non-female specific. Within the body of research which examines specific women's health concerns, childlessness status is usually treated as an intermediate variable, i.e. a variable that is a part of the casual pathway.

The invisibility of the effects of childlessness in non-childless-centric research sets up a contradiction between what the evidence suggests in the childless-centric research (i.e. childlessness is associated with health determinants) and what is being addressed in the non-childless-centric health research (i.e. that childlessness is not sufficiently important to consider). There is a need for the inclusion of childlessness in health research to recognise this distinct population and the potential health sequelae for those who remain childless.

Examples of childlessness inclusive research

The inclusion of childlessness within the non-childless-centric health research to date has been limited. This section draws on examples of where childlessness status has been considered and accounted for in relation to non-female-specific health conditions.

A comprehensive search of the literature resulted in only a limited number of studies which had considered the effects of childlessness on health outcomes for non-female-specific health conditions. These studies mainly included 'childlessness' as a study factor or covariate and controlled for the effects using regression modelling. Here the term 'controlled for' refers to the inclusion of variables in regression models to account for the variance they contribute to the outcome of interest. No studies were found that considered 'childlessness' as a potential confounder or effect modifier. However, where childlessness was accounted for in the analysis, the findings generally support those from the childless-centric research: that childlessness is associated with health determinants and outcomes.

A cross-sectional study of 203 women in Brazil aimed to determine the association between the maternal experience and changes in adiposity, and found that nulliparous women (a woman who has not ever given birth) had lower body mass index (BMI) and percentage body fat when compared to women with children (Rodrigues and Da Costa 2001). In this study, parity (the number of times that a woman has ever given birth) was classified as a covariate and included in the analysis (along with other covariates) to test whether these covariates had an effect on the outcomes of interest (BMI, waist-to-hip ratio) after removing the variance for which the covariates accounted. These findings support the evidence from the childless-centric research that increasing parity is associated with increasing body weight among women. This is important, as being overweight or obese are known risk factors for a range of health outcomes, for example heart disease.

A cross-sectional study nested within the Health, Ageing and Body Composition Study of 504 women, which aimed to examine the effect of parity on cardiovascular disease prevalence, found that nulliparous women have a reduced prevalence of cardiovascular disease when compared to parous women (Catov et al. 2008). This study suggests that childlessness is a protective factor against cardiovascular disease for women. However, census-based longitudinal data from Israel suggests that cardiovascular disease mortality is higher for nulliparous and grand multi-gravid women (women who have had five or more pregnancies) aged 45–64 years than for parous women (Jaffe et al. 2011). These data suggest that the risks associated with cardiovascular disease among women may function through non-pregnancy-related mechanisms, and that social or lifestyles factors rather than biological determinants may be contributing to this excess in risk.

The different ways in which parity was measured or treated within the analysis in the two studies cited above may partially explain the different findings. However, these studies do demonstrate the need to include a measure of 'childlessness' status in non-female-specific health research, as analysis by women as a homogenous group could potentially mask those women most at risk. The evidence from the childless-centric research adds support to this notion. For example, a study on the association between number of children and coronary heart disease was conducted to determine if coronary heart disease risk was related to the biological effects of pregnancy or adverse lifestyle risk factors associated with parenting. The study found similar patterns of risk for coronary heart disease for both men and women and suggest that those with at least two children recorded the lowest level of risk, with risk increasing for each subsequent child but also increasing for those with no children.

These findings may demonstrate that lifestyle factors lead to increased risk of coronary heart disease, and that lifestyle may vary across family size (Lawlor et al. 2003). Similarly, Hardy et al. (2007) found that any association between the number of children and coronary heart disease risk factors was a result of lifestyle factors rather than the biological effects of pregnancy. However, in both of these studies, the number of children was the outcome factor of interest and other known risk factors (e.g. socio-economic status, cigarette smoking, physical activity, BMI) were controlled. So, while these two studies have demonstrated a difference in coronary heart disease risk, most studies on coronary heart disease and women have failed to consider motherhood/ childlessness status as a potential confounding variable or effect modifier.

The example studies discussed briefly here have shown that childlessness should be considered in health research and can contribute to a more rigorous approach to life-course research. A woman's motherhood/childlessness status does impact on health outcomes and as such should be included as a variable in health research. However, even when childlessness has been accounted for in analyses of health risks and determinants, the full range of ways in which a woman may be considered childless or a mother has not been adequately or inclusively considered. This is taken up in the next section.

Defining childlessness in an inclusive way

If childlessness status is to be included within health research in a meaningful way, an important consideration is then: how do we best measure childlessness? Childlessness has mainly been measured in biological terms. For example, gravidity (the number of times that a woman has ever been pregnant) and parity (the number of times that a woman has ever given birth, regardless of the outcome of that birth e.g. the child was born alive or was stillborn) are the two main ways in which childlessness has been measured. Within these biological definitions, nulligravida is therefore a woman who has never been pregnant and a nulliparous woman can then be considered a woman who has not ever given birth. Parity is the term most frequently used to describe how childlessness status has been measured, with limited consideration given to the role of social childlessness. This is also problematic in the context of the findings in the previous section, which emphasised that the differences found between childless and non-childless women were better accounted for by social and lifestyle explanations rather than biological mechanisms tied to pregnancy.

Biological determinations of childlessness consider women who have given birth but have outlived their child (whether that be the result of a stillbirth or death at a later age) to be 'mothers' rather than 'childless'. If a woman has not ever assumed the role of mother, but is parous, does that render her childless or is she still a mother? The childless-centric research has demonstrated that health outcomes associated with childlessness are not limited to the biology of pregnancy but also the social consequences of being a woman without children. So while these biological definitions are helpful and may be of particular importance in research that hypothesises that the biology of pregnancy may be a part of the causal pathway, they do not account for the social definitions of childlessness. Social definitions of childlessness distinguish between those who have not biologically borne children but who have assumed the role of mother, including being a foster or adoptive mother, or a step-mother (biologically childless but socially a mother), and those who have never assumed a mother role (biologically and socially childless).

This raises a challenge to health researchers' understanding of what it means to be a woman without children. Is it biological? Social? Or is it both? Here it is posited that being a woman without children is both biological and social, and most importantly should be identified by the woman herself, particularly for gravid or parous women who have never assumed a mothering role. Therefore, in research, childlessness should be defined in multiple ways in order to account for both the biological and social definitions of what it means to be a woman without children.

Recommendations for inclusive practice

All health research across the life-course should include a measure of childlessness status which accounts for both biological and social definitions of childlessness. Table 18.1 demonstrates the range of questions that need to be asked in order to identify a woman's childlessness status.

As you can see, the questions have been divided into ways in which to measure biological and social childlessness. In the biological column it is clear that it is insufficient to simply ask about past gravidity or parity, but rather the number of current children also needs to be included. This then accounts for women who have had a child but may have given the child up for adoption, or placed the child in the foster system (or other care) or whose child died. The social column considers the other ways in which women may have children other than as a result of reproduction. This then accounts for women who have fostered, adopted a child or have step-children. The final item in this column cuts across both the biological and the social as is concerned with women's self-identification of whether or not they have ever assumed the role of mother. A final question which should be considered is, 'Do you identify as a woman who does not have any children?' This allows women to self-identify their status as a woman with or without children and in combination with the responses women can then be classified in one of three ways:

1. childless
2. childless mother
3. mother (either a biological or social mother, or both).

Table 18.1 Examples of ways in which to measure childlessness for inclusive health research practice

Biological		Social	
Item	Response options	Item	Response options
Have you ever been pregnant?	Yes No	Are you currently or have you ever been a step-mother?	Yes – I am currently a step-mother
			Yes – I have been a step-mother in the past
			No
How many times have you been pregnant?	0 1 2 3 4 5 6 or more	Are you currently or have you ever been a foster mother (that is, you have fostered children)?	Yes – I am currently a foster mother
			Yes- I have previously been a foster mother
			No
How many children have you ever given birth to?	0 1 2 3 4 5 6 or more	Have you adopted child(ren)?	Yes No
How many children do you currently have?	0 1 2 3 4 5 6 or more	Have you ever assumed the role of mother?	Yes No

Conclusions

This chapter has demonstrated that health differentials exist between women with and without children, yet childlessness status is rarely routinely considered in health research across the life-course. Where it is considered, measures of childless and mother are mainly based on a measure of parity, rather than considering the range of ways in which a woman may be childless or indeed be a mother. This approach neglects to account for the range of childlessness and mothering positions and women's own self-identification of her status as a woman with or without children. Health research across the life-course should consider the potential effects of childlessness status on health determinants and outcomes. As this chapter has demonstrated, childlessness has both positive and negative health implications for women which may be a result of both biological and/or social processes associated with mothering/childlessness status. The inclusion of more comprehensive measures of childlessness status, that is measures that go beyond parity, will result in a more rigorous approach to life-course research and address the contradictions evident between the childless-centric research and the non–childless-centric research.

19 Inclusion in participatory research

What were the whitefellas doing in an Aboriginal health project?

Sarah Barter-Godfrey, Sarah Pollock and Ann Taket

We acknowledge and respect the traditional custodians of the land on which this work was written and developed, the Wurundjeri peoples of the Kulin nations and Elders past and present. As we share knowledge, learning and research within this chapter, we also pay respect to the knowledge embedded forever within the Aboriginal custodianship of country.

Throughout the body of this chapter the term 'community' in relation to Australian work should be understood to mean 'Aboriginal and/or Torres Strait Islander community'; in discussing the work we did, we introduce later the particular nature of the community we worked with.

Introduction

Health research in indigenous communities, like many interactions between such communities and white-dominated institutions, has a chequered history leading to a three-fold decrement: suspicion and resistance to research that is seen as coming from outside of the community (Johnstone 2007; Cochran et al. 2008); a shortage of research generators and leaders within the community; and cumulative gaps in the research evidence base, both in terms of coverage of topics and in terms of meeting the priorities of the community (Pyett and Vichealth Koori Research and Community Development Unit 2002; Cochran et al. 2008; Pyett et al. 2008; Kendall et al. 2011). Additionally, these decrements have been mistakenly located as problems being caused from within the community, rather than recognising that these are outcomes of wider contextual, historical and institutional factors and failings (Pyett and Vichealth Koori Research and Community Development Unit 2002; d'Abbs and Brady 2004; Cochran et al. 2008; Pyett et al. 2008; Pholi et al. 2009; Kendall et al. 2011). Good research, as culturally appropriate, inclusive of community voices and meeting the needs and priorities of the community, is necessary in an increasingly evidence-based-practice culture within policy and health settings. Culturally safe research with and for indigenous communities has the potential to be empowering, and to bring community voices, views and experiences into the influential realm of 'evidence' (see, for example, Kendall et al. 2011). This process of developing safe, appropriate and inclusive research is not straightforward: the decrements are recursive, with a shortage of connections between the community, its priorities and research. However, as the Healing Stories project that we discuss here has shown, it is possible to develop culturally safe participatory research by working with Elders from within the community and with leaders from within white institutions, in a spirit of reconciliation. The methods and findings of Healing Stories have been reported elsewhere (Firebrace et al. 2009, 2010), with an emphasis on the voices from the community; this chapter explores some of the 'behind the scenes' processes, from the perspective of the white researchers working from within white-dominated institutions.

After briefly describing the Healing Stories project, this chapter reflects on three parts of the participatory research process: getting started, leading together, and working together. The first of these considers laying the foundations for participatory research, working with Elders and leaders, and planning for inclusion, examining participatory research as a recognisable research design, with potential for rigour, cultural safety and inclusion. The second explores developing participatory methods, working with communities, and opportunities and choices for inclusion. The third examines the process of being participatory, working together and engaging in inclusion across the long-term commitment to the project.

Working to support indigenous research projects does not erase the identity or personal history of white researchers, however, it does challenge them to work with themselves; you have to start where you are (see also Subreen-duth and Rhee 2010; Chapman 2011). Ideas from within the academy can be transferrable, particularly those from the syllabi of inclusion, equity and human rights, and working with ideas already understood within the context of one's own learning can help to build practices that are culturally congruent with participatory methods and can withstand robust self-interrogation in the moments of meaning-making that arise in cross-cultural research. The chapter authors reflect on ideas that helped construct and deconstruct meaning in the management of the personal aspects of being a part of Healing Stories, as bearers of culture, as active participants in reconciliation-spirited research and as whitefellas in blackfella research. The term 'whitefella' is used to refer to the non-Aboriginal people and 'blackfella' for people of Aboriginal or Torres Strait islander origin/identity; this usage was common within our work. The chapter concludes by reflecting on the shared journey, and the lessons learned.

Health and research in indigenous communities in Australia: Putting us into context

As in many countries, there exist substantial health disparities across Australia, with higher mortality in remote and regional areas compared to metro or urban areas, and higher mortality in the lowest socio-economic quintiles (Phillips 2009; AIHW 2010). There are also disparities between social and cultural groups, in measures of health, economics and representation. Historically and consistently across contemporary assessments, Aboriginal and Torres Strait Islander (ATSI) populations in Australia have experienced poorer health outcomes, shorter life expectancy, lower economic security and attainment, and less representation in state and federal level institutions (Johnstone 1996; Anderson et al. 2006; Gunstone 2008; McCalman et al. 2009; Vos et al. 2009; Marmot 2011). This persistence of poor health and poor access to the determinants of good health has become colloquially referred to as 'the gap' which must be 'closed', with an emphasis on seven 'blocks': early childhood, schooling, health, economic partnership, healthy homes, safe communities and governance and leadership, all of which must be improved for ATSI Australians (COAG 2008) in order to achieve equality of life expectancy and quality of life.

Following the Talimba report of 1986, 'special group' status for ATSI peoples has been established in research practice in Australia (NHMRC 1991, 2007). This special status effectively reclassified health research with ATSI communities as 'high risk', and placed greater checks and balances on the research approval and delivery process. This aimed to disrupt and prevent poor research practices that had previously occurred, in which ATSI communities had been open to exploitation, misrepresentation and insensitive treatment, and the potential for conflict between practices that are typical in Western scientific research but which may be culturally inappropriate (NHMRC 1991). Current regulations require (in addition to the usual ethical requirements of merit, integrity, justice and beneficence): reciprocity, respect, equality, responsibility, valuing survival and protection, spirit and integrity (NHMRC 2007).

Taking these trends together, we can see a three-fold change to the research context. First, increasing importance was placed on research within health service, policy and delivery settings, through the rise of 'evidence-based practice' (Walshe and Rundall 2001; Fineout-Overholt et al. 2005). However, the universities and other institutions that produce evidence for practice tend to not be representative of ATSI communities. Second, there was an increasing recognition (COAG 2008) of the need to improve the health and social circumstances of ATSI communities and individuals in response to well-documented health and social disparities. Together, these first two trends have created an increased demand by state and federal institutions for research into ATSI health. Thirdly, there was an increasing recognition of the need to perform research in culturally appropriate and inclusive ways with and for ATSI communities. This creates a demand being placed on underserved communities to take part in research, but at the same time promotes the inclusion of those communities' interests and priorities through participative strategies.

Upstream changes to research governance, increased power sharing and the changing dynamics of research control in Australia have fostered a general cultural shift in academia towards embracing more culturally appropriate research methods, and, in particular, participatory methods have flourished. There is now an established pattern of success of participatory methods, across a range of health topics, research types and ATSI communities (for example, de Crespigny et al. 2004; Tsey et al. 2004; Couzos et al. 2005; Kelly 2006; Pyett et al. 2008; Kildea et al. 2009; Mooney-Somers and Maher 2009; Bulman and Hayes

2011). Across these examples, and in particular from authors who have reflected on the research process as well as outcomes, emerges a body of principles that is core to the appropriate and successful delivery of participatory health research with ATSI communities, including: shared values, respect, holism, partnerships, ownership and control, empowerment and working towards meeting the needs of the community. There are also repeated calls for highlighting solutions and resiliency, not just reinforcing 'bad news' or supporting negative stereotypes of ATSI communities (Ritchie 2010). Healing Stories was a project that fitted within this wider context as a locally developed participatory research project, which built qualitative research methods around storytelling and which put the community's voice, through spoken word and artwork, at the core of the data, analysis and reporting.

Healing stories: Origins and overview

The origin of Healing Stories lies with Aunty Shirley Firebrace, an Aboriginal Elder; Aunty is the term used to denote a female Aboriginal Elder, the corresponding term for male Elders is Uncle. During her time working as the Aboriginal Patient and Peer Support Officer at a large metropolitan hospital in Melbourne, she met Sarah Pollock (at the time working as Executive Manager of Research and Social Policy at a large community services organisation in Melbourne). They started a conversation about community members' wishes for their experiences of health services and access to be heard, and how research/researchers might support that. The Ngarra Jarra Strategic Plan for Aboriginal consumers of the hospital's services auspiced Aunty Shirley to act as an advocate for the community members she worked with and, in this capacity, she suggested that Aboriginal people and families were provided with the opportunity to tell their stories. All those things that Aunty Shirley heard every week from her clients were often dismissed as 'anecdote' because they were not being talked about in 'authorised' forms of evidence. Sometimes they had been lost because they did not fit within predetermined fields of review and improvement typical of whitefella organisations. These elided important dimensions of Aboriginal holistic notions of health. These conversations and mutual rapport grew, and soon included two more people, Uncle Reg Blow, an Aboriginal elder and community leader (at the time working as CEO of an Aboriginal healing centre in north-east Melbourne), and Ann Taket (a professor and head of a research centre at a major university in Melbourne). A fifth person, Sarah Barter-Godfrey, also working at the university, joined the team to provide liaison between the different components of the project.

Through these conversations the project slowly took shape: the focus would be on the local urban community's voices and their stories of using and not using health services, within a context of their stories of healing. The 'community' was understood to be those geographically linked to (presently living, working or using services locally) north-east Melbourne who might identify culturally as belonging to, or having ties to, other countries and communities, and that as a consequence of the Stolen Generation may not yet have fully worked out who and where their Aboriginality came from. The Stolen Generations were the children of Australian ATSI descent who were removed from their families by the Australian Federal and State government agencies and church missions, under acts of their respective parliaments. The removals occurred in the period between approximately 1869 to the 1970s.

Both of the Aboriginal Elders who led Healing Stories were 'off country'. In other words, the country where their mob (the term used to denote a linked group of people, linked by particular language or extended family) were traditional owners and custodians was not the same land where they lived day-to-day. However, both kept strong ties to their mob and countries. Both had established community leadership roles within the locality and through organisations that served multiple mobs and parts of ATSI communities. As the study progressed it became increasingly important to recognise that the community who took part in Healing Stories was a small and underrepresented component of a diverse ATSI population. They lived and worked in urban areas, often with some but not all family living close by, but were also typically living 'off country'. Urban Aboriginal populations are generally underrepresented in health research foci; a recent literature review indicated that, although more than half of the Australian Aboriginal population live in urban areas, research with urban populations represented only 11 per cent of recent Aboriginal health research publications (Eades et al. 2010). Partly because of the changes to ways ATSI health research is approved, with an (appropriate and needed) expectation that Elders and traditional community leaders are engaged in the research process, Aboriginal people living 'off country' and away from their mob's cultural and community leaders are particularly underrepresented in research. The Healing Stories project was therefore different from other forms of participatory research where there is a clear and well-defined Aboriginal community, with clear and well-defined ways of approaching and working within that community, and instead worked in a massively underserved community where many different Aboriginal identities and mobs were represented and respected.

A community reference group was established at the beginning of the project, drawing on community members and Elders, who worked to develop the priorities, research materials, direction, pace and strategies of the specific elements of the research project. A 'working methods' document, outlining these priorities and strategies was developed and formed an agreement between the researchers and community members about how they would work together. Researchers from within the community were trained alongside research assistants from the university and community services organisation, with an emphasis on capacity building and flexibility. Community researchers were paid for both the training sessions and any subsequent work they did on the project, including interviewing and transcribing the data. The project ran, at varying pace and intensity, over five years. Major decisions were guided by the Elders and in consultation with the community reference group. Interim findings and drafts of reports were shared with participants, some of whom joined the reference group as well, and all reports were discussed in community consultation lunches and subsequently revised before being distributed outside of the participant and reference groups. Versions of project documents, written in plain language and using, where possible, visual symbols and other materials drawn from indigenous culture were also offered to community members. Copies of all final reports were sent to those participants who wanted them and to all members of the research team.

By the end of the five years, two projects had been completed: the original Healing Stories story-telling project, which collected, shared and learned from individual stories of healing and health services; and a supplementary project called Talking it Up, which used group discussions to explore the community's view on health policy, and produced a review of the policies governing Aboriginal health in Victoria at the state and federal level. A report from Talking it Up, including a brief review of principles of good practice in Aboriginal health research, alongside findings from the community discussions and policy analysis, was launched in 2009, following community consultation and approval. The final report from Healing Stories came out in 2010, also after consultation, revision and approval, followed by the story bank, a permanent collection of the stories that participants submitted to be held communally. For both elements, conclusions and recommendations were written by participants with input from the reference group, to ensure that the 'take home message' came from within the community. Inclusion was therefore built into the delivery of the research products (findings, reports) and design (deciding what to do at each stage) as much as in the day-to-day conduct of the data collection (training researchers from within the community and involving community members in the research team). The following sections reflect on some of the ways we worked with and through challenges, and how we worked together to support inclusion in our research practices.

Getting started

Setting out on participatory research entails a process of decentring power within the research relationship. There was a three-way pull. Firstly, there was a pull away from trying to dominate or assuming a didactic role. Secondly there was a pull for us as whitefellas towards being able to gain the knowledge that blackfellas hold, counterbalanced by not wanting to use that knowledge inappropriately. Thirdly, however, was a pull towards wanting to share knowledge and ideas, to build capacity, and to build an expertise that complemented the knowledge, wisdom and preferences of the community leaders and reference group. Across the project we realised how important circles were to Healing Stories, in depicting holism and interconnectedness, and in performing community business. It is also possible to describe decentring in terms of circles. Rather than coming to a participatory relationship, each with one's own circle of expertise and trying to create a Venn diagram in which others' circles abut and encroach on your own and the point of most overlap becomes the common group view, it was instead more of a process of jointly drawing a circle between us, with each attached at the edge, and placing in the circle one's own knowledge, alongside, informed by and shaped within the context of the rest of the conversation. In this way, decentring of power, like other processes of empowerment, is not a zero-sum activity, but is a productive creation of new ways of working for everyone involved. At the heart of our decentring process was the notion, or spirit, of reconciliation; a perspective on research collaboration as a site of reconciliation was posited by Aunty Shirley early in the research process and reinforced through our discussions as a team and with community members

Reconciliation begins with an honest recognition of historical and perpetuated wrongs and harms, accepting that legacies exist and in turn accepting that how people behave and treat others has consequences that extend far beyond the moment of interaction. On this last point, there is also an opportunity for social change and healing: sharing power and knowledge, building trust and transparency, and developing new supportive and fair ways of working together create moments in which opportunities for reconciliation can occur. These are small, localised opportunities, but are essential for the 'undoing' of colonisation and the 'doing' of reconciliation. Setting the foundations for reconciliation was important for creating circumstances in which people in the community might want to be included in the research, and was essential for building sufficient trust and openness to make the research project accessible. Inclusion is not merely providing technical ways to fit in, but a process of facilitating engagement in ways that are meaningful, wanted and achievable.

Decentring in participatory research also entails letting go of some research assumptions about how the research process is going to proceed, and moving away from standardised models towards more responsive, flexible ways of applying principles of enquiry to meet the requirements of the specific project and people (see also Firebrace et al. 2001; Kaplan-Myrth 2005; Edwards and Taylor 2008; de la Barra et al. 2009; Rowse 2009;). The notion of 'bricolage' in qualitative research (Denzin and Lincoln 1998), roughly translating from the French as 'do it yourself', was a useful parallel here, and brought some textbook legitimacy to a sense of not knowing all the details of the project before we embarked (something which much of the scientific method would discourage and locate in the margins as sources of error or bias). The purpose was not to defer to the textbook over the demands of the community, but to draw on relevant concepts to help fit our work within the spectrum of social enquiry, and to justify why our encouragement and support for flexible methods could be viewed dispassionately as maintaining basic ethical standards of 'merit'.

Knowledge was a key part of the research relationship, and provided a reason for our (whitefella) involvement; however, it was not the only element of what we brought to the project. We are all bearers of culture, and each of the team brought a complex web of cultural perspectives, expectations and identities. The privileges we carried into the research relationship were not arithmetically compiled from our whiteness and education and various other advantages (or disadvantages), but were intersectional across a wide range of socially conse-quential dimensions of who we are and how we live. As one of the reference group put it, 'just because you're privileged doesn't mean you're any better or worse than anyone else'. The collective process of working out how we worked together and articulating this in our 'working methods' document took time, but recognising from the beginning that we would be working in ways that we were not used to, and with a commitment that these changes would not be detrimental to anyone in the group (rejecting zero-sum notions of power) opened up more opportunities of finding a 'good' way of working. The process of saying 'we don't know that yet', compatible with participatory designs, and open to including a range of perspectives, also allowed us to grow into roles and strengths that were only potential or were unknown at the outset.

Leading together

Respect was central to the Healing Stories project. Respect for culture and Country; respect for Elders past, present and future; respect for individuals but also for collective experience and community; and respect that the people who came into the circles in which Healing Stories existed would choose for themselves whether to be included and in what ways. The design and provision of choice was one expression of this respect, and also represented one of the ways in which we set aside trying to make assumptions about how the research project should run. For example, the process of capacity building included training research assistant interviewers within the community, drawing on male and female, aboriginal and non-aboriginal, older and younger people. Partici-pants could choose, from a list of possible interviewers, whether to be inter-viewed by someone of the same or different gender, by someone who was also Aboriginal or from the whitefella institutions, and whether to be interviewed using artwork as a point of discussion or to 'have a yarn' (to talk to someone). Across the project every possible combination of gender/Aboriginality/story style was chosen by at least one interviewee. That is not to suggest that people might not have taken part if that one combination was not available, but does emphasise that offering choices was meaningful for this particular community.

Choice was also important in the ways 'participation' was constructed. For Healing Stories, participation was personal, not prescribed. It was possible to be in the reference group and not be interviewed, to train to be an interviewer but not continue with the project, to tell your story but not contribute to the story bank, to come along to the community lunches but not take part in any individual activities, to attend some but not all parts of the project, etc. The five researchers, including the three chapter authors and two Aboriginal elders, were the only people who worked on all aspects of the project; for the com-munity there were multiple points of contact and each was a choice of whether or not to participate, how, how much, how long for and when. This fluidity of inclusion was another expression of our respect for the community in which we were working, while the consistency at the core of the research leadership meant that the project could be sustained over a longer period of time, something we found necessary in building trusting relationships. Working towards the priorities of the community meant that we did not assume that a research project would ever be a priority over family and cultural business.

Choice and flexibility additionally supported capacity building within the community, as people took up different positions within the project at different times, according to their availability and preferences which changed over time, and in response to their experiences within the project. Having been interviewed, some participants then wanted to become interviewers; having held back early on, but attending community lunches associated with the project, some people then wanted to be involved later; seeing the Talking it Up part of the programme encouraged some people to get involved in the story telling part of the research. This fluidity was tempered by a very specific process of ensuring control over one's story. Stories were transcribed and sent to participants, not just for 'checking' but for articulated approval, with specific options for choosing to include the story in the project or not (taking part in an interview did not necessarily mean opting into the research analysis or story bank), and whether to commit the story to the story bank for sharing within the community (agreeing to have your story in the project did not necessarily mean that your story ended up in the story bank). Multiple points of contact for inclusion were complemented and balanced by multiple points in which each participant had to choose to opt in, with no assumptions that contact with the project automatically conferred commitment to the next phase or component of the research. Leadership was therefore shared between the research team, but also increasingly shared with the participants, further decentring the control over the research process.

Working together: Looking back, looking forward

> If you have come to help me, you are wasting your time. But if you have come because your liberation is bound up with mine, then let us walk together . . .
>
> (Aboriginal activists group, Queensland, 1970s, Lila Watson, Australian Aboriginal woman, in response to mission workers)

In the final section of this chapter we want to offer some reflections on our key learnings from this work. First of all, reflecting back, we found all of the principles mentioned earlier in the chapter (shared values, respect, holism, partnerships, ownership and control, empowerment and working towards meeting the needs of the community) pertinent throughout our journey, see also Firebrace et al. (2001), de Crespigny et al. (2004), Kelly (2006), Edwards and Taylor (2008), Pyett et al. (2008) and Kendall et al. (2011).

Secondly, joint decision-making, shared but with the final decision being made by Elders, was vital in joint ownership and keeping the knowledge within the community. As a result of this, the project became part of community life, and the community determined how much attention could be paid to it at any point. This offered us whitefellas a chance to participate in many aspects of community life, something that we each learnt a lot from and developed as individuals through.

The work that we did together enabled us to create evidence out of the collective experience that can be heard and valued within whitefella settings, rather than devalued as anecdote. This evidence serves as a basis for the promotion of change in services that should be available and accessible to the community, and avoids emphasising problems or barriers as being within or emergent from the community.

At the conclusion of the project, we agreed that we would/will work together in the future as and when appropriate; we offer the metaphor that we are all on the bus together, and the journey continues. It seems to us that an agreement like that is only possible when everyone takes out more than they put in and, as whitefellas working in this project, we were each enriched by our experiences. The quote that begins this section can be read as a comment on our whitefella positionality in several different ways. Firstly, it decentres us as researchers. Secondly, it requires us to recognise and acknowledge our privileged whitefella position and actively work for its ending. For us, this rests on our value base of seeking social justice for all.

Part VII

Conclusion

20 Implementing the social inclusion agenda

Beth R. Crisp, Ann Taket, Melissa Graham and Lisa Hanna

Introduction

This book has explored what is known about what works, and why, in practising social inclusion in the variety of fields or contexts that deal with human health and wellbeing. While recognising the influence of professionals in service planning, delivery and evaluation, we have also explored how, despite its extensive diversity, the wider community can practise inclusion. In Chapters 2 to 19, the book's various contributing authors have gone beyond identifying mechanisms and processes of exclusion to considering how to work towards inclusion. These chapters provide a diverse range of exemplars of inclusive practice, and illustrate some of the challenges that remain.

In a book of this length, it has not been possible to be comprehensive in detailed coverage of each specific group that finds itself excluded in particular circumstances, and we want to acknowledge this explicitly. In Chapter 1, we scoped social inclusion practice and illustrated the different bodies of work originating from around the globe that have provided important knowledge about how to practice social inclusion. While the academic literature is still dominated by research carried out in high-income countries, we have drawn on the grey literature to try to redress this balance and ensure the knowledge gained from work in low- and middle-income countries is represented.

Undoubtedly the issues identified as warranting attention and the methods for practising inclusion vary depending on the particular setting and a wide variety of contextual factors, including history. Nevertheless, some modes of inclusive practice are more directly transferable, such as the social group for teenagers with High Functioning Autism described by Gill et al.. in Chapter 14, which was developed in Melbourne, Australia, after one of the participants had experienced a similar group in Sweden. Practising social inclusion is not necessarily straightforward, and there are always likely to be barriers or issues which need to be addressed irrespective of the country, the professional training and allegiances of workers seeking to promote inclusion, the population(s) being worked with, and the methods of working.

The emphasis of many social inclusion policies has been economic participation (Bhalla and Lapeyre 1997; Sullivan 2002). However in keeping with the understanding of social inclusion set out in Chapter 1, and as several chapters in this book have directly argued, social inclusion requires that the human rights of individuals and communities are actively recognised and respected in all aspects of their lives (Room 1999). In some instances an inclusive approach can successfully be mandated by regulation, such as the ethical requirements for involvement of research involving Aboriginals and Torres Strait Islanders in Australia which were outlined by Barter-Godfrey et al. in Chapter 19. Conversely, regulations which seek to protect vulnerable individuals can end up disenfranchising them. Foster and Freeman (Chapter 17) found those who were socially excluded were willing to participate in research but declined when required to sign an informed consent form.

As Barter-Godfrey and Shelley have noted in Chapter 2, there is a significant challenge posed when different groups have needs and values in diametric opposition to each other. In other words, how do we meet the needs of one marginalised group or population without displacing the needs of those whom the *status quo* may be supporting? In settings where there is no choice of provider, such as in rural areas (Teliska 2005) or where there is a monopoly of one organisation providing all services within a region (Roshelli 2009), this may be particularly problematic.

A new paradigm

This book has demonstrated a range of ways in which social inclusion can be practised. While some will require what Crisp and Ross have referred to in Chapter 4 as 'courageous stands', and sometimes completely subverting existing paradigms, as Furlong argued in Chapter 8 there is much that may be achieved by individual workers in how they relate to clients which does not need organisational sanctions. Nevertheless, social inclusion is most likely to be achieved when the overall culture of a community or organisation is aligned with this aim. Stagnitti et al. discussed 'a whole-school' approach in Chapter 6 to promoting social inclusion, including staff commitment to improvement, a redesigned physical layout of teaching spaces, a change in educational philosophy and teaching methods, identifying effective uses of technology to support the new curriculum, and ensuring children feel valued for their contributions to the school community. This suite of innovations mutually reinforced each other and worked together to promote social inclusion. Likewise, organisations and communities will much more effectively be perceived as socially inclusive if their policies and procedures, service design and delivery, community relations and research are all aligned with the aim of practising social inclusion, rather than just individual elements being inclusive. This was demonstrated by Wesley Mission Victoria, which developed a 'Social Inclusion and Belonging' policy that sought to influence agency practice at all levels (Chapter 5).

Practising social inclusion is not always going to be straightforward, and obstacles which must be negotiated will almost certainly emerge. Nevertheless, we hope that whatever field or type of work or community involvement readers are engaged in, they will recognise there are many benefits to be gained by practising in a socially inclusive manner, even though the challenges to working inclusively with diverse groups of people may sometimes seem overwhelming.

Inclusive professional practice

Professional practice can reinforce social inequalities, promoting the needs of professionals and institutions, and effectively excluding recognition of the needs of those individuals and communities whom they are supposed to serve. While it may occur by chance, inclusive professional practice often emerges in response to critical reflection about who is favoured by the systems and structures. In Chapter 16, Wilson and Campain have argued that reflection needs to occur on an ongoing basis. An intention to be socially inclusive does not, however, guarantee this will occur, as Layton and Wilson have noted in Chapter 3 in respect of the Victorian Aids and Equipment Program (VAEP). In particular, they note how inclusionary aims can be lost when policies are translated into operational guidelines. Although lack of social connectedness is a key factor in social exclusion (Taket et al. 2009a), the priorities of the VAEP exclude funding for any equipment which primarily facilitates participation in recreational or leisure activities. A narrow focus on needs was also discussed in Chapter 4 by Crisp and Ross, who reflect on the fact that, with the exception of sexually transmissible infections, the occupational health and safety needs of commercial sex workers have generally been ignored.

Practising social inclusion involves recognition of needs outside the mainstream. This can include those not generally regarded as having particular needs, including childless women in a pronatalist society (Chapter 18). Some groups may have particular needs which can be easily overlooked or ignored, and stigmatisation reinforced as a result. For example, in Chapter 7, Goldingay and Stagnitti recognise that young people in the criminal justice system who exhibit concerning behaviours are much more likely than the general population to be living with some form of learning disability, and this needs to be recognised in service design.

Rather than providing services or doing research *on* a community, professionals working in partnership *with* communities may be a more inclusive way of working. In this vein, in Chapter 16 Wilson and Campain have described an initiative in which adults with intellectual disabilities were engaged as co-researchers who undertook data collection. Methodologies such as community-based participatory research, as outlined in Chapter 15 by Dolwick Grieb et al., may be a much more effective way of both delivering interventions and evaluating their efficacy. Barter-Godfrey et al. (Chapter 19) note how working in partnership decreases suspicion about, and resistance to, participating in community research projects and helps ensure work is conducted in the best interests of the community.

Practising social inclusion may also require taboo subjects to be addressed. Health and welfare workers in many Western countries are frequently ambivalent towards, or even actively avoid, discussion of religion in their professional practice (Crisp 2010b). However, it is increasingly recognised that 'service users need opportunities to discuss their religious and spiritual beliefs, and the strengths, difficulties and needs that arise from them' (Furness and Gilligan 2010: 44). In Chapter 9, Makhoul et al. note the importance of these discussions in working with Lebanese clients who identify as homosexual or transsexual.

Several chapters emphasise the need for spaces which can be experienced as a safe place or sanctuary by socially excluded people. This was noted in Chapter 10 by Lennon et al. regarding street-based sex workers attending the St Kilda Gatehouse, in Chapter 9 by Makhoul et al. in regard to homosexual and transsexual clients attending a clinic, and in Chapter 13 by Hanna and Moore about the need for a gendered space in which older women could meet in the community. Although the needs of each group were different, in each instance what was critical was the opportunity which was enabled for individuals to be recognised as 'relational, social beings' (Furlong, Chapter 8).

In Chapter 19, Barter-Godfrey et al. suggest that for practitioners seeking to work more inclusively, a starting point is critical reflection on oneself, identifying assumptions about privilege which militate against inclusive practice. The growing canon of literature specifically on inclusion and exclusion is obviously relevant, as is current thinking in related areas such as equity and human rights. However, even if professionals have a desire to practise in a more socially inclusive way, and even if the context is supportive of such changes, they may need assistance to do so. For example, in Chapter 9, Makhoul et al. note that it is rare for physicians in Lebanon to receive any education about homosexuality in their medical training; however, ongoing education can fill this gap. Also, as reported in Chapter 6 by Stagnitti et al., a range of professional development activities were critical in achieving the successful redevelopment of a school.

When possible, consultation with service users and other stakeholders should also occur. As described by Pollock and Taket in Chapter 5, the extensive client consultations undertaken by Wesley Mission Victoria revealed that aspects of supposedly inclusive practice had unintended consequences. For example, some of the professional language used by agency staff was perceived as impersonal and reinforced a sense of distance between staff and service users. Conversely, as Furlong (Chapter 8) demonstrates, an inclusive approach to mental health practice is one in which the practitioner deliberately seeks, from the outset, to engage a depressed client where they are at. However, taking such an approach may be counter to workers' professional training.

It is not just the language which professionals use to describe programme aims and procedures which is potentially exclusionary. For example, in choosing to refer to the participants in their services as 'therapees', Makhoul et al. in Chapter 9 wanted to avoid terms that may reinforce the exclusion experienced by those they work with. Appropriate terminology is a vexed issue which crosses national and professional borders (McLaughlin 2009).

Inclusive practice encourages the voices and experiences of community members, particularly those not generally privileged, to be heard. Moreover, community voices should be regarded as 'evidence' rather than dismissed as 'anecdote'. Yet, for people not accustomed to having their voices heard, let alone their view sought, it is not sufficient for workers to adopt a more open attitude to service users. As Makhoul et al. note in Chapter 9, their Lebanese maternity patients also needed to be provided with information about the different options available in maternity care, prior to being able to make informed decisions about treatment. These patients also needed to be made aware that hospital staff actively wanted their views regarding what care they would receive. This was often in stark contrast with the patient's previous contacts with health care systems which they had experienced as intimidating and uninterested in their views.

Inclusive communities

While much of the focus of this book has been concerned with the work of professional practitioners in health, welfare, education or public policy, the efforts of any member of a community can result in that community being more inclusive. The examples presented in Chapters 11 and 13, both dealing with older people, focus on building and strengthening relationships in the community, and were achieved with relatively modest funding. Moreover, as social isolation, disconnectedness and stress have negative health consequences for many older people (Cornwell and Waite 2009), small investments in activities to promote social inclusion may actually be cost-effective.

Although use of volunteers in programmes such as Do Care (Chapter 11) and Comfort Zone (Chapter 14) both reduces costs and places service users on a more even level with the professionals who service these groups, careful screening and training of both participants and volunteers is essential, as is having procedures in place to safeguard all those involved. Nevertheless, as research into Do Care (Chapter 11) found, the strict boundaries which many professionals put in place with regard to their interactions with clients are not necessarily appropriate in relationships between volunteers and community members, and there should not be barriers to genuine friendships developing.

Making connections does not only facilitate a sense of belonging but may also be crucial in enabling individuals to effectively navigate their way through complex organisations and bureaucracies. This was certainly the case for some of the first-year university students discussed by Crisp and Fox in Chapter 12. However, even in much smaller and less complex organisations or groups, newcomers can readily be daunted, not just by formal rules and regulations, but by lacking a nuanced understanding of the organisational history or culture, or 'habitus' (Bourdieu 1993). Including newcomers may not only require efforts to understand who they are, but also to ensure they are provided with information in ways which are appropriate and meaningful, which may not necessarily reflect current practice. In other words, we need to appreciate how our habitus or organisational practices are understood by the outsiders we are seeking to attract.

Inclusive groups or programmes typically value diversity. The women who participated in the group described in Chapter 13 by Hanna and Moore, clearly valued the group's diversity, with many delighting in new friendships with women from other ethnic groups. The need to find a place of acceptance is particularly an issue for people with a disability. As Gill et al. note in Chapter 14, for those who are marginalised within the wider community, finding a place of support within their own community is essential both for the wellbeing of individuals and also enabling them to cope better in other social contexts. Nevertheless, it is worth remembering that even within marginalised communities there may be individuals or groups whose views or experiences differ from the rest of the community, and hence care must be taken not to treat communities as homogenous entities.

While there are some groups, including people with disabilities, where the experience of exclusion is readily recognised, the needs of family members and carers can readily be overlooked. Hence, groups such as Comfort Zone (Chapter 14) not only provided opportunities for social interaction for children with high-functioning ASD but also much-needed opportunities for their families to meet and support each other.

An agenda for the future

In *Realizing the Future We Want for All*, the UN (2012: 1) recommended 'A vision . . . that rests on the core value of human rights, equality and sustainability' which included goals and targets for 'inclusive social development'. While many of the chapters in this book report on work seeking to address this goal at a local or regional level, such efforts underpin national and global initiatives to promote social inclusion of marginalised individuals and groups. Nevertheless, the approaches used in promoting social inclusion need to be tailored to the needs and issues of particular settings and rather than attempting to implement a generic policy or program initiative (UN 2012).

When inclusive practice is not the norm, radical transformation of the various systems which impinge on how individuals, organisations and/or communities run their affairs may be required. A starting point is the recognition that addressing social inclusion is not just good for the wellbeing of marginalised individuals and groups, but also for the wider community. At an organisational level, participation and inclusion have been linked with what are often deemed desirable characteristics such flexibility, diversity and resilience (Béné et al. 2012).

Changes in behaviour will need to be accompanied by a change of culture which enables *status quo* beliefs, identities and stereotypes that promote exclusion to be challenged and overturned (Béné et al. 2012). While it is often claimed that the costs of transforming a system are greater than maintaining the *status quo* (Béné et al. 2012), in some contexts it has been proposed that the insistence of outsiders such as funding bodies on inclusive approaches, such as participatory decision-making, can itself be a form of tyranny. This is particularly so if groups are not enabled to effectively challenge any powerful elites who may disproportionately benefit from so-called 'participatory processes' (Cooke and Kothari 2001).

A key agenda item will be recognising social inclusion as a human right. While Ghandi famously refused the convention of referring to people from the lowest class of Hinduism as 'untouchables', on the basis that this failed to recognise their humanity (Radcliffe 2012), services specifically aimed at providing for marginalised individuals and groups have often traditionally involved some form of charity or patronage. This can reinforce experiences of exclusion, especially if accompanied by expectations of gratefulness by recipients (Ramsland 1992). Hence, realising the social inclusion agenda, especially in respect of addressing poverty, will also require inclusive economic development. Given that poverty is widespread, even in many of the richest countries in the world (UN 2012), human rights values need to underpin domestic policies and programmes as well as international aid and development. These include expectations that people will be treated with dignity, not be discriminated against on the basis of beliefs or other personal characteristics, and be afforded the rights to live safely with access to food, water, health care and shelter, as well as the right to work and earn an income (UN 2012).

Importantly, there needs to be recognition that efforts to promote social inclusion must take into account lived realities of social exclusion at the local level, which are often 'complex, diverse, dynamic, uncontrollable and unpredictable' (Chambers 2010: 3). Yet the solutions proposed by many professionals and organisations are too simplistic and fail to recognise these factors (Chambers 2010).

As Chambers (2010) has argued, commencing our efforts to promote social inclusion cannot wait the often long periods of time it takes to obtain evaluative data from randomised controlled trials. We already know enough to get started. At the end of Chapter 1, we identified some key messages from the literature which could provide guidance to individuals and organisations seeking to be inclusive in their practice. Subsequent chapters have highlighted: the importance of authentic and trusting relationships; the ability of language to challenge or reinforce social exclusion; the need to analyse power relations in the socio-economic–political–cultural context, to challenge the political and economic *status quo*; and the necessity for flexible and adaptable methods and processes. Furthermore, as we have discussed in this chapter, social inclusion practice requires a rights-based approach.

Finally, resourcing and support for inclusionary practice continues to be essential, but is too often an obstacle. Such resources need to be carefully targeted to ensure increased resources actually benefit those who are most excluded (Przeworski 2008). In some situations this may require a change in funding paradigms, from those which primarily provide resources to cover direct costs such as staffing, to also providing resourcing to marginalised individuals or groups which would enable them to participate in projects or programmes which aim to enhance their experience of social inclusion (Osmani 2008).

Achieving social inclusion is a continuing challenge which will require ongoing political will and support from all levels of the community. Undoubtedly, some initiatives to promote social inclusion will be more effective in achieving this goal than others, and there will be ongoing need to critically reflect and identify factors influencing both success and failure (Blair 2008). In researching and writing this book we have taken encouragement from the volume of knowledge that is rapidly accumulating and can be put to very real and immediate use in supporting social inclusion in multiple domains. It is our hope that this book will encourage further critical reflection as to what practising social inclusion entails, and inspire further research by a wide range of practitioners exploring issues associated with socially inclusive practice.

References

Abbott-Chapman, J. and Edwards, J. (1999) 'Student services in the modern university: responding to changing student needs', *Journal of the Australian and New Zealand Student Services Association*, 13: 1–21.

Abell, S., Ashmore, J., Beart, S., Brownley, P., Butcher, A., Clarke, Z., Combes, H., Francis, E., Hayes, S., Hemmingham, I., Hicks, K., Ibraham, A., Kenyon, E., Lee, D., McClimens, A., Collins, M., Newton, J. and Wilson, D. (2007) 'Including everyone in research: the Burton Street Research Group', *British Journal of Learning Disabilities*, 35: 121–4.

Abelson, J., Lomas, J., Eyles, J., Birch, S. and Veenstra, G. (1995) 'Does the community want devolved authority? Results of deliberative polling in Ontario', *Canadian Medical Association Journal*, 153: 403–12.

Abma, J. and Martinez, G. (2006) 'Childlessness among older women in the United States: trends and profiles', *Journal of Marriage and the Family*, 68: 1045–56.

Abrams, D. and Christian, J. (2007) 'A relational analysis of social exclusion', in D. Abrams, J. Christian and D. Gordon (eds) *Multidisciplinary Handbook of Social Exclusion Research*, Chichester: John Wiley and Sons.

Abrams, L.S. (2000) 'Guardians of virtue: the social reformers and the "girl problem", 1890–1920', *Social Service Review*, 74: 436–52.

Abrams, L.S. and Curran, L. (2000) 'Wayward girls and virtuous women: social workers and female delinquency in the progressive era', *Affilia: Journal of Women and Social Work*, 15: 49–64.

ABS (1999) *Older People, Australia: a social report*, Canberra: Australian Bureau of Statistics.

ABS (2003) *Disability, Ageing and Carers, Australia: summary of findings, 2003*, Canberra: Australian Bureau of Statistics.

ABS (2007) *1986, 1996 and 2006 Census of Population and Housing Customised Tables*, Canberra: Australian Bureau of Statistics.

ABS (2008) *Australian Social Trends 2008: how many children have women in Australia had?* Canberra: Australian Bureau of Statistics.

ABS (2010) *Australian Social Trends December 2010*, Canberra: Australian Bureau of Statistics.

Adami, H.O., Hansen, J., Jung, B. and Rimsten, A.J. (1980) 'Age at first birth, parity and risk of breast cancer in a Swedish population', *British Journal of Cancer*, 42: 651–8.

Aday, R.H., Kehoe, G.C. and Farney, L.A. (2006) 'Impact of senior center friendships on aging women who live alone', *Journal of Women and Aging*, 18: 57–73.

ADB (1996) *Framework for Mainstreaming Participatory Development Processes into Bank Operations*, Manila: Asian Development Bank.

ADB (2003) *Poverty and Social Development Papers No. 6*, Manila: Asian Development Bank.

Adimora, A.A. and Schoenbach, V.J. (2005) 'Social context, sexual networks, and racial disparities in rates of sexually transmitted infections', *Journal of Infectious Diseases*, 191: S115–22.

AEDI (2009) *A Snapshot of Early Childhood Development in Australia Australian: Early Development Index (AEDI) national report 2009* (re-issue 2011), Canberra: Australian Government Department of Education, Employment and Workplace Relations. Online. Available HTTP: <http://video.rch.org.au/aedi/National_Report-March_2011_Reissue_final.pdf> (accessed 18 March 2013).

AEDI (2012) *Australian Early Development Index Community Profile Ballarat, Victoria*, Canberra: Australian Government Department of Education, Employment and Workplace Relations. Online. Available HTTP: <http://www.reports.aedi.org.au/community-profile/vic/2012/20570.pdf> (accessed 22 April 2013).

Agger, A. and Larsen, J.N. (2009) 'Exclusion in area-based urban policy programmes', *European Planning Studies*, 17 (7): 1085–99.

Ahari, S.S., Habibzadeh, S., Yousefi, M., Amani, F. and Abdi, R. (2012) 'Community based needs assessment in an urban area: a participatory action research project', *BMC Public Health*, 12: 161.

AIHW (2010) *Australia's Health 2010: the twelfth biennial health report of the Australian Institute of Health and Welfare*, Canberra: Australian Institute of Health and Welfare.

AIPC (2008) *The Active Service Model: a conceptual and empirical review of recent Australian and international literature (1996–2007)*, Bundoora Victoria: Australian Institute for Primary Care, La Trobe University.

Alaszewski, A. (1999) 'Towards the creative management of risk: perceptions, practices and policies', *British Journal of Learning Disabilities*, 30: 56–62.

Albrecht, G., Seelman, K. and Bury, M. (eds) (2001) *Handbook of Disability Studies*, Thousand Oaks, CA: Sage.

Alegría, M., Wong, Y., Mulvaney-Day, N., Nillni, A., Proctor, E., Nickel, M., Jones, L., Green, B., Koegel, P., Wright, A. and Wells, K.B. (2011) 'Community-based partnered research: new directions in mental health services research', *Ethnicity and Disease* 21 (Suppl 1): 8–16.

Alexander, F.G. and French, T.M. (1946) *Psychoanalytic Therapy: principles and applications*, New York: Ronald.

Alexander, P. (1998) 'Sex work and health: a question of safety in the workplace', *Journal of the American Medical Women's Association*, 53: 77–82.

Allali, F., Maaroufi, H., Aichaoui, S.E., Khazani, H., Saoud, B., Benyahya, B., Abouqal, R. and Hajjaj-Hassouni, N. (2007) 'Influence of parity on bone mineral density and peripheral fracture risk in Moroccan postmenopausal women', *Maturitas*, 57: 392–8.

Allsop, J. and Taket, A.R. (2003) 'Evaluating user involvement in primary health care', *International Journal of Healthcare Technology and Management*, 5: 34–44.

Althusser, L. (2006) *Philosophy of the Encounter: later writings, 1978–1987*, London: Verso.

Amin, A. (2002) *Ethnicity and the Multicultural City: living with diversity. Report for the Department of Transport, Local Government and the Regions and the ESRC Cities Initiative*, University of Durham. Online. Available HTTP: <http://red.pucp.edu.pe/ridei/wp-content/uploads/biblioteca/Amin_ethnicity.pdf> (accessed 18 March 2013).

Anderson, I., Crengle, S., Leialoha Kamaka, M., Chen, T., Palafox, N. and Jackson-Pulver, L. (2006) 'Indigenous health in Australia, New Zealand, and the Pacific', *The Lancet*, 367: 1775–85.

Anderson, W.F., Matsuno, R.K., Sherman, M.E., Lissowska, J., Gail, M.H., Brinton, L.A., Yang, X.R., Peplonska, B., Chen, B.E., Rosenberg, P.S., Chatterjee, N., Szeszenia-Dabrowska, N., Bardin-Mikolajczak, A., Zatonski, W., Devesa, S.S. and García-Closas, M. (2007) 'Estimating age-specific breast cancer risks: a descriptive tool to identify age interactions', *Cancer Causes and Control*, 18: 439–47.

Andover, M.S., Schatten, H.T., Crossman, D.M. and Donovick, P.J. (2011) 'Neuropsychological function in prisoners with and without self-injurious behaviours: implications for the criminal justice system.' *Criminal Justice and Behaviour*, 38: 1103–14.

Anghel, R. and Ramon, S. (2009) 'Service users and carers' involvement in social work education: lessons from an English case study', *European Journal of Social Work*, 12: 185–99.

Annells, M. (2006) 'Triangulation of qualitative approaches: hermeneutical phenomenology and grounded theory', *Journal of Advanced Nursing*, 56: 55–61.

Anon (n.d.). Online. Available HTTP: <http://www.cloverquotes.com/quote/by/anonymous/114-butterfuly-caterpillar-coccoon-does-education-emerge-faster> (accessed 18 March 2013).

Ansley, F. and Gaventa, J. (1997) 'Researching for democracy and democratizing research', *Change*, 29: 46–53.

Apfelbacher, C., Loerbroks, A., Matterne, U., Strassner, T., Büttner, M. and Weisshaar, E. (2009) 'Informed consent affects prevalence estimates in an epidemiological study on chronic pruritus: lessons learned from a pretest', *Annals of Epidemiology*, 19: 745–6.

Arendall, T. (2000) 'Conceiving and investigating motherhood: the decade's scholarship', *Journal of Marriage and the Family*, 62: 1192–207.

Arimoto, Y. (2012) 'Participatory rural development in 1930s Japan: the economic rehabilitation movement', *Developing Economies*, 50: 170–92.

Arneil, B. (2009) 'Disability, self-image, and modern political theory', *Political Theory*, 37: 218–42.

Arnot, A. (2002) 'Legalisation of the sex industry in the State of Victoria, Australia: the impact of prostitution law reform on the working and private lives of women in the legal sex industry', Unpublished Masters Thesis, University of Melbourne, Australia.

Arnot, D., Jepsen, S. and Kilama, W. (2000) 'Health research ethics in Africa', *Parasitology Today*, 16: 136–7.

Arnstein, S.R. (1969) 'A ladder of citizen participation', *Journal of the American Institute of Planners*, 35: 216–24.

AT Collaboration (2009) *Assistive Technology*. Online. Available HTTP: <http://www.ilcnsw.asn.au/home/what_we_do/at_collaboration/> (accessed 1 April 2013).

Ataöv, A. and Haider, J. (2006) 'From participation to empowerment: critical reflections on a participatory action research project with street children in Turkey', *Children, Youth and Environments*, 16: 127–52.

Atkinson, A.B., Cantillon, B., Marlier, E. and Nolan, B. (2005) *Taking Forward the EU Social Inclusion Process: an independent report commissioned by the Luxembourg Presidency of the Council of the European Union*. Online. Available HTTP: <http://travail-emploi.gouv.fr/IMG/pdf/final_report.pdf> (accessed 18 March 2013).

Australian Government (2009) *The Australian Public Service Social Inclusion Policy Design and Delivery Toolkit*, Canberra: Social Inclusion Unit, Department of the Prime Minister and Cabinet.

Australian Government (2010) *Australian Social Inclusion Board Annual Report 2010*, Canberra: Department of the Prime Minister and Cabinet. Online. Available HTTP: <http://www.socialinclusion.gov.au/sites/www.socialinclusion.gov.au/files/publications/pdf/asib-board-annual-repor-2010.pdf> (accessed 18 March 2013).

Australian Government (2012) *Social inclusion*. Online. Available HTTP: <http://www.socialinclusion.gov.au> (accessed 18 March 2013).

Australian Government (n.d.) *About The Social Inclusion Agenda. Australian Government.* Online. Available HTTP: <http://www.socialinclusion.gov.au/about> (accessed 18 March 2013).

Australian Institute of Health and Welfare National Perinatal Statistics Unit (2009) *Australia's Mothers and Babies 2007*, Perinatal Statistics Series, 23, Sydney: Australian Institute of Health and Welfare.

Australian Social Inclusion Board (2010) *Social Inclusion in Australia: how Australia is faring*, Canberra: Department of the Prime Minister and Cabinet, Commonwealth of Australia.

Autism Victoria (2009) *Diagnosis and Definitions.* Online. Available HTTP: <http://www.autismvictoria.org.au/diagnosis> (accessed 18 March 2013).

Bacchi, C.L. (2007) 'The ethics of problem representation: widening the scope of the ethical debate', *Policy and Society*, 26: 5–19.

Bacchi, C.L. (2009) *Analysing Policy: what's the problem represented to be?* Frenchs Forest, New South Wales: Pearson.

Bailey, A. (2010) 'Comparison of language complexity of children who attend a school with a play based curriculum and children who attend a traditional school', Unpublished Honours thesis, School of Health and Social Development, Deakin University, Australia.

Balffour, T.D. (2011) 'Addressing health and social disparities through community-based participatory research in rural communities: challenges and opportunities for social work', *Contemporary Rural Social Work*, 3 (3): 4–16.

Ballinger, G.J. (2003) 'Bridging the gap between A Level and degree: some observations on managing the transitional stage in the study of English literature', *Arts and Humanities in Higher Education*, 2: 99–109.

Bandura, A. (1994) 'Social cognitive theory and the exercise over HIV infection', in R.J. Di Clemente and J.L. Peterson (eds) *Preventing AIDS: theories and methods of behavioral intervention*, New York: Plenum.

Baptcare (2011) Home page. Online. Available HTTP: <http://www.baptcare.org.au/Pages/default.aspx> (accessed 18 March 2012).

Barbour, R. (2009) *Introducing Qualitative Research: a student guide to the craft of doing qualitative research*, London: Sage.

Barnard, M.A. (1993) 'Violence and vulnerability: conditions of work for streetworking prostitutes', *Sociology of Health and Illness*, 15: 683–705.

Barnes, C. (2003) 'What a difference a decade makes: reflections on doing "emancipatory" disability research', *Disability and Society*, 18: 3–17.

Barnes, C. and Mercer, G. (1997) 'Breaking the mould? An introduction to doing disability research', in C. Barnes and G. Mercer (eds) *Doing Disability Research*, Leeds: The Disability Press.

Baron-Cohen, S. (1996) *Mindblindness*, Cambridge, MA: MIT Press.

Barter-Godfrey, S. and Taket, A. (2009) 'Othering, marginalisation and pathways to exclusion in health', in A. Taket, B.R. Crisp, A. Nevill, G. Lamaro, M. Graham and S. Barter-Godfrey (eds) *Theorising Social Exclusion*, London: Routlege.

Bartram, B. (2008) 'Supporting international students in higher education: constructions, cultures and clashes', *Teaching in Higher Education*, 13: 657–68.

Bastian, L.A., West, N.A., Corcoran, C. and Munger, R.G. (2005) 'Number of children and the risk of obesity in older women', *Preventive Medicine*, 40: 99–104.

Bauman, Z. (2001) *The Individualized Society*, Cambridge: Polity Press.

Bauman, Z. (2003) *Liquid Love: on the frailty of human bonds*, Cambridge: Polity Press.

Bautista, C.T., Pando, M.A., Reynaga, E., Marone, R., Sateren, W.B., Montano, S.M., Sanchez, J.L. and Avila, M.M. (2009) 'Sexual practices, drug use behaviors, and prevalence of HIV, syphilis, hepatitis B and C, and HTLV-1/2 in immigrant and non-immigrant female sex workers in Argentina', *Journal of Immigrant and Minority Health*, 11: 99–104.

Beal, C. (2006) 'Loneliness in older women: a review of the literature', *Issues in Mental Health Nursing*, 27: 795–813.

Beare, H. (2001) *Creating the Future School*, New York: Routledge.

Beauchamp, T. (2011) 'Informed consent: its history, meaning and present challenges', *Cambridge Quarterly of Healthcare Ethics*, 20: 515–23.

Beckman, L.J. and Houser, B.B. (1982) 'The consequences of childlessness on the social-psychological well-being of older women', *Journal of Gerontology*, 37: 243–50.

Bedell, G.M. and Dumas, H.M. (2004) 'Social participation of children and youth with acquired brain injuries discharged from inpatient rehabilitation: a follow-up study', *Brain Injury*, 18: 65–82.

Bedini, L.A. (2000) 'Just sit down so we can talk: perceived stigma and the pursuit of community recreation for people with disabilities', *Therapeutic Recreation Journal*, 34: 55–68.

Bell, S., Delbanco, T., Anderson-Shaw, L., McDonald, T. and Gallagher, T. (2011) 'Accountability for medical error: moving beyond blame to advocacy', *Chest*, 140: 519–26.

Béné, C., Godfrey Wood, R., Newsham, A. and Davies, M. (2012) *Resilience: new utopia or new tyranny? Reflection about the potentials and limits of the concept of resilience in relation to vulnerability reduction programs*, IDS Working Paper 405, Brighton: Institute of Development Studies, University of Sussex.

Berk, L., Jorm, A.F., Kelly, C.M., Dodd, S. and Berk, M. (2011) 'Development of guidelines for caregivers of people with bipolar disorder: a Delphi expert consensus study', *Bipolar Disorders*, 13: 556–70.

Berkman, L. and Glass, T. (2000) 'Social integration, social networks, social support and health', in L. Berkman and I. Kawachi (eds) *Social Epidemiology*, New York: Oxford University Press.

Berrington, A. (2004) 'Perpetual postponers? Women's, men's and couple's fertility intentions and subsequent fertility behaviour', *Population Trends*, 117: 9–19.

Beswick, A.D., Rees, K., Dieppe, P., Ayis, S., Gooberman-Hill, R., Horwood, J. and Ebrahim, S. (2008) 'Complex interventions to improve physical function and maintain independent living in elderly people: a systematic review and meta-analysis', *The Lancet*, 371: 725–35.

Bhalla, A. and Lapeyre, F. (1997) 'Social exclusion: towards an analytical and operational framework', *Development and Change*, 28: 413–33.

Bhutta, A. (2004) 'Beyond informed consent', *Bulletin of the World Health Organization*, 82: 771–8.

Bickenbach, J., Chatterji, S., Bradley, E. and Ustun, T. (1999) 'Models of disablement, universalism and the International Classification of Impairments, Disabilities and Handicaps', *Social Science and Medicine*, 48: 1173–87.

Biddlecom, A. and Martin, S. (2006) 'Childless in America', *Contexts*, 5 (4): 54.

Bigby, C. and Frawley, P. (2010) 'Reflections on doing inclusive research in the "Making Life Good in the Community" study', *Journal of Intellectual and Developmental Disability*, 35: 53–61.

Binswanger-Mkhize, H.P., de Regt, J.P. and Spector, S. (eds) (2010) *Local and Community Driven Development*, Washington, DC: World Bank.

Bishop, R. (1996) *Collaborative research stories: Whakawhanaungatnaga*, Wellington, New Zealand: Dunmore Press.

Blair, H. (2008) 'Innovations in participatory local governance', in *Participatory Governance and the Millennium Development Goals*, New York: United Nations.

Blaudeau, T.E., Hunter, G.R., St-Onge, M.-P., Gower, B.A., Roy, J.L.P., Bryan, D.R., Zuckerman, P.A. and Darnell, B.E. (2008) 'IAAT, catecholamines, and parity in African-American and European-American women', *Obesity*, 16: 797–803.

Bletsas, A. (2007) 'Contesting representations of poverty: ethics and evaluation', *Policy and Society*, 26 (3): 65–83.

Bletzer K.V. (2003) 'Risk and danger among women-who-prostitute in areas where farmworkers predominate', *Medical Anthropology Quarterly*, 17: 251–8.

Blumer, H. (1986) *Symbolic Interactionism: perspective and method*, San Francisco, CA: University of California Press.

Boal, A. (1998) *Legislative Theatre*, London: Routledge.

Boateng, A. (2009) 'A mixed methods analysis of social capital of Liberian refugee women in Ghana', *Journal of Sociology and Social Welfare*, 36: 59–81.

Boddingtom, B. and Didham, R. (2009) 'Increases in childlessness in New Zealand', *Journal of Population Research*, 26: 131–51.

Boscolo, L. and Bertrando, P. (1996) *Systemic Therapy with Individuals*, London: Karnac.

Boszormenyi-Nagy, I. (1974) 'Ethical and practical implications of intergenerational family therapy', *Psychotherapy and Psychosomatics*, 24: 261–8.

Botros, S.M., Abramov, Y., Miller, J.-J.R., Sand, P.K., Gandhi, S., Nickolov, A. and Goldberg, R.P. (2006) 'Effect of parity on sexual function: an identical twin study', *Obstetrics and Gynecology*, 107: 765–70.

Bourdieu, P. (1977) *Outline of a theory of practice*, Cambridge: Cambridge University Press.

Bourdieu, P. (1993) *Sociology in Question*, London: Sage Publications.

Boushey, H., Fremstad, S., Gragg, R. and Waller, M. (2007) *Social Inclusion for the United States*, Centre for Economic Policy and Research. Online. Available HTTP: <http://www.inclusionist.org/files/socialinclusionusa.pdf> (accessed 18 March 2013).

Bradley, C. (2009) 'Emergency contraception and physicians' rights of conscience: a review of current legal standards in Wisconsin', *Wisconsin Medical Journal*, 108: 156–60.

Brehaut, J., Fergusson, D., Kimmelman, J., Shojania, K., Saginur, R. and Elwyn, G. (2010) 'Using decision aids may improve informed consent for research', *Contemporary Clinical Trials*, 31: 218–20.

Breland-Noble, A.M., Bell, C.C., Burriss, A., Poole, K.H. and The AAKOMA Project Adult Advisory Board. (2012) 'The significance of strategic community engagement in recruiting African American youth and families for clinical research', *Journal of Child and Family Studies*, 21: 273–280.

Brewer, J.D. (2003) 'Philosophy of social research', in Miller, R.L. and J.D. Brewer, J.D. (eds) *The A-Z of Social Research*, London: Sage Publications.

Bridges, M. (2006) 'Activating the corrective emotional experience', *Journal of Clinical Psychology*, 62: 551–68.

Bromell, D. and Hyland, M. (2007) *Social Inclusion and Participation: a guide for policy and planning*, Wellington: Social Inclusion and Participation Group, Ministry of Social Development, New Zealand.

Brooks, F. (2008) 'Nursing and public participation in health: an ethnographic study of a patient council', *International Journal of Nursing Studies*, 45: 3–13.

Bryant, J., Saxton, M., Madden, A., Bath, N. and Robinson, S. (2008a) 'Consumer participation in the planning and delivery of drug treatment services: the current arrangements', *Drug and Alcohol Review*, 27: 130–7.

Bryant, J., Saxton, M., Madden, A., Bath, N. and Robinson, S. (2008b) 'Consumers' and providers' perspectives about consumer participation in drug treatment services: is there support to do more? What are the obstacles?', *Drug and Alcohol Review*, 27: 138–44.

Bryant, W., Vacher, G., Beresford, P. and McKay, E. (2010) 'The modernisation of mental health day services: participatory action research exploring social networking,' *Mental Health Review Journal*, 15 (3): 11–21.

Buckmaster, L. and Thomas, M. (2009) *Social inclusion and social citizenship: towards a truly inclusive society*, Canberra: Parliament of Australia. Online. Available HTTP: <http://parlinfo.aph.gov.au/parlInfo/search/display/display.w3p;adv=yes;orderBy=customrank;page=0;query=social%20inclusion%20citizenship;rec=1;resCount=Default> (accessed 18 March 2013).

Buerki, R. (2008) 'The conscience clause in American pharmacy: an historical overview', *Pharmacy In History*, 50: 107–18.

Buettner, P. and Muller, R. (2011) *Epidemiology*, South Melbourne, Victoria: Oxford University Press.

Bulman, J. and Hayes, R. (2011) 'Mibbinbah and Spirit healing: fostering safe, friendly spaces for Indigenous males in Australia', *International Journal of Men's Health*, 10: 6–25.

Burgess, M.M. (2007) 'Proposing modesty for informed consent', *Social Science and Medicine*, 65: 2284–95.

Burgess-Allen, J. and Owen-Smith, V. (2010) 'Using mind mapping techniques for rapid qualitative data analysis in public participation processes', *Health Expectations*, 13: 406–15.

Burland, K. and Pitts, S. (2007) 'Becoming a music student: investigating the skills and attitudes of students beginning a music degree', *Arts and Humanities in Higher Education*, 6: 289–308.

Burnett, L. (2009) 'An institution-wide approach to retaining and supporting first year students', in Australian Learning and Teaching Council (eds) *ALTC First Year Experience Curriculum Design Symposium 2009*. Brisbane: Queensland University of Technology. Online. Available HTTP: <http://www.fyecd2009.qut.edu.au/resources/FYE_ShowcaseAbstracts_17Mar09_final.pdf> (accessed 18 March 2013).

Butler, J.P. (1990) *Gender Trouble: feminism and the subversion of identity*, New York: Routledge.

Cacioppo, J. and Patrick, W. (2008) *Loneliness: human nature and the need for social connection*, New York: W.W. Norton.

Cameron, L. and Murphy, J. (2007) 'Obtaining consent to participate in research: the issues involved in including people with a range of learning and communication disabilities', *British Journal of Learning Disabilities*, 35: 113–20.

Campain, R. and Wilson, E. (2010) *Food Court Friends: building relationships through research*, Melbourne: Scope (Vic).

Campbell, J. and Davidson, G. (2009) 'Coercion in the community: a situated approach to the examination of ethical challenges for mental health social workers', *Ethics and Social Welfare*, 3: 249–63.

Cancedda, A. and McDonald, N. (2011) *Evaluation of the European Year 2010 for Combating Poverty and Social Exclusion*, Rotterdam: Ecorys Nederlands BV for the European Commission – DG Employment, Social Affairs and Inclusion.

Cannold, L. (2004) 'Declining marriage rates and gender inequity in social institutions: towards an adequately complex explanation for childlessness', *People and Place*, 12: 1–11.

Cannold, L. (2005) *What, No Baby? Why women are losing the freedom to mother, and how they can get it back*, Fremantle: Curtin University Books and Fremantle Arts Centre Press.

Cappo, D. (2009) *People and Community at the Heart of Systems and Bureaucracy: South Australia's social inclusion initiative*, Adelaide: Government of South Australia.

Carmien, S., Dawe, M., Fischer, G., Gorman, A., Kintson, A. and Sullivan, J.F., Jr. (2005) 'Socio-technical environments supporting people with cognitive disabilities using public transportation', *Transactions on Human–Computer Interaction (ToCHI)*, 12: 233–62.

Carnaby, S. Roberts, B., Lang, J. and Nielsen, P. (2011) 'A flexible response: person-centred support and social inclusion for people with learning disabilities and challenging behaviour', *British Journal of Learning Disabilities*, 39: 39–45.

Carr, W. and Kemmis, S. (1986) *Becoming Critical: education, knowledge and action research*, Geelong, Victoria: Deakin University Press.

Carroll, K.M., Ball, S.A., Nich, C., Martino, S., Frankforter T.L., Farentinos, C., Kunkel, L.E., Mikulich-Gilbertson S.K., Morgenstern, J., Obert, J.L., Polcin, D., Snead, N. and Woody, G.E. (2006) 'Motivational interviewing to improve treatment engagement and outcome in individuals seeking treatment for substance abuse: a multisite effectiveness study', *Drug and Alcohol Dependence*, 81: 301–12.

Carter, B. and McGoldrick, M. (1999) 'Coaching at various stages in the life-cycle', in B. Carter and M. McGoldrick (eds) *The Expanded Family Life Cycle*, Boston, MA: Allyn and Bacon,

Cashin, C., Scheffler, R., Felton, M., Adams, N. and Miller, L. (2008) 'Transformation of the California mental health system: stakeholder-driven planning as a transformational activity', *Psychiatric Services*, 59: 1107–14.

Cashman, S.B., Adeky, S., Allen, A.J., Corburn, J., Israel, B.A., Montaño, J., Rafelito, A., Rhodes, S.D., Swanston, S., Wallerstein, N. and Eng, E. (2008) 'The power and the promise: working with communities to analyze data, interpret findings, and get to outcomes', *American Journal of Public Health*, 98: 1407–17.

Catalani, C. and Minkler, M. (2010) 'Photovoice: a review of the literature in health and public health', *Health Education and Behavior*, 37: 424–57.

Catlin, J.H. (2008) 'Accessibility for all: a case study of the access living headquarters', *Topics in Stroke Rehabilitation*, 15: 97–102.

Catov, J.M., Newman, A.B., Sutton-Tyrrell, K., Harris, T.B., Tylavsky, F., Visser, M., Ayonayon, H.N. and Ness, R.B. (2008) 'Parity and cardiovascular disease risk among older women: how do pregnancy complications mediate the association?', *Annals of Epidemiology*, 18: 873–9.

Catroppa C., Anderson, V.A., Muscara, F., Morse, S.A., Haritou, F., Rosenfeld, J.V. and Heinrich, L.M. (2009) 'Educational skills: long-term outcome and predictors following paediatric traumatic brain injury', *Neuropsychological Rehabilitation*, 19: 716–32.

CDC (2010a) *HIV and AIDS Among African American Youth*, Atlanta, GA: US Centers for Disease Control and Prevention. Online. Available HTTP: <http://www.cdc.gov/nchhstp/newsroom/docs/HIVamongBlackYouthFactSheet-FINAL-508c.pdf> (accessed 18 March 2013).

CDC (2010b) *HIV Among Gay, Bisexual and Other Men Who Have Sex with Men (MSM)*, Atlanta, GA: US Centers for Disease Control and Prevention. Online. Available HTTP: <http://www.cdc.gov/hiv/topics/msm/pdf/msm.pdf> (accessed 18 March 2013).

CDC (2011a) *HIV Surveillance Report 2009*, Atlanta, GA: US Centers for Disease Control and Prevention. Online. Available HTTP: <http://www.cdc.gov/hiv/surveillance/resources/reports/2009report/index.htm> (accessed 18 March 2013).

CDC (2011b) *Sexually Transmitted Disease Surveillance 2010*, Atlanta: US Centers for Disease Control and Prevention. Online. Available HTTP: <http://www.cdc.gov/std/stats10/surv2010.pdf> (accessed 18 March 2013).

Cemlyn, S. (2008) 'Human rights practice: possibilities and pitfalls for developing emancipatory social work', *Ethics and Human Welfare*, 2: 222–42.

Center for Universal Design. (1997). *The Principles of Universal Design: Version 2.0* (updated 30 May 2011). Online. Available HTTP: <http://www.ncsu.edu/project/design-projects/udi/center-for-universal-design/the-principles-of-universal-design> (accessed 18 March 2013).

Chamberlain, J. M. (2011) 'The hearing of fitness to practice cases by the General Medical Council: current trends and future research agendas', *Health, Risk and Society*, 13: 561–75.

Chambers, R. (1983) *Rural Development: putting the last first*, London: Longman.

Chambers, R. (1994) *The Origins and Practice of Participatory Rural Appraisal*, Amsterdam: Elsevier.

Chambers, R. (2010) *Paradigms, Poverty and Adaptive Pluralism*, Brighton: Institute of Development Studies, IDS Working Paper 344.

Chapman, C. (2011) 'Resonance, intersectionality, and reflexivity in critical pedagogy (and research methodology)', *Social Work Education*, 30: 723–44.

Chessie, K. (2009) 'Health system regionalization in Canada's provincial and territorial health systems: do citizen governance boards represent, engage, and empower?', *International Journal of Health Services*, 39: 705–24.

Chou, K.-L. and Chi, I. (2004) 'Childlessness and psychological well-being in Chinese older adults', *International Journal of Geriatric Psychiatry*, 19: 449–57.

Christensen, J. (2012) 'Telling stories: exploring research storytelling as a meaningful approach to knowledge mobilization with Indigenous research collaborators and diverse audiences in community-based participatory research', *Canadian Geographer*, 56: 231–42.

Christie, H., Tett, L., Cree, V.E., Hounsell, J. and McCune, V. (2008) '"A real rollercoaster of confidence and emotions": learning to be a university student', *Studies in Higher Education*, 33: 567–81.

City of Port Phillip (2011) *Street Sex Work: information sheet*. Online. Available HTTP: <http://www.portphillip.vic.gov.au/default/Factsheet_Street_Sex_Work_FINAL.pdf> (accessed 18 March 2013).

Clatts, M.C., Giang, L.M., Goldsamt, L.A. and Yi, H. (2007) 'Male sex work and HIV risk among young heroin users in Hanoi, Vietnam', *Sexual Health*, 4: 261–7.

Cleary, M., Horsfall, J., Hunt, G.E., Escott, P. and Happell, B. (2011) 'Continuing challenges for the mental health consumer workforce: a role for mental health nurses?', *International Journal of Mental Health Nursing*, 20: 438–44.

Clegg, S., Bradley, S. and Smith, K. (2006) '"I've had to swallow my pride": help seeking and self-esteem', *Higher Education Research and Development*, 25: 101–13.

Coad, J., Flay, J., Aspinall, M., Bilverstone, B., Coxhead, E. and Hones, B. (2008) 'Evaluating the impact of involving young people in developing children's services in an acute hospital trust', *Journal of Clinical Nursing*, 17: 3115–22.

COAG (2008) *Closing the Gap in Indigenous Disadvantage.* Council of Australian Governments. Online. Available HTTP: <http://www.coag.gov.au/closing_the_gap_in_indigenous_disadvantage> (accessed 18 March 2013).

Coalition for Disability Rights (2006) *Call to Political Parties – 2006 Victorian state election*, Melbourne: Coalition for Disability Rights.

Cochran, P.A.L., Marshall, C.A., Garcia-Downing, C., Kendall, E., Cook, D., McCubbin, L. and Cover, R.M.S. (2008) 'Indigenous ways of knowing: implications for participatory research and community', *American Journal of Public Health*, 98: 22–7.

Cohen, J. and Burg, E. (2003) 'On the possibility of a positive-sum game in the distribution of health care resources', *The Journal of Medicine And Philosophy*, 28: 327–38.

Colgan, S., Moodie, M. and Carter, R. (2010) *The Economic Study*, Melbourne: Deakin University.

Collier, P.J. and Morgan, D.L. (2008) '"Is that paper really due today?" Differences in first generation and traditional college students' understanding of faculty expectations', *Higher Education*, 55: 425–46.

Collishaw, S., Maughan, B., Goodman, R. and Pickles, A. (2004) 'Time trends in adolescent mental health', *Journal of Child Psychology and Psychiatry*, 45: 1350–62.

Colomb, C. (2011) 'Urban regeneration and policies of "social mixing" in British cities: a critical assessment', *Architecture, City and Environment*, 17: 223–43.

Commission of the European Communities (2005) *Working Together, Working Better: a new framework for the open co-ordination of social protection and inclusion policies in the European Union.* Communication from the Commission to the Council, the European Parliament, the European Economic and Social Committee and the Committee of the regions. Brussels.

Commonwealth of Australia (1992) *National Mental Health Policy*, Canberra: Australian Government Publishing Service.

Commonwealth of Australia (2008) *National Mental Health Policy*, Canberra: Commonwealth of Australia.

Commonwealth of Australia (2011) *2010–2020 National Disability Strategy*, Canberra: Attorney General's Department.

Community Health Scholars Program (2002) *Stories of Impact*, Ann Arbor: Kellogg Health Scholars. Online. Available HTTP: <http://www.kellogghealthscholars.org/about/ctrack_impact_scholars_book.pdf> (accessed 18 March 2013).

Cone-Wesson, B. (2005) 'Prenatal alcohol and cocaine exposure: influences on cognition, speech, language, and hearing', *Journal of Communication Disorders*, 38: 279–302.

Cook, T. and Wills, J. (2012) 'Engaging with marginalized communities: the experiences of London health trainers', *Perspectives in Public Health*, 132: 221–27.

Cooke, B. and Kothari, U. (eds) (2001) *Participation: the new tyranny?* London: Zed Books.

Coomber, R. (2002) 'Signing your life away? Why research ethics committees (REC) shouldn't always require written confirmation that participants in research have been informed of the aims of a study and their rights – the case of criminal populations', *Sociological Research Online*, 7 (1). Online. Available HTTP: <http://www.socresonline.org.uk/7/1/coomber.html> (accessed 18 March 2013).

Cooper, R., Hardy, R. and Kuh, D. (2008) 'Timing of menarche, childbearing and hysterectomy risk', *Maturitas*, 61: 317–22.

Corbie-Smith, G., Tomas, S., Williams, M. and Moody-Ayers, S. (1999) 'Attitudes and beliefs of African Americans toward participation in medical research', *Journal of General Internal Medicine*, 14: 537–46.

Corker, M. and Shakespeare, T. (eds) (2002) *Disability Postmodernity: embodying disability theory*, New York: Continuum.

Cornwall, A. (2006) 'Historical perspectives on participation in development', *Commonwealth and Comparative Politics*, 44: 62–83.

Cornwell, E.Y. and Waite, L.J. (2009) 'Social disconnectedness, perceived isolation, and health among older adults', *Journal of Health and Social Behaviour*, 50: 31–48.

Corrigan, O. (2003) 'Empty ethics: the problem with informed consent', *Sociology of Health and Illness*, 25: 768–92.

Corrigan, P.W., Watson, A.C. and Barr, L. (2006) 'The self-stigma of mental illness: implications for self–esteem and self–efficacy', *Journal of Social and Clinical Psychology*, 25: 875–84.

Cotterell, P., Harlow, G., Morris, C., Beresford, P., Hanley, B., Sargeant, A., Sitzia, J. and Staley, K. (2011) 'Service user involvement in cancer care: the impact on service users', *Health Expectations*, 14: 159–69.

Couzos, S., Lea, T., Murray, R. and Culbong, M. (2005) '"We are not just participants – we are in charge": The NACCHO ear trial and the process for Aboriginal community-controlled health research', *Ethnicity and Health*, 10: 91–111.

Crawford, M., Aldridge, T., Bhui, K., Rutter, D., Manley, C., Weaver, T., Tyrer, P. and Fulop, N. (2003) 'User involvement in the planning and delivery of mental health services: a cross-sectional survey of service users and providers', *Acta Psychiatrica Scandinavica*, 107: 410–4.

Crawford, M.J., Rutter, D., Manley, C., Weaver, T., Bhui, K., Fulop, N. and Tyrer, P. (2002) 'Systematic review of involving patients in the planning and development of health care', *British Medical Journal*, 325: 1263–5.

Cree, V., Hounsell, J., Christie, H., McCune, V. and Tett, L. (2009) 'From further education to higher education: social work students' experiences of transition to an ancient, research-led university', *Social Work Education*, 28: 887–901.

Crews, D.E. and Zavotka, S. (2006) 'Aging, disability, and frailty: implications for universal design', *Journal of Physiological Anthropology*, 25: 113–8.

Crisp, B.R. (2010a) 'Belonging, connectedness and social exclusion', *Journal of Social Inclusion*, 1: 123–32.

Crisp, B.R. (2010b) *Spirituality and Social Work*, Farnham: Ashgate.

Crisp, B.R. and Barber, J.G. (1997) 'The prevention of AIDS among injecting drug users', *British Journal of Social Work*, 27: 255–74.

Crossan, B. Field, J., Gallacher, J. and Merrill, B. (2003) 'Understanding participation in learning for non-traditional adult learners: learning careers and the construction of learning identities', *British Journal of Sociology of Education*, 24: 55–67.

CSCI (2007a) *Guidance for Inspectors: experts by experience*, London: Commission for Social Care Inspection.

CSCI (2007b) *Experts by Experience in Regulatory Inspections 2006/07 (Excluding Domicili-ary Care) Evaluation Report*, London: Commission for Social Care Inspection.

CSCI (2009) *Experts by Experience*, London: Commission for Social Care Inspection.

CSDH (2008) *Closing the Gap in a Generation: health equity through action on the social deter-minants of health: final report of the Commission on Social Determinants of Health*, Geneva: World Health Organization.

Culyer, A. J. (1995) 'Need: the idea won't do but we still need it', *Social Science and Medicine*, 40: 727–30.

Cummins, B. (2005) 'Measuring health and subjective wellbeing: vale, quality-adjusted life-years', in L. Manderson (ed.) *Rethinking Wellbeing*, Perth: Australia Research Institute.

Curtis, S.E. and Taket, A.R. (1996) *Health and Societies: changing perspectives*, London: Arnold.

d'Abbs, P.H. and Brady, M. (2004) 'Other people, other drugs: the policy response to petrol sniffing among Indigenous Australians', *Drug and Alcohol Review*, 23: 253–60.

Dalla, R. (2002) 'Night moves: a qualitative investigation of street-level sex work', *Psychology of Women Quarterly*, 30: 276–90.

Daly, M. (2007) 'Whither EU social policy: an account and assessment of developments in the Lisbon social inclusion process', *Journal of Social Policy*, 37: 1–19.

Dandona R., Dandona, L., Kumar, G.A., Gutierrez, J.P., McPherson, S., Samuels, F., Bertozzi, S.M. and the ASCI FPP Study Team (2006) 'Demography and sex work characteristics of female sex workers in India', *BMC International Health and Human Rights* 6: 5. Online. Available HTTP: <http://www.biomedcentral.com/1472-698X/6/5> (accessed 18 March 2013).

Daniluk, J. (2001) 'Reconstructing their lives: a longitudinal, qualitative analysis of the transition to biological childlessness for infertile couples', *Journal of Counseling and Development*, 79: 439–49.

Davies, A.F. (1988) *The Human Element: three essays in political psychology*, Fitzroy, Victoria: McPhee Gribble.

Davis, T.W.D. (2009) 'The politics of human rights and development: the challenge for official donors', *Australian Journal of Political Science*, 44: 173–92.

Davis-Floyd, R., Barclay, L., Davis, B. and Tritten, J. (2009) *Birth Models that Work*. Berkeley, CA: University of California Press.

Day, A. (2008) 'Emergency contraception: when the pharmacist conscience clause restricts access', *Nursing For Women's Health*, 12: 343–6.

Day, A., Howells, K. and Rickwood, D. (2003) *The Victorian Juvenile Justice Rehabili-tation Review*. Online. Available HTTP: <http://www.aic.gov.au/en/publications/previous%20series/other/41–60/victorian%20juvenile%20justice%20rehabilitation%20review.html> (accessed 15 September 2011).

De Couvreur, L. and Goossens, R. (2011) 'Design for (every)one: co-creation as a bridge between universal design and rehabilitation engineering', *CoDesign*, 7: 107–21.

de Crespigny, C., Emden, C., Kowanko, I. and Murray, H. (2004) 'A "partnership model" for ethical Indigenous research', *Collegian*, 11 (4): 7–13.

de la Barra, S.L., Redman, S. and Eades, S. (2009) 'Health research policy: a case study of policy change in Aboriginal and Torres Strait Islander health research', *Australia and New Zealand Health Policy*, 6 (2).

de las Nueces, D., Hacker, K., DiGirolamo, A. and Hicks, L.S. (2012) 'A systematic review of community-based participatory research to enhance clinical trials in racial and ethnic minority groups', *Health Services Research*, 47: 1363–86.

de Leeuw, E. (2012) 'Healthy Cities deserve better', *The Lancet*, 380: 1306–7.

de Leeuw, E., McNess, A., Crisp, B. and Stagnitti, K. (2008) 'Theoretical reflections on the nexus between research, policy and practice', *Critical Public Health*, 18: 5–20.

DeJong, J., Akik, C., El Kak, F., Osman, H. and El Jardali, F. (2010) 'The safety and quality of childbirth in the context of health systems: mapping maternal mealth provision in Lebanon', *Midwifery*, 26: 549–57.

Delman, J. (2012) 'Participatory action research and young adults with psychiatric disabilities', *Psychiatric Rehabilitation Journal* 35: 231–4.

Denzin, N.K. and Lincoln, Y.S. (1998) 'Entering the field of qualitative research', in N.K. Denzin and Y.S. Lincoln (eds) *The Landscape of Qualitative Research: theories and issues*, Thousand Oaks, CA: Sage.

Department of Work and Pensions (2008) *Working Together. UK national action plan on social inclusion*, London: Department of Work and Pensions.

DePoy, E. and Gilson, S.F. (2010) *Studying Disability: multiple theories and responses*, Thousand Oaks, CA: Sage.

Dever, M. (2005) 'Baby talk: the Howard Government, families, and the politics of difference', *Hecate*, 31: 45–61.

DHS (2010a) *The Victorian Aids and Equipment Program*. Melbourne: Department of Human Services.

DHS (2010b) *Disability, Mental Health and Medication – implications for practice and policy*. Melbourne: Department of Human Services. Online. Available HTTP: <http://www.dhs.vic.gov.au/about-the-department/documents-and-resources/reports-publications/disability,-mental-health-and-medication-implications-for-practice-and-policy> (accessed 18 March 2013).

Disability Investment Group (2009) *The Way Forward: a new disability policy framework for Australia*, Canberra: Department of Families Housing, Community Services and Indigenous Affairs.

Djernes, J.K. (2006) 'Prevalence and predictors of depression in populations of elderly: a review', *Acta Psychiatrica Scandinavica*, 113: 372–87.

DoH (2000) *National Cancer Plan: a plan for investment, a plan for reform*, London: Department of Health.

DOHA (1998) *Consumer Focus Collaboration*, Canberra: Commonwealth Department of Health and Aged Care.

DOHA (2002) *National Mental Health Report 2002: seventh report. Changes in Australia's mental health services in the first two years of the second National Mental Health Plan 1998–2000*, Canberra: Commonwealth Department of Health and Ageing.

DOHA (2004) *National Mental Health Report 2004: eighth report. Summary of changes in Australia's mental health services under the national mental health strategy 1993–2002*, Canberra: Commonwealth Department of Health and Ageing.

Doidge, N. (2010) *The Brain that Changes Itself: stories of personal triumph from the frontiers of brain science*, Melbourne: Scribe.

Dominelli, L. (2005) 'Social inclusion in research: reflecting on a research project involving young mothers in care' *International Journal of Social Welfare*, 14: 13–22.

Doyle, M. and Timonen, V. (2010) 'Lessons from a community-based participatory research project: older people's and researchers' reflections', *Research on Aging*, 32: 244–63.

Dumbaugh, E. (2008) 'Designing communities to enhance the safety and mobility of older adults: a universal approach', *Journal of Planning Literature*, 23: 17–36.

Durbach, N. (2002) 'Class, gender, and the conscientious objector to vaccination, 1898–1907', *Journal of British Studies*, 41: 58–83.

Durey, R. (2009) *Women and Ageing (Gender Impact Assessment No. 10)*, Melbourne: Women's Health Victoria.

Dyer, C. (1988) 'Receptionists may not invoke conscience clause', *British Medical Journal*, 297: 1493–4.

Dyer, J. (2008) *Fertility of American women: 2006, population reports*, Washington DC: US Census Bureau, Department of Commerce.

Eades, S., Taylor, B., Bailey, S., Williamson, A., Craig, J. and Redman, S. (2010) 'The health of urban Aboriginal people: insufficient data to close the gap', *The Medical Journal of Australia*, 193: 521–4.

Earle-Richardson, G., Sorensen, J., Brower, M., Hawkes, L. and May J. J. (2009) 'Community collaborations for farmworker health in New York and Maine: process analysis of two successful interventions', *American Journal of Public Health*, 99: S584–7.

Echeverría, S., Diez-Roux, A.V., Shea, S., Borrell, L.N. and Jackson, S. (2008) 'Associations of neighbourhood problems and neighbourhood social cohesion with mental health and health behaviors: the Multi-Ethnic Study of Atherosclerosis', *Health and Place*, 14: 853–65.

Edwards, C., Gandini, L. and Forman, G. (1998) *The Hundred Languages of Children: the Reggio Emilia approach advanced reflections*, 2nd edn, Westport CT: Ablex Publishing.

Edwards, T. and Taylor, K. (2008) 'Decolonising cultural awareness', *Australian Nursing Journal*, 15 (10): 31–3.

Efstathiou, N., Ameen, J. and Coll, A.M. (2008) 'A Delphi study to identify healthcare users' priorities for cancer care in Greece', *European Journal of Oncology Nursing*, 12: 362–71.

Eisenmajer, R. (2006) *Imagine having Asperger's Syndrome: a first consultation* [video-recording], Glen Iris, Victoria: PerformArts.

El Kak, F. (2009) Homophobia in clinical services in Lebanon a physician survey, Unpublished Report, Beruit: American University of Beirut.

El-Bassel, N., Wiitte, S.S., Wada, T., Gilbert, L. and Wallace, J. (2001) 'Correlates of partner violence among female street-based sex workers: substance abuse, history of childhood abuse and HIV risks', *AIDS Patient Care and STDs*, 15: 41–51.

Elliot, A. and Lemert, C. (2006) *The New Individualism: the emotional costs of globalization*, London: Routledge.

Ellis, A. (2006) 'What is special about religion?', *Law and Philosophy: An International Journal for Jurisprudence and Legal Philosophy*, 25: 219–41.

Elmore-Meegan, M., Conroy, R. and Agala, B. (2004) 'Sex workers in Kenya, numbers of clients and associated risks: an exploratory survey', *Reproductive Health Matters*, 12 (23): 50–7.

Eng, E., Rhodes, S.D. and Parker, E.A. (2009) 'Natural helper models to enhance a community's health and competence', in R.J. Di Clemente, R.A. Crosby and M.C. Kegler (eds) *Emerging Theories in Health Promotion Practice and Research*, Volume 2, San Francisco, CA: Jossey-Bass.

English, F.W. and Hill, J.C. (1994) *Total Quality Education: transforming schools into learning places*, Thousand Oaks, CA: Corwin Press.

Eshbaugh, E.M. (2009) 'The role of friends in predicting loneliness among older women living alone', *Journal of Gerontological Nursing*, 35: 13–6.

European Agency for Safety and Health at Work (2003) *Gender Issues in Safety and Health at Work: a review*, Luxembourg: Office for Official Publications of the European Communities.

European Parliament (2000a) *European Council – Nice 7–10 December 2000: conclusions of the presidency*. Online. Available HTTP: <http://www.europarl.europa.eu/summits/nice1_en.htm> (accessed 18 March 2013).

European Parliament (2000b) *Lisbon European Council 23 and 24 March 2000: presidency conclusions*. Online. Available HTTP: <http://www.europarl.europa.eu/summits/lis1_en.htm> (Accessed 18 March 2013).

Ewing-Cobbs, L., Barnes, M.A. and Fletcher, J.M. (2003) 'Early brain injury in children: development and reorganization of cognitive function', *Developmental Neuropsychology*, 24: 669–704.

Fallon, S., Smith, J., Morgan, S., Stoner, M. and Austin, C. (2008) '"Pizza, patients and points of view": involving young people in the design of a post registration module entitled the adolescent with cancer', *Nurse Education in Practice*, 8: 140–7.

Fang, X., Li, X., Yang, H., Hong, Y., Stanton, B., Zhao, R., Dong, B., Liu, W., Zhou, Y. and Liang, S. (2008) 'Can variation in HIV/STD-related risk be explained by individual SES? Findings from female sex workers in a rural Chinese county', *Health Care for Women International*, 29: 316–35.

Farley, M., Cotton, A., Lynne, J., Zumbeck, S., Spiwak, F., Reyes, M.E., Alvarez, D. and Sezgin, U. (2003) 'Prostitution and trafficking in nine countries: an update on violence and posttraumatic stress disorder', *Journal of Trauma Practice*, 2: 33–74.

Farmer, J., Philip, L., King, G., Farrington, J. and MacLeod, M. (2010) 'Territorial tensions: misaligned management and community perspectives on health services for older people in remote rural areas', *Health and Place*, 16: 275–83.

Farquhar, P. and Pollock, S. (2011) *'It's a Well-being Thing': understanding what wellbeing means and how it is experienced by socially isolated people in later-middle and older age living in the growth suburbs of metropolitan Melbourne*, Melbourne: Wesley Mission Victoria.

Farrugia, S. and Hudson, J. L. (2006) 'Anxiety in adolescents with Asperger syndrome: negative thoughts, behavioural problems, and life interference', *Focus on Autism and Other Developmental Disabilities*, 21: 25–35.

Fawaz, M. and Peillin, I. (2003) Urban Slums Reports: the case of Beirut, Lebanon', in *Understanding Slums: case studies for the global report on human settlements*. Online. Available HTTP: <http://www.ucl.ac.uk/dpu-projects/Global_Report/pdfs/Beirut_bw.pdf> (accessed 18 March 2013).

Fenge, L. (2010) 'Striving towards inclusive research: an example of participatory action research with older lesbians and gay men', *British Journal of Social Work*, 40: 878–94.

Fernández-Esquer, M.E. (2003) 'Drinking for wages: alcohol use among Cantineras', *Journal of Studies on Alcohol*, 64: 160–6.

Fick, N. (2005) *Coping with Stigma, Discrimination and Violence: sex workers talk about their experiences*, Cape Town: Sex Worker Education and Advocacy Taskforce. Online. Available HTTP: <http://www.heart-intl.net/HEART/120606/coping.pdf> (accessed 18 March 2013).

Finch, J. (1984) '"It's great to have someone to talk to": the ethics and politics of interviewing women', in C. Bell and H. Roberts (eds) *Social Researching*, London: Routledge and Kegan Paul.

Finch, J.B. (1887) *The People Versus the Liquor Traffic: speeches of John B. Finch delivered in the prohibition campaigns of the United States and Canada*, New York: Funk and Wagnalls.

Fineout-Overholt, E, Melnyk, B. and Schultz, A (2005) 'Transforming health care from the inside out: advancing evidence-based practice in the 21st century', *Journal of Professional Nursing*, 21: 335–44.

Firebrace, S., Blow, R., Pollock, S., Taket, A. and Barter-Godfrey, S. (2009) *Talking it up! Project report: Aboriginal voices in the formulation of health policy that works*, Melbourne: Wesley Mission Victoria.

Firebrace, S., Blow, R., Pollock, S., Taket, A. and Barter-Godfrey, S. (2010) *Healing Stories: experiences of health services by Aboriginal people living in NE Melbourne, Final report*, Melbourne: Wesley Mission Victoria.

Firebrace, S., Hammond, M., Bell, B., Mathison, P., Watson, A. and Hurley, B. (2001) 'Improving Koori Access to Darebin Community Health Service', *Australian Journal of Primary Health*, 7 (1): 120–3.

Fitzgerald, M.M., Kirk, G.D. and Bristow, C.A. (2011) 'Description and evaluation of a serious game intervention to engage low secure service users with serious mental illness in the design and refurbishment of their environment', *Journal of Psychiatric and Mental Health Nursing*, 18: 316–22.

Flaskerud, J.H. and Winslow, B. (1998) 'Conceptualizing vulnerable populations' health related research', *Nursing Research*, 47 (2): 69–78.

Fletcher, T., Glasper, A., Prudhoe, G., Battrick, C., Coles, L., Weaver, K. and Ireland, L. (2011) 'Building the future: children's views on nurses and hospital care', *British Journal of Nursing*, 20: 39–45.

Flynn, D. (2008) 'Pharmacist conscience clauses and access to oral contraceptives', *Journal of Medical Ethics*, 34: 517–20.

Folch, C., Esteve, A., Sanclemente, C., Martró, E., Lugo, R., Molinos, S., Gonzalez, V., Ausina, V. and Casabona, J. (2008) 'Prevalence of HIV, *Chlamydia trachomatis*, and *Neisseria gonorrhoeae* and risk factors for sexually transmitted infections among immigrant female sex workers in Catalonia, Spain', *Sexually Transmitted Diseases*, 35: 178–83.

Foucault, M. (1976) 'Two lectures', in C. Gordon (ed.) (1980) *Power/Knowledge*, Brighton: Harvester.

Fox, J. (1987) *The Essential Moreno: writings on psychodrama, group method and spontaneity*, New York: Springer.

Fox, M., Martin, P. and Green, G. (2007) *Doing Practitioner Research*, London: Sage.

Francis, S.A. and Liverpool, J. (2009) 'A review of faith-based HIV prevention programs', *Journal of Religion and Health*, 48: 6–15.

Freeman, M. (2008) *Examination of the Asperger Syndrome Profile in Children and Adolescents: behaviour, mental health and temperament*, Guelph: University of Guelph.

Freire, P. (1972) *Pedagogy of the Oppressed*, London: Penguin.

Freire, P. (1973) *Education for Critical Consciousness*, New York: Seabury Press.

Freire, P. (1990) *Pedagogy of the Oppressed*, New York: Continuum.

Frejka, T. and Sobotka, T. (2008) 'Overview chapter 1. Fertility in Europe: diverse, delayed and below replacement', *Demographic Research*, 19: 15–45.

Furlong, M. (2009) 'Reconstituting the social: is the vocabulary of health and well-being colonizing how "the social" is understood?', *Arena Magazine*, 103: 34–40.

Furlong, M. (2010) 'Sovereign selves or social beings?: The practitioner's role in constructing the subjectivity and sociality of the consumer', *Newparadigm*, Autumn: 50–7.

Furlong, M. (2013) *Strengthening the Client's Relational Base*, Bristol: Policy Press.

Furman, B. and Ahola, T. (1995) *Solutions Talk: hosting therapeutic conversations*, New York: W.W. Norton.

Furness, S. and Gilligan, P. (2010) *Religion, Belief and Social Work: making a difference*, Bristol: Policy Press.

Gagnon, S., Nagle, R. and Nickerson, A. (2007) 'Parent and teacher ratings of peer interactive play and socio-emotional development of preschool children at risk', *Journal of Early Intervention*, 29: 228–42.

Galanti, M.R., Ivarsson, B.H., Helgason, A.R. and Gilljam, H. (2002) 'Smoking cessation: gender on the agenda', *Drugs: Education, Prevention and Policy*, 9: 71–84.

Gale, T. and Tranter, D. (2011) 'Social justice in higher education policy: an historical and conceptual account of student participation, *Critical Studies in Education*, 52: 29–46.

Gallie, D. (2004) 'Unemployment, poverty, and social isolation: an assessment of the current state of social exclusion theory', in D. Gallie (ed.) *Resisting Marginalization: unemployment experience and social policy in the European Union*, Oxford: Oxford University Press.

Galvin, J., Froude, E.H. and McAleer, J. (2010) 'Children's participation in home, school and community life after acquired brain injury', *Australian Occupational Therapy Journal*, 57: 118–26.

Gauld, R. (2010) 'Are elected health boards an effective mechanism for public participation in health service governance?', *Health Expectations*, 13: 369–78.

Gaventa, J. and Barrett, G. (2010) *So What Difference Does it Make? Mapping the outcomes of citizen engagement*, Brighton: Institute of Development Studies, IDS Working Paper 347.

Gawith, L. and Abrams, P. (2006) 'Long journey to recovery for Kiwi consumers: recent developments in mental health policy and practice in New Zealand', *Australian Psychologist*, 41: 140–8.

Gaynor, S., Weersing, V., Kolko, D., Birmaher, B., Heo, J. and Brent, D. (2003) 'The prevalence and impact of large sudden improvements during adolescent therapy for depression: a comparison across cognitive–behavioral, family, and supportive therapy', *Journal of Consulting and Clinical Psychology*, 71: 386–93.

Geene, R., Huber, E., Hundertmark-Mayser, J., Moller-Bock, B. and Thiel, W. (2009) 'Development, situation and perspective of self-help support in Germany', *Bundesgesundheitsblatt-Gesundheitsforschung-Gesundheitsschutz*, 52 (1): 11–20.

Gilchrist, G., Gruer, L. and Atkinson, J. (2005) 'Comparison of drug use and psychiatric morbidity between prostitute and non-prostitute female drug users in Glasgow, Scotland', *Addictive Behaviors*, 30: 1019–23.

Gill, J. and Liamputtong, P. (2011) 'Being a mother of a child with Asperger's syndrome and stigma', *Health Care for Women International*. 32: 708–22.

Gill, J. and Liamputtong, P. (2013) 'Walk a mile in my shoes: the lived experience as mothers of children with Asperger's Syndrome', *Qualitative Social Work*. 12: 41–56.

Gillespie, R. (1999) 'Voluntary childlessness in the United Kingdom', *Reproductive Health Matters*, 7 (13): 43–53.

Gillespie, R. (2003) 'Childfree and feminine: understanding the gender identity of childless women', *Gender and Society*, 17: 122–36.

Giorcelli, L.R. (1996) 'An impulse to soar: sanitisation, silencing and special education', *Australasian Journal of Special Education*, 20, 5–11.

Glasson, J. and Wood, G. (2009) 'Urban regeneration and impact assessment for social sustainability', *Impact Assessment and Project Appraisal*, 27: 283–90.

Gledhill, S., Abbey, J. and Schweitzer, R. (2008) 'Sampling methods: methodological issues involved in the recruitment of older people into a study of sexuality', *Australian Journal of Advanced Nursing*, 26 (1): 84–94.

Global Extension of Social Security (n.d.) *Social Inclusion and Poverty Reduction in Mexico (Vivir Mejor strategy)*. Online. Available HTTP: <http://www.socialsecurityextension.org/gimi/gess/ShowTheme.do?tid=2670> (accessed 18 March 2013).

Goggin, G. and Newell, C. (eds) (2005) *Disability in Australia: exposing a social apartheid*, Sydney: University of New South Wales Press.

Gomperts, R. (2002) 'Women on waves: where next for the abortion boat?', *Reproductive Health Matters*, 10 (19): 180–3.

Göncü, A. and Perone, A. (2005) 'Pretend play as a lifespan activity', *Topoi*, 24: 137–47.

Goodman, R. (1997) 'The Strengths and Difficulties Questionnaire: a research note', *Journal of Child Psychology and Psychiatry*, 38: 581–6.

Gordis, L. (2009) *Epidemiology*, Philadelphia: Saunders Elsevier.

Gordon, C. (1980) 'Afterword', in C. Gordon (ed.) *Power/knowledge*, Brighton: Harvester.

Gott, M., Stevens, T., Small, N. and Ahmedzai, S. (2000) *User Involvement in Cancer Care: exclusion and empowerment*, Bristol: The Policy Press.

Government of Ireland (2007) *National Action Plan for Social Inclusion 2007–2016*, Dublin: Government of Ireland.

Government of South Australia (2004) *South Australia's Strategic Plan. Creating opportunity*. Online. Available HTTP: <http://saplan.org.au/media/BAhbBlsHOgZmS-SIhMjAxMS8wOS8yOC8yMV8yNF8zOF83OTlfZmlsZQY6BkVU/21_24_38_799_file> (accessed 18 March 2013).

Government of South Australia (2007) *South Australia's Strategic Plan 2007*. Online. Available HTTP: <http://saplan.org.au/media/BAhbBlsHOgZmSSIhMjAxMS-8wOS8wNy8wM181OF80M18xMDBfZmlsZQY6BkVU/03_58_43_100_file> (accessed 18 March 2013).

Government of the People's Republic of China and United Nations Development Programme (2004) *Capacity Building to Support Pro-poor Fiscal Reform in China*. Online. Available HTTP: <http://www.undp.org.cn/projectdocs/39815.pdf> (accessed 18 March 2013).

GPC (2010) *Guidance on the Provision of Pharmacy Services Affected by Religious and Moral beliefs, September 2012*, London: General Pharmaceutical Council. Online. Available HTTP: <http://www.pharmacyregulation.org/sites/default/files/Guidance%20on%20the%20provision%20of%20pharmacy%20services%20affected%20by%20religious%20moral%20beliefs%20g.pdf> (accessed 18 March 2013)

Graham, M., Hill, E., Shelley, J. and Taket, A. (2011) 'An examination of the health and wellbeing of childless women: a cross-sectional exploratory study in Victoria, Australia', *BMC Women's Health*, 11: 47.

Gray, D. (2002) 'Everybody just freezes. Everybody is just embarrassed: felt and enacted stigma among parents of children with high functioning autism', *Sociology of Health and Illness*, 24: 734–49.

Green, C.R., Mihic, A.M. Nikkel, S.M., Stade, B.C., Rasmussen, C., Munoz, D.P. and Reynolds, J.N. (2008) 'Executive function deficits in children with foetal alcohol spectrum disorders (FASD) measured using the Cambridge Neuropsychological

Tests Automated Battery (CANTAB)', *Journal of Child Psychology and Psychiatry*, 50: 688–97.

Green, J. (2005) 'Refusal clauses and the Weldon Amendment', *Journal of Legal Medicine*, 26: 401–15.

Green, L.W. and Mercer, S.L. (2001) 'Can public health researchers and agencies reconcile the push from funding bodies and the pull from communities?', *American Journal of Public Health*, 91: 1926–9.

Grenfell, A. (2009) 'Enhancing FYE using system-generated student study plans that adhere to a university-wide curriculum model', In Australian Learning and Teaching Council (eds) *ALTC First Year Experience Curriculum Design Symposium 2009*. Brisbane: Queensland University of Technology. Online. Available HTTP: <http://www.fyecd2009.qut.edu.au/resources/FYE_ShowcaseAbstracts_17Mar09_final.pdf> (accessed 18 March 2013).

Griffith, M.D., Campbell, B., Allen, O.J, Robinson, J.K and Stewart, K.S. (2010a) 'YOUR Blessed Health: An HIV-prevention program bridging faith and public health communities', *Public Health Reports*, 125: 4–11.

Griffith, M.D., Pichon, C.L, Campbell B. and Allen O.J. (2010b) 'YOUR Blessed Health: a faith-based CBPR approach to addressing HIV/AIDS among African Americans', *AIDS Education and Prevention*, 22: 203–17.

Griffiths, D.S., Winstanley, D. and Gabriel, Y. (2005) 'Learning shock: the trauma of return to formal learning', *Management Learning*, 36: 275–97.

Groneberg, D.A., Molliné, M. and Kusma, B. (2006) 'Sex work during the world cup in Germany', *The Lancet*, 368: 840–1.

Grundy, E. and Kravdal, Ø. (2008) 'Reproductive history and mortality in late middle age among Norwegian men and women', *American Journal of Epidemiology*, 167: 271–79.

Grundy, E. and Kravdal, Ø. (2010) 'Fertility history and cause-specific mortality: a register-based analysis of complete cohorts of Norwegian woman and men', *Social Science and Medicine*, 70: 1847–57.

Grundy, E. and Tomassini, C. (2005) 'Fertility history and health in later life: a record linkage study in England and Wales', *Social Science and Medicine*, 61: 217–28.

Guest, G., Bunce, A. and Johnson, L. (2006) 'How many interviews are enough? An experiment with data saturation and variability', *Field Methods*, 18: 59–82.

Guillemin, M. and Gillam, L. (2004) 'Ethics, reflexivity, and "ethically important moments" in research', *Qualitative Inquiry*, 10: 261–80.

Gunderson, E.P., Lewis, C.E., Murtaugh, M.A., Quesenberry, C.P., West, D.S. and Sidney, S. (2004) 'Long-term plasma lipid changes associated with a first birth: the Coronary Artery Risk Development in Young Adults Study', *American Journal of Epidemiology*, 159: 1028–39.

Gunderson, E.P., Jacobs, D.R., Jr., Chiang, V., Lewis, C.E., Tsai, A., Quesenberry, C.P., Jr. and Sidney, S. (2009) 'Childbearing is associated with higher incidence of the metabolic syndrome among women of reproductive age controlling for measurements before pregnancy: the CARDIA study', *American Journal of Obstetrics and Gynecology*, 201 (2): 177.e1–9.

Gunstone, A. (2008) 'Reconciliation and Australian Indigenous health in the 1990s: a failure of public policy', *Journal of Bioethical Inquiry*, 5: 251–63.

Guttmacher Institute (2011) *States Enact Record Number of Abortion Restrictions in First Half of 2011*. Online. Available HTTP: <http://www.guttmacher.org/media/inthenews/2011/07/13/index.html> (accessed 18 March 2013).

Guttmacher Institute (2012) *State Policies in Brief: Refusing to Provide Health Services, January 2012*. Online. Available HTTP: <http://www.guttmacher.org/statecenter/spibs/spib_RPHS.pdf> (accessed 18 March 2013).

Haddad, S. (2002) 'Cultural diversity and sectarian attitudes in postwar Lebanon', *Journal of Ethnic and Migration Studies*, 28: 291–306.

Hagland, C. (2009) *Getting to Grips with Asperger Syndrome: understanding adults on the autism spectrum*, London: Jessica Kingsley.

Hair, H.J. and O'Donoghue, K. (2009) 'Culturally relevant, socially just social work supervision: becoming visible through a social constructionist lens', *Journal of Ethnic and Cultural Diversity in Social Work*, 18: 70–88.

Haldeman, D. (2004) 'When sexual and religious orientation collide: considerations in working with conflicted same-sex attracted male clients', *The Counseling Psychologist*, 32: 691–715.

Happell, B. and Roper, C. (2003) 'The role of a mental health consumer in the education of postgraduate psychiatric nursing students: the students' evaluation', *Journal of Psychiatric and Mental Health Nursing*, 10: 343–50.

Harcourt, C. and Donovan, B. (2005) 'The many faces of sex work', *Sexually Transmitted Infections*, 81: 201–6.

Harcourt, C., van Beek, I., Heslop, J., McMahon, M. and Donovan, B. (2001) 'The health and welfare needs of female and transgender sex workers in New South Wales', *Australian and New Zealand Journal of Public Health*, 25: 84–9.

Harcourt, C., Egger, S. and Donovan, B. (2005) 'Sex work and the law', *Sexual Health*, 2: 121–8.

Hardy, R., Lawlor, D.A., Black, S., Wadsworth, M.E.J. and Kuh, D. (2007) 'Number of children and coronary heart disease risk factors in men and women from a British birth cohort', *British Journal of Obstetrics and Gynaecology*, 114: 721–30.

Harris Helm, J. and Beneke, S. (2003) *The Power of Projects: meeting contemporary challenges in early childhood classrooms – strategies and solutions*, New York: Teachers College Press.

Harris, M.A., Nilan, P.M. and Kirby, E.R. (2010) 'Risk and risk management for Australian sex workers', *Qualitative Health Research*, 21: 386–98.

Harris, P. (1994) 'Understanding pretence', in C. Lewis and P. Mitchell (eds) *Children's Early Understanding of Mind: origins and development*. Hillsdale, NJ: Lawrence Erlbaum Associates.

Hartmann, E. (2001) 'Understandings of information literacy: the perceptions of first year undergraduate students at the University of Ballarat', *Australian Academic and Research Libraries*, 32: 110–22.

Hasson, F., Keeney, S. and McKenna, H. (2000) 'Research guidelines for the Delphi survey technique', *Journal of Advanced Nursing*, 32: 1008–15.

Hassouneh, D., Alcala-Moss, A. and McNeff, E. (2011) 'Practical strategies for promoting full inclusion of individuals with disabilities in community-based participatory intervention research', *Research in Nursing and Health*, 34: 253–65.

Hawes, D.J. and Dadds, M.R. (2004) 'Australian data and psychometric properties of the Strengths and Difficulties Questionnaire', *Australian and New Zealand Journal of Psychiatry*, 38: 644–51.

Hawkes, S., Collumbien, M., Platt, L., Lalji, N., Rizvi, N., Andreasen A., Chow, J., Muzaffar, R., ur-Rehman, H., Siddiqui, N., Hasan, S. and Bokhari, A. (2009) 'HIV and other sexually transmitted infections among men, transgenders and women sell-ing sex in two cities in Pakistan: a cross-sectional prevalence survey', *Sexually Transmitted Infections*; 85: ii8–16.

Hawthorne, G., Richardson, J. and Osborne, R. (1999) 'The Assessment of Quality of Life (AQoL) instrument: a psychometric measure of health related quality of life', *Quality of Life Research*, 8: 209–24.

Hayashi, K., Fairbairn, N., Suwannawong, P., Kaplan, K., Wood, E. and Kerr, T. (2012) 'Collective empowerment while creating knowledge: a description of a community-based participatory research project with drug users in Bangkok, Thailand', *Substance Use and Misuse*, 47: 502–10.

Health Protection Agency (2010) *Survey of Prevalent HIV Infections Diagnosed (SOPHID) Data Tables 2010*, London: Centre for Infections, Health Protection Agency. Online. Available HTTP: <www.hpa.org.uk/webc/HPAwebFile/HPAweb_C/1221482342808> (accessed 18 March 2013).

Health Protection Agency (2012) *United Kingdom New HIV Diagnoses to end of June 2012*, London: HIV/STI Department, Health Protection Agency. Online. Available HTTP: <www.hpa.org.uk/webc/HPAwebFile/HPAweb_C/12379720242135> (accessed 18 March 2013).

Heard, G. (2006) 'Pronatalism under Howard', *People and Place*, 14: 12–25.

Hedges, F. (2005) *An Introduction to Systemic Therapy with Individuals: a social constructivist approach*, Basingstoke: Palgrave Macmillan.

HELEM (2013) Home page. Online. Available HTTP: <http://www.helem.net> (accessed 18 March 2013).

Henderson, S., Kendall, E. and See, L. (2011) 'The effectiveness of culturally appropriate interventions to manage or prevent chronic disease in culturally and linguistically diverse communities: a systematic literature review', *Health and Social Care in the Community*, 19: 225–49.

Henry, J., Sloane, M. and Black-Pond, C. (2007) 'Neurobiology and neurodevelopmental impact of childhood traumatic stress and prenatal alcohol exposure', *Language, Speech and Health Services in Schools*, 38: 99–108.

Hernandez-Medina, E. (2010) 'Social inclusion through participation: the case of the participatory budget in São Paulo', *International Journal of Urban and Regional Research*, 34: 512–32.

Hickey, S. and Mohan, G. (eds) (2005) *Participation: from tyranny to transformation? Exploring new approaches to participation in development*, London: Zed Books.

Hickie, I., Groom, G., McGorry, P., Davenport, T. and Luscombe, A. (2005) 'Australian mental health reform: time for real outcomes', *Medical Journal of Australia*, 182: 401–6.

Hillock, S. (2012) 'Conceptualisations and experiences of oppression: gender differences', *Affilia*, 27: 38–50.

Hines, J.M. (2012) 'Using an anti-oppressive framework in social work practice with lesbians', *Journal of Gay and Lesbian Social Services*, 24: 23–39.

Hitch, D., Larkin, H., Watchorn, V. and Ang, S. (2011) 'Community mobility in the context of universal design: interprofessional collaboration and education', *Australian Occupational Therapy Journal*, 59 (5): 375–83.

HMG (2000) *The NHS Plan: a plan for investment, a plan for reform*, London: HMSO.

HMG (2001) *Health and Social Care Act 2001*, London: HMSO.

HMG (2002) *National Health Service Reform and Health Care Professions Act 2002*, London: HMSO.

HMG (2007) *The Equality Act (Sexual Orientation) Regulations 2007*. Online. Available

HTTP: <http://www.legislation.gov.uk/uksi/2007/1263/contents/made> (accessed 18 March 2013).

Hoem, J.M., Neyer, G. and Andersson, G. (2006) 'Education and childlessness: the relationship between educational field, educational level, and childlessness among Swedish women born in 1955–59', *Demographic Research*, 14: 331–80.

Hoeyer, K., Dahlager, L. and Lynöe, N. (2005) 'Conflicting notions of research ethics: the mutually challenging traditions of social scientists and medical researchers', *Social Science and Medicine*, 61: 1741–9.

Holdcroft, A. (2007) 'Gender bias in medical research: how does it affect evidence-based medicine?', *Journal of the Royal Society of Medicine*, 100: 2–3.

Holland, J., Ruedin, L., Scott-Villiers, P. and Sheppard, H. (2012) 'Tackling the governance of socially inclusive service delivery', *Public Management Review*, 14: 181–96.

Holloway, R., Shonasimova, S., Ngari, M. and Chiaji, A. (2009) 'Lessons from the work of the Aga Khan Foundation in promoting good local governance in Tajiki-stan, Kenya and Tanzania', in C. Malena (ed.) *From Political Won't to Political Will: building support for participatory governance*, Sterling, VA: Kumarian Press.

Holton, S., Fisher, J. and Rowe, H. (2010) 'Motherhood: is it good for women's men-tal health?', *Journal of Reproductive and Infant Psychology*, 28: 223–39.

Hong, G. (1998) 'Logistics and researchers as legitimate tools for "doing" intercultural research: a rejoinder to Günther', *Culture and Psychology*, 4: 81–90.

Hong, Y., Fang, X., Li, X., Liu, Y., Li, M. and Tai-Seale, T. (2010) 'Self-perceived stigma, depressive symptoms and suicidal behaviours among female sex workers in China', *Journal of Transcultural Nursing*, 21: 29–34.

Horowitz, C.R., Robinson, M. and Seifer, S. (2009) 'Community-based participatory research from the margin to the mainstream: are researchers prepared?', *Circulation*, 119: 2633–42.

Howard, B., Cohn, E. and Orsmond, G. L. (2006) 'Understanding and negotiating friendships: perspectives from an adolescent with Asperger syndrome', *Autism*, 10: 619–27.

Howard, C. (2007) *Contested Individualization: debates about contemporary personhood*, New York: Palgrave Macmillan.

Huang, H. and Coker, A. (2010) 'Examining issues affecting African American partici-pation in research studies', *Journal of Black Studies*, 40: 619–36.

Hubbard, G., Kidd, L., Donaghy, E., McDonald, C. and Kearney, N. (2007) 'A review of literature about involving people affected by cancer in research, policy and plan-ning and practice', *Patient Education and Counselling*, 65: 21–33.

Hudson, K.D. (2012) 'Bordering community: reclaiming ambiguity as a transgressive landscape of knowledge', *Affilia*, 27: 167–79.

Hughes, C. and Leekam, S. (2004) 'What are the links between theory of mind and social relations? Review, reflections and new directions for studies of typical and atypical development', *Social Development*, 13: 590–619.

Hull, N.E.H. (2010) *Roe v. Wade: the abortion rights controversy in American history,* 2nd edn, Lawrence, KS: University Press of Kansas.

Huntington, I. and Robinson, W. (2007) 'The many ways of saying yes and no: reflec-tions on the research coordinator's role in recruiting research participants and obtain-ing informed consent', *Ethics and Human Research*, 29 (3): 6–10.

IASSW and IFSW (2004) *Global Standards for the Education and Training of the Social Work Profession*, International Association of Schools of Social Work and International

Federation of Social Work. Online. Available HTTP: <http://www.ifsw.org/cm_data/GlobalSocialWorkStandards2005.pdf> (accessed 18 March 2013).

Ife, J. (2002) *Community Development: community-based alternatives in an age of globalisation*, Frenchs Forest, New South Wales: Pearson Education.

Illingworth, K., Knight, T., Pollock, S. and Durham, J. (2009) *Mental Health in the Independently Living Elderly and the Role of Volunteer Befriending: evaluation of the Wesley Do Care program*, Melbourne: School of Psychology, Deakin University for Wesley Do Care.

ISO (2007) *ISO 9999 Assistive products for persons with disability: classification and terminology*, Geneva: International Organisation for Standardization.

Israel, B.A., Schulz, A.J., Parker, E.A. and Becker, A.B. (1998) 'Review of community-based research: assessing partnership approaches to improve public health', *Annual Review of Public Health*, 19: 173–202.

Israel, B.A., Eng, E., Schulz, A.J. and Parker, E.A. (2005) 'Introduction to methods in community-based participatory research for health', in B.A. Israel, E. Eng, A.J. Schulz and E.A. Parker (eds) *Methods in Community-Based Participatory Research for Health*, San Francisco, CA: Jossey-Bass.

Israel, B.A., Coombe, C.M., Cheezum, R.R., Schulz, A.J., McGranaghan, R.J., Lichtenstein, R., Reyes, A.G., Clement, J., and Burris, A. (2010) 'Community-based participatory research: a capacity-building approach for policy advocacy aimed at eliminating health disparities', *American Journal of Public Health*, 100: 2094–102.

Itzin, C., Taket, A. and Barter-Godfrey, S. (2010a) *Domestic and Sexual Violence and Abuse: tackling the health and mental health effects*, London: Routledge.

Itzin, C., Taket, A. and Barter-Godfrey, S. (2010b) *Domestic and Sexual Violence and Abuse: findings from a Delphi expert consultation on therapeutic and treatment interventions with victims survivors and abusers, children adolescents and adults*, Melbourne: Deakin University. Online. Available HTTP: <http://www.dh.gov.uk/en/Publicationsandstatistics/Publications/PublicationsPolicyAndGuidance/DH_123971> (accessed 18 March 2013).

Jacklin, A. and Le Riche, P. (2009) 'Reconceptualising student support: From "support" to "supportive"', *Studies in Higher Education*, 34: 735–49.

Jackson, M., Hardy, G., Persson, P. and Holland, S. (2011) *Acquired brain injury in the Victorian prison system*, Corrections Research Paper Series No. 4. Online. Available HTTP: <http://www.justice.vic.gov.au/home/prisons/research+and+statistics/acquired+brain+injury+in+the+victorian+prison+system> (accessed 18 March 2013).

Jacquez, F., Vaughn, L.M. and Wagner, E. (2012) 'Youth as partners, participants or passive recipients: a review of children and adolescents in community-based participatory research (CBPR)', *American Journal of Community Psychology*, DOI: 10.1007/s10464–012–9533–7.

Jaffe, D., Eisenbach, Z. and Manor, O. (2011) The effect of parity on cause-specific mortality among married men and women, *Maternal and Child Health Journal*, 15: 376–85.

Janzen, R., Nelson, G., Trainor, J. and Ochocka, J. (2006) 'A longitudinal study of mental health consumer/survivor initiatives: part 4 – benefits beyond the self? A quantitative and qualitative study of system-level activities and impacts', *Journal of Community Psychology*, 34: 285–303.

Jarrold, C., Boucher, J. and Smith, P. (1993) 'Symbolic play in autism: a review', *Journal of Autism and Developmental Disorders*, 23: 281–307.

Jeal, N. and Salisbury, C. (2004) 'Self-reported experiences of health services among female street-based prostitutes: a cross sectional study', *British Journal of General Practice*, 54: 515–9.

Jiménez, J., Puig, M., Sala, A.C., Ramos, C.J., Castro, E., Morales, M., Santiago, L. and Zorrilla, C. (2011) 'Felt stigma in injection drug users and sex workers: focus group research with HIV-risk populations in Puerto Rico', *Qualitative Research in Psychology*, 8: 26–39.

Johanson, R., Newborn, M. and Macfarlane, A. (2002) 'Has the medicalisation of childbirth gone too far?', *British Medical Journal*, 324: 892–5.

Johner, R. and Maslany, G. (2011) 'Paving a path to inclusion', *Journal of Community Health*, 36: 150–7.

Johnstone, M.J. (2007) 'Research ethics, reconciliation, and strengthening the research relationship in Indigenous health domains: an Australian perspective', *International Journal of Intercultural Relations*, 31: 391–406.

Johnstone, P. (1996) 'Aboriginal health: a discussion of some current issues', *Australian Health Review*, 19 (4): 43–54.

Jones, A. and May, J. (1992) *Working in Human Service Organisations: a critical introduction*, Melbourne: Longman Cheshire.

Jones, H. (2009) *Equity in Development: why it is important and how to achieve it*, London: Overseas Development Institute.

Jones, J. (1981) *Bad Blood: the Tuskegee syphilis experiment – a tragedy of race and medicine*, New York: The Free Press.

Jones, P.S. (2003) 'Urban regeneration's poisoned chalice: is there an impasse in (community) participation-based policy?', *Urban Studies*, 40 (3): 581–601.

Jones, S. (2012) 'Working with immigrant clients: perils and possibilities', *Families in Society*, 93: 47–53.

Jonsson, U. (2003) *Human Rights Approach to Development Programming*, Nairobi: UNICEF.

Jørgensen, M.B. (2011) 'Understanding the research–policy nexus in Denmark and Sweden: the field of migration and integration', *British Journal of Politics and International Relations*, 13 (1): 93–109.

Joseph, S. (1997) 'The public/private – the imagined boundary in the imagined nation/ state/community: the Lebanese case', *Feminist Review*, 57: 73–92.

Justice, L. and Pullen, P. (2003) 'Promising interventions for promoting emergent literacy skills: three evidence based approaches', *Topics in Early Childhood Special Education*, 23: 99–113.

Kabakian-Khasholian, T., Campbell, O., Shediac-Rizkallah, M. and Ghorayeb, F. (2000) 'Women's experiences of maternity care: satisfaction or passivity?', *Social Science and Medicine*, 51: 103–13.

Kane, L. (2001) *Popular Education and Social Change in Latin America*, London: Latin American Bureau.

Kaplan-Myrth, N. (2005) 'Sorry Mates: reconciliation and self-determination in Australian aboriginal health', *Human Rights Review*, 6 (4): 69–83.

Katz, D.L., Murimi, M., Gonzalez, A., Njike, V. and Green, L.W. (2011) 'From controlled trial to community adoption: the multi-site translational community trial', *American Journal of Public Health*, 101 (8): e17–27.

Keene, J. (2001) *Clients with Complex Needs: interprofessional practice*, Oxford: Blackwell Science.

Kellogg Foundation (2004) *Logic Model Development Guide*, Battle Creek, MI: W.K. Kellogg Foundation.

Kelly, J. (2006) 'Is it Aboriginal friendly? Searching for ways of working in research and practice that support Aboriginal women', *Contemporary Nurse: Healthcare across the Lifespan*, 22: 317–326.

Kemeny, M.E., Arnold, R. and Marge, M. (2011) 'I can do it, you can do it: a community development approach to health promotion for individuals with disabilities', *Community Development*, 42: 137–51.

Kendall, E., Sunderland, N., Barnett, L., Nalder, G. and Matthews, C. (2011) 'Beyond the rhetoric of participatory research in Indigenous communities', *Qualitative Health Research*, 21: 1719–28.

Kendig, H., Dykstra, P., Van Gaalen, R. and Melkas, T. (2007) 'Health of aging parents and childless individuals', *Journal of Family Issues*, 28: 1457–86.

Kennard, B.D., Clarke, G.N., Weersing, V.R., Asarnow, J.R., Shamseddeen, W., Porta, G., Berk, M., Hughes, J.L., Spirito, A., Emslie, G.J., Keller, M.B., Wagner, K.D. and Brent, D.A. (2009) 'Effective components of TORDIA cognitive–behavioral therapy for adolescent depression: preliminary findings', *Journal of Consulting and Clinical Psychology*, 77: 1033–41.

Kennedy, G., Judd, T., Churchward, A., Gray, K. and Krause, K. (2008) 'First year students' experiences with technology: are they really digital natives?', *Australasian Journal of Educational Technology*, 24: 108–22.

Khalaf, S. (2001) *Cultural Resistance: global and local encounters in the Middle East*, London: Saqi Books.

Kildea, S., Barclay, L., Wardaguga, M. and Dawumal, M. (2009) 'Participative research in a remote Australian Aboriginal setting', *Action Research*, 7: 143–63.

Kiltzman, R. (2006) 'Complications of culture in obtaining informed consent', *The American Journal of Bioethics*, 6: 20–1.

Kimberley, H. and Simons, B. (2009) *The Brotherhood's Social Barometer: living the second fifty years*, Fitzroy, Victoria: Brotherhood of St Laurence.

Kimberlin, S. (2009) 'Political science theory and disability', *Journal of Human Behavior in the Social Environment*, 19: 26–43.

King, A. (2011) 'Service user involvement in methadone maintenance programmes: the "philosophy, the ideal and the reality"', *Drugs: Education, Prevention, and Policy*, 18: 276–84.

Kingsnorth, S., Gall, C., Beayni, S. and Rigby, P. (2011) 'Parents as transition experts? Qualitative findings from a pilot parent-led peer support group', *Child: Care, Health and Development*, 37: 833–40.

Kitchin, R. (1998) 'Out of place, knowing one's place: space, power and the exclusion of disabled people', *Disability and Society*, 13: 343–56.

Klasen, S. (n.d.), *Social Exclusion, Children, and Education: conceptual and measurement issues*, Department of Economics, University of Munich. Online. Available HTTP: <http://www.oecd.org/dataoecd/19/37/1855901.pdf> (accessed 18 March 2013).

Klein, H. (2004) 'Health inequality, social exclusion and neighbourhood renewal: can place-based renewal improve the health of disadvantaged communities', *Australian Journal of Primary Health*, 10 (3): 110–9.

Kligerman, N. (2007) 'Homosexuality in Islam: a difficult paradox', *Macalester Islam Journal*, 2 (3): 53–64.

Klin, A, Volkmar, F.R. and Sparrow, S.S. (2000) *Asperger Syndrome*, New York: The Guilford Press.

Knapp, M.L.G. (2009) *Aging in Place in Suburbia: a qualitative study of older women*, Unpublished PhD thesis, Antioch University New England, USA.

Koropeckyj-Cox, T. (1998) 'Loneliness and depression in middle and old age: are childless more vulnerable?', *Journal of Gerontology: Social Sciences*, 53B: S303–11.

Koster, R., Baccar, K. and Lemelin, R.H. (2012) 'Moving from research ON, to research WITH and FOR indigenous communities: a critical reflection on community-based participatory research', *Canadian Geographer*, 56: 195–210.

KPMG (2006) *Final Report of the Review of the Aids and Equipment Program*, Melbourne: KPMG.

Krause, K.L., Hartley, R., James, R. and McInnis, C. (2005) *The First Year Experience in Australian Universities: findings from a decade of studies*, Canberra: Department of Education, Science and Training.

Krieger, N. (1999) 'Embodying inequality: a review of concepts, measures, and methods for studying health consequences of discrimination', *International Journal of Health Services: Planning, Administration, Evaluation*, 29: 295–352.

Kubitskey, B.W., Vath, R.J., Johnson, H.J., Fishman, B.J. Konstantopoulos, S. and Park, G.J. (2012) 'Examining study attrition: implications for experimental research on professional development', *Teaching and Teacher Education*, 28: 418–27.

Kulkin, H., Chauvin, E. and Percle, G. (2000) 'Suicide among gay and lesbian adolescents and young adults', *Journal of Homosexuality*, 40: 1–29.

Kunz, P.A. (2009) *Social Experiences of Adolescents with High Functioning Autism and/or Asperger's Syndrome – their perceptions and the views of their caregivers: an exploratory study*, Chicago, IL: Loyola University.

Kurtz, S.P., Surratt, H.L., Kiley, M.C. and Inciardi, J.A. (2005) 'Barriers to health and social services for street-based sex workers', *Journal of Health Care for the Poor and Underserved*, 16: 345–61.

Kwon, S., Rideout, C., Tseng, W., Islam, N., Cook, W.K., Ro, M. and Trinh-Shevrin, C. (2012) 'Developing the community empowered research training program: building research capacity for community-initiated and community-driven research', *Progress in Community Health Partnerships*, 6: 43–52.

Lather, P. (1986) 'Issues of validity in openly ideological research: between a rock and a soft place', *Interchange*, 17 (4): 63–84.

Laurakeet, S. (2011) *Your Fee-Fees End Where my Body Begins*. Online. Available HTTP: <http://shakespearessister.blogspot.com/2011/04/your-fee-fees-end-where-my-body-begins.html> (accessed 18 March 2013).

Lavalette, M. and Mooney, G. (2000) *Class Struggle and Social Welfare*, London: Routledge.

Lawlor, D.A., Emberson, J.R., Ebrahim, S., Whincup, P.H., Wannamethee, S.G., Walker, M. and Smith, G.D. (2003) 'Is the association between parity and coronary heart disease due to biological effects of pregnancy or adverse lifestyle risk factors associated with child-rearing? Findings from the British Women's Heart and Health Study and the British Regional Heart Study', *Circulation*, 107: 1260–4.

Lawrence, J. (2002) 'The "deficit discourse" shift: university teachers and their role in helping first year students persevere and succeed in the new university culture', Paper presented at *6th Pacific Rim, First Year in Higher Education Conference*, 8–10 July 2002. Online. Available HTTP: <http://www.fyhe.com.au/past_papers/abstracts02/LawrenceAbstract.htm> (accessed 18 March 2013).

Lawson, W. (2006) 'Typical development, learning styles, single attention and associated cognition in autism (SAACA)', *Good Practice in Autism*, 7: 61–70.

Lawson, W. (2010) *The Passionate Mind: how people with autism learn*. London: Jessica Kingsley.

Layton, N. and Wilson, E. (2010) *The Equipment Study*, Melbourne: Deakin University.

Layton, N., Wilson, E., Colgan, S., Moodie, M. and Carter, R. (2010) *The Equipping Inclusion Studies: Assistive Technology Use and Outcomes in Victoria*, Melbourne: Deakin University.

Learmonth, E. (2010) *Sense of Community of Older People (Service Users of Wesley Mission)*, Unpublished Honours thesis, School of Health and Social Development, Deakin University, Australia.

Learmonth, E., Taket, A. and Hanna, L. (2012) 'Ways in which 'community' benefits frail older women's wellbeing: "… we are much happier when we feel we belong"', *Australasian Journal on Ageing*, 31 (1): 60–3.

Leathwood, C. and O'Connell, P. (2003) '"It's a struggle": the construction of the "new student" in higher education', *Journal of Education Policy*, 18: 597–615.

Lee, D., Binger, A., Hocking, J. and Fairley, C. (2005) 'The incidence of sexually transmitted infections among frequently screened sex workers in a decriminalized and regulated system in Melbourne', *Sexually Transmitted Infections*, 81: 434–6.

Lehmann, W. (2007) '"I just didn't feel like I fit in": the role of habitus in university drop-out decisions', *The Canadian Journal of Higher Education*, 37: 89–110.

Leiter, V. (2011) 'Bowling together: foundations of community among youth with a disability', in R.K. Scotch, A.C. Carey, S.N. Barnartt and B.M. Altman (eds) *Disability and Community: research in social science and disability*, Volume 6, Bingley: Emerald Group Publishing.

Letherby, G. (1999) 'Other than mother and mothers as others: the experience of motherhood and non-motherhood in relation to "infertility" and "involuntary childlessness"', *Women's Studies International Forum*, 22: 359–72.

Leung, T.T.F. (2008) 'Accountability to welfare service users: challenges and responses of service providers', *British Journal of Social Work*, 38: 531–45.

Levin, E. (2004) *Involving Service Users and Carers in Social Work Education*, Bristol: Policy Press.

Levine, P. (1994) 'Venereal disease, prostitution and the politics of empire: The case of British India', *Journal of the History of Sexuality*, 4: 579–602.

Levitas, R., Pantazis, C., Fahmy, E., Gordon, D., Lloyd, E. and Patsios, D. (2007) *The Multi-Dimensional Analysis of Social Exclusion*, Bristol: Department of Sociology and School for Social Policy, University of Bristol.

Lewis, F.M. and Murdoch, B.E. (2011) 'Language function in a child following mild traumatic brain injury: evidence from pre-and post-injury language testing', *Developmental Neurorehabilitation*, 14: 348–54.

Liamputtong, P. (2007) *Researching the Vulnerable: a guide to sensitive research methods*, London: Sage Publications.

Liamputtong, P. (2013) *Qualitative Research Methods*, 4th edn, Melbourne: Oxford University Press.

Liamputtong, P. and Kitisriworapan, S. (2012) 'Deviance, difference and stigma as social determinants of health', in P. Liamputtong, R. Fanany and G. Verrinder (eds) *Health, Illness and Well-being: perspectives and social determinants*, Melbourne: Oxford University Press.

Lincoln, Y.S. and Tierney, W.G. (2004) 'Qualitative research and Institutional Review Boards', *Qualitative Inquiry*, 10: 219–34.

Lindsey, E.W. and Colwell, M.J. (2003) 'Preschoolers' emotional competence: links to pretend and physical play', *Child Study Journal*, 33: 39–52.

Linhart, Y., Shohat, T., Amitai, Z., Gefen, D., Srugo, I., Blumstein, G. and Dan, M. (2008) 'Sexually transmitted infections among brothel-based sex workers in Tel-Aviv area, Israel: high prevalence of pharyngeal gonorrhoea', *International Journal of STD and AIDS*, 19: 656–9.

Litva, A., Canvin, K., Shepherd, M., Jacoby, A. and Gabbay, M. (2009) 'Lay perceptions of the desired role and type of user involvement in clinical governance', *Health Expectations*, 12: 81–91.

Lloyd, C.E, Johnson, M.R.D., Mughal, S., Sturt, J.A, Collins, G.S, Roy, T., Bibi, R. and Barnett, A.H. (2008) 'Securing recruitment and obtaining informed consent in minority ethnic groups in the UK', *BMC Health Services Research*, 8 (68). Online. Available HTTP: <http://www.biomedcentral.com/1472-6963/8/68> (accessed 18 March 2013).

Loff, B., Gaze, B. and Fairley, C. (2000) 'Prostitution, public health, and human rights law', *The Lancet*, 356: 1764.

Lorenzo,T. (2008) '"We are also travellers": an action story about disabled women mobilising for an accessible public transport system in Khayelitsha and Nyanga, Cape Metropole, South Africa', *South African Journal of Occupational Therapy*, 38 (1): 32–40.

Lorway, R., Reza-Paul, S. and Pasha, A. (2009) 'On becoming a male sex worker in Mysore: sexual subjectivity, "empowerment", and community-based HIV prevention research', *Medical Anthropology Quarterly*, 23: 142–60.

Lowman, J. (2000) 'Violence and the outlaw status of (street) based prostitution in Canada', *Violence Against Women*, 6: 987–1011.

Lui, C.W., Everingham, J.A., Warburton, J., Cuthill, M. and Bartlett, H. (2009) 'What makes a community age-friendly: a review of international literature', *Australasian Journal on Ageing*, 28: 116–21.

Lutz, B. and Bowers, B. (2005) 'Disability in everyday life', *Qualitative Health Research*, 15: 1037–54.

McCalman, J., Smith, L., Anderson, I., Morley, R. and Mishra, G. (2009) 'Colonialism and the health transition: aboriginal Australians and poor whites compared, Victoria, 1850–1985', *The History of The Family*, 14: 253–65.

McClimens, A. (2008) 'This is my truth, tell me yours: exploring the internal tensions within collaborative learning disability research', *British Journal of Learning Disabilities*, 36: 271–6.

MacColl, E. (1949) *Dirty Old Town*, Vanguard VS-9110. Online. Available HTTP: <http://www.wirz.de/music/washfrm.htm> (accessed 18 March 2013).

McCormack, C. and Collins, B (2010) 'Can disability studies contribute to client centred occupational therapy practice?', *British Journal of Occupational Therapy*, 73: 339–42.

McCrady, B. and Bux, D. (1999) 'Ethical issues in informed consent with substance abusers', *Journal of Consulting and Clinical Psychology*, 67: 186–93.

McCullough, L., McGuire, A. and Whitney, S. (2007) 'Consent: informed, simple, implied and presumed', *The American Journal of Bioethics*, 7 (12): 49–50.

McCune L. (1995) 'A normative study of representational play at the transition to language', *Child Development*, 31: 198–206.

MacDonald, S. and Wiseman-Hakes, C. (2010) 'Knowledge translation in ABI rehabilitation: a model for consolidating and applying the evidence for cognitive-communication interventions', *Brain Injury*, 24: 486–508.

McEwan, M. (2007) *MREWYB*. Online. Available HTTP: <http://shakespearessister.blogspot.com/2007/03/mrewyb.html> (accessed 18 March 2013).

McEwan, M. (2011) *Feminism 101: helpful hints for dudes, part 2*. Online. Available HTTP: <http://shakespearessister.blogspot.com/2011/02/feminism-101-helpful-hints-for-dudes_15.html> (accessed 18 March 2013).

McGee, C.L., Bhorkquist, O.A., Price, J.M., Mattson, S.N. and Riley, E.P. (2009) 'Social information processing skills in children with histories of heavy prenatal alcohol exposure', *Journal of Abnormal Child Psychology*, 37: 817–30.

McGrath, M. (1989) 'Consumer participation in service planning – the AWS experience', *Journal of Social Policy*, 18: 67–89.

McKenna, S.A., Iwasaki, P.G., Stewart, T. and Main, D.S. (2011) 'Key informants and community members in community-based participatory research: one is not like the other', *Progress in Community Health Partnerships*, 5: 387–97.

Mckeown, M., Malihi-Shoja, L., Hogarth, R., Jones, F., Holt, K., Sullivan, P., Lunt, J., Vella, J., Hough, G., Rawcliffe, L. and Mather, M. (2012) 'The value of involvement from the perspective of service users and carers engaged in practitioner education: not just a cash nexus', *Nurse Education Today*, 32: 178–84.

McLaughlin, K. (2005) 'From ridicule to institutionalisation: anti-oppression, the state and social work', *Critical Social Policy*, 25: 283–305.

McLaughlin, H. (2009) 'What's in a name: "Client", "Patient", "Customer", "Consumer", "Expert by Experience", "Service User" – what's next?', *British Journal of Social Work*, 39: 1101–17.

McLean, S.A.M (2010) *Autonomy, Consent and the Law*. London: Routledge-Cavendish.

MacLeavy, J. (2009) ' (Re) analysing community empowerment: Rationalities and technologies of government in Bristol's new deal for communities', *Urban Studies*, 46 (4): 849–75.

McMichael, C. and Manderson, L. (2004) 'Somali women and well-being: social networks and social capital among immigrant women in Australia', *Human Organization*, 63: 88–99.

McMillan, F.V., Browne, N., Green, S. and Donnelly, D. (2009) 'A card before you leave: participation and mental health in Northern Ireland', *Health and Human Rights*, 11 (1): 61–72.

Macpherson, S. (2008) 'Reaching the top of the ladder? Locating the voices of excluded young people within the participation debate', *Policy and Politics*, 36, 361–79.

Magalhaes, M.G. (2007) 'Comorbidities in older patients with HIV: a retrospective study', *Journal of the American Dental Association*, 138: 1468–75.

Maginn, P.J. (2007) 'Towards more effective community participation in urban regeneration: the potential of collaborative planning and applied ethnography', *Qualitative Research*, 7: 25–43.

Mahood, L. and Littlewood, B. (1994) 'The "vicious" girl and the "street-corner" boy: sexuality and the gendered delinquent in the Scottish child-saving movement 1850–1940', *Journal of the History of Sexuality*, 4: 549–78.

Maidment, J. and Macfarlane, S. (2011) 'Crafting communities: promoting inclusion, empowerment, and learning between older women', *Australian Social Work*, 64: 283–98.

Malena, C. (2009) 'Participatory governance: where there is lack of will, is there a way?', in C. Malena (ed.) *From Political Won't to Political Will: building support for participatory governance*, Sterling, VA: Kumarian Press.

Manderson, L. (2010) 'Social capital and inclusion: locating wellbeing in the community', *Australian Cultural History*, 28: 233–52.

Månsson, S.-A. and Hedin, U.-C. (1999) 'Breaking the Matthew effect – on women leaving prostitution', *International Journal of Social Welfare*, 8: 67–77.

Manthorpe, J., Moriarty, J., Hussein, S., Sharpe, E., Stevens, M., Orme, J., MacIntyre, G., Green Lister, P. and Crisp, B.R. (2010) 'Changes to admissions work arising from the new social work degree in England', *Social Work Education*, 29: 704–14.

Marcham, A. J. (1971) 'A question of conscience: the church and the "conscience clause" 1860–70', *Journal of Ecclesiastical History*, 22: 237–49.

Marmot, M. (2004) *Status Syndrome: how your social standing directly affects your health*, London: Bloomsbury.

Marmot, M. (2011) 'Social determinants and the health of Indigenous Australians', *Medical Journal of Australia*, 194: 512–3.

MARSA (2011) *Marsa Sexual Health Center Beirut Lebanon*. Online. Available HTTP: <http://www.youtube.com/watch?v=PKQJcbokBaw> (accessed 18 March 2013).

MARSA (2013) *Home page*. Online. Available HTTP: <http://www.marsa.me/> (accessed 18 March 2013).

Marsh, P. and Doel, M. (2005) *The Task-Centred Book*, London: Routledge.

Martin, S. (2004) 'Reconceptualising social exclusion: A critical response to the neo-liberal welfare reform agenda and the underclass thesis', *Australian Journal of Social Issues*, 39: 79–94.

Martina, C.M.S. and Stevens, N.L. (2006) 'Breaking the cycle of loneliness? Psychological effects of a friendship enrichment program for older women', *Aging and Mental Health*, 10: 467–75.

Martinez-Brawley, E.E. and Zorita, P.M.B. (2011) 'Immigration and social work: contrasting practice and education', *Social Work Education*, 30: 17–28.

Maryland Department of Health and Mental Hygiene (2009) *Baltimore City HIV/AIDS Epidemiological Profile Fourth Quarter 2009*. Online. Available HTTP: <http://ideha.dhmh.maryland.gov/chse/pdf/BaltimoreCityHIVEpiProfile12–2009.pdf> (accessed 18 March 2013).

Maslen, S. (2008) *Social Determinants of Women's Health and Wellbeing in the Australian Capital Territory*, Mawson, ACT: Women's Centre for Health Matters.

Mason, S. (2005) 'Offering African Americans opportunities to participate in clinical trials research: how social workers can help', *Health and Social Work*, 30: 296–304.

Massad, J. (2002) 'Re-orienting desire: the gay international and the Arab world' *Public Culture*, 14: 361–85.

Mayhew, S., Collumbien, M., Qureshi, A., Platt, L., Rafiq N., Faisel, A., Lalji, N. and Hawkes, S. (2009) 'Protecting the unprotected: mixed-methods research on drug use, sex work and rights in Pakistan's fight against HIV/AIDS', *Sexually Transmitted Infections*, 85: ii31–6.

Mayo, M. and Rooke, A. (2006) *Active Learning for Active Citizenship: an evaluation report*, London: Togetherwecan.

Maziak, W. (2009) 'The crisis of health in a crisis ridden region', *International Journal of Public Health*, 54: 349–55.

Megret, F. (2008) 'The Disabilities Convention: towards an holistic concept of rights', *The International Journal of Human Rights*, 12: 261–77.

Meyrick, J.D. (2003) 'The Delphi method and health research', *Health Education*, 103: 7–16.

Michaelson, M. T. (2008) 'Inclusion and social justice for gay, lesbian, bisexual, and transgender members of the learning community in Queensland state schools' *Australian Journal of Guidance and Counselling*, 18: 76–83.

Michigan Department of Community Health (2007) *Profiles of Genesee County Health Department, 2007.* Lansing, Michigan: Michigan Department of Community Health.

Middleton, P., Stanton, P. and Renouf, N. (2004) 'Consumer consultants in mental health services: addressing the challenges', *Journal of Mental Health*, 13: 507–18.

Milewa, T., Dowswell, G. and Harrison, S. (2002) 'Partnership, power and the "new" politics of community participation in British health care', *Social Policy and Administration*, 36: 796–809.

Mill, J.S. (1858/1991) 'On Liberty', in *On Liberty and Other Essays*, Oxford: Oxford University Press.

Miller, T. and Bell, L. (2002) 'Consenting to what? Issues of access, gatekeeping and "informed consent"', in M. Mauthnre, M. Birch, J. Jessop and T. Miller (eds) *Ethics in Qualitative Research*, London: Sage.

Miller, T. and Boulton, M. (2007) 'Changing constructions of informed consent: qualitative research and complex social worlds', *Social Science and Medicine*, 65: 2199–211.

Miller, V., VeneKlasen, L. and Clark, C. (2005) 'Rights-based development: linking rights and participation – challenges in thinking and action', *IDS Bulletin*, 36 (1): 31–40.

Milner, P. and Kelly, B. (2009) 'Community participation and inclusion: people with disabilities defining their place,' *Disability and Society*, 24: 47–62.

Minichiello, V., Mariño, R., Browne, J., Jamieson, M., Peterson, K., Reuter, B. and Robinson, K. (1999) 'A profile of the clients of male sex workers in three Australian cities', *Australian and New Zealand Journal of Public Health*, 23: 511–8.

Minkler, M. (2004) 'Ethical challenges for the "outside" researcher in community-based participatory research', *Health Education and Behavior*, 31: 684–97.

Minkler, M. (ed.) (2012) *Community Organizing and Community Building for Health and Welfare*, 3rd edn, New Brunswick, NJ: Rutgers University Press.

Minkler, M. and Wallerstein, N. (eds) (2008) *Community-Based Participatory Research for Health: from process to outcomes*, San Francisco, CA: Wiley.

Miranti, R., McNamara, J., Tanton, R. and Yap, M. (2009) 'A narrowing gap? Trends in childlessness of professional women in Australia 1986–2006', *Journal of Population Research*, 26: 359–79.

Mishtal, J. (2009) 'Matters of "conscience": the politics of reproductive healthcare in Poland', *Medical Anthropology Quarterly*, 23: 161–83.

Mistra, G., Mahal, A. and Shah, R. (2000) 'Protecting the rights of sex workers: the Indian experience', *Health and Human Rights*, 5: 88–115.

Mitchell, W., Franklin, A., Greco, V. and Bell, M. (2009) 'Working with children with learning disabilities and/or who communicate non-verbally: research experiences and their implications for social work education, increased participation and social inclusion', *Social Work Education*, 28: 309–24.

Mladenov, T. (2012) 'Personal assistance for disabled people and the understanding of human being', *Critical Social Policy*, 32: 242–61.

Mohammed, S.A., Walters, K.L., LaMarr, J., Evans-Campbell, T. and Fryberg, S. (2012) 'Finding middle ground: negotiating university and tribal community interests in community-based participatory research', *Nursing Inquiry*, 19: 116–27.

Mohan, G. (2001) 'Participatory development', in V. Desai and R. Potter, (eds) *The Arnold Companion to Development Studies*, London: Hodder.

Monash University. (2010) *AQoL-6D Population Norms.* Online. Available HTTP: <http://www.aqol.com.au/choice-of-an-instrument/56.html> (accessed 18 March 2013).

Mooney-Somers, J. and Maher, L. (2009) 'The Indigenous Resiliency Project: a worked example of community-based participatory research', *New South Wales Public Health Bulletin*, 20 (7–8): 112–8.

Moore, J., Hanna, L., Mutisya, T. (2011) *Women connecting*, Unpublished report, Burwood, Australia: School of Health and Social Development, Deakin University.

Moreau, M.-P. and Leathwood, C. (2006) 'Balancing paid work and studies: Working (-class) students in higher education', *Studies in Higher Education*, 31: 23–42.

Morgan, S. and Hemming, M. (1999) 'Balancing care and control: risk management and compulsory community treatment', *Mental Health and Learning Disabilities Care*, 21: 19–21.

Moriarty, J., MacIntyre, G., Manthorpe, J., Crisp, B.R., Orme, J., Green Lister, P., Cavanagh, K., Stevens, M., Hussein, S. and Sharpe, E. (2010) '"My expectations remain the same. The student has to be competent to practise": practice assessor perspectives on the new social work degree qualification in England', *British Journal of Social Work*, 40: 583–601.

Morse, J. (1995) 'The significance of saturation', *Qualitative Health Research*, 5: 147–9.

Mowbray, C., Moxley, D. and Collin, M.E. (1998) 'Consumers as mental health providers: first-person accounts of benefits and limitations', *Journal of Behavioral Health Services and Research*, 25: 397–412.

Moxley, D.P., Raider, M.C. and Cohen, S.N. (1989) 'Specifying and facilitating family involvement in services to persons with developmental disabilities', *Child and Adolescent Social Work*, 6: 301–12.

Mubyazi, G.M. and Hutton, G. (2012) 'Reality of community participation in health planning, resource allocation and service delivery: a review of the reviews, primary publications and grey literature', *Rwanda Journal of Health Sciences*, 1: 51–65.

Mulligan, M. (2006) *Creating Community Supplement: social profiles of local communities*, Melbourne: Global Institute, RMIT.

Mumvuma, T. (2009). Building political will for participatory budgeting in rural Zimbabwe: the case of Mutoko Rural District Council, in C. Malena (ed.) *From Political Won't to Political Will: building support for participatory governance*, Sterling, VA: Kumarian Press.

Munro, E. (2010) 'Learning to reduce risk in child protection', *British Journal of Social Work*, 40: 1135–51.

Murphy, E. and Dingwall, R. (2007) 'Informed consent, anticipatory regulation and ethnographic practice', *Social Science and Medicine*, 65: 2223–34.

Murray, D.M. (1998) *Design and Analysis of Group-Randomized Trials*, New York: Oxford University Press.

Murray, R. (2012) 'Sixth Sense: the disabled children and young people's participation project', *Children and Society*, 26: 262–7.

Mutisya, T. (2011) *Women Connecting: exploring women's friendship in a multicultural setting*, Unpublished Master of Public Health thesis, School of Health and Social Development, Deakin University, Australia.

Myhill, W., Cogburn, D., Samant, D., Addom, B. and Blanck, P. (2008) 'Developing accessible cyberinfrastructure-enabled knowledge communities in the National Disability Community: theory, practice and policy', *Assistive Technology*, 20: 157–74.

National People with Disabilities and Carers Council (2009) *Shut Out: the experience of people with disabilities and their families in Australia – National Disability Strategy Consultation Report*, Canberra: Commonwealth Government.

National Social Inclusion Programme (2009) *Vision and Progress: social inclusion and mental health.* Online. Available HTTP: <http://ec.europa.eu/health/mental_health/eu_compass/reports_studies/report_vision_and_progress_en.pdf> (accessed 18 March 2013).

Neighbourhood Renewal (2010) *Action areas.* Online. Available HTTP: <http://www.dhs.vic.gov.au/about-the-department/plans,-programs-and-projects/projects-and-initiatives/housing-and-accommodation/neighbourhood-renewal> (accessed 18 March 2013).

Nelson, W.A. and Dark, C.K. (2003) 'Evaluating claims of conscience', *Healthcare Executive*, 18 (2): 54–5.

Neuhauser, L., Rothschild, B., Graham, C., Ivey, S.L. and Konishi, S. (2009) 'Participatory design of mass health communication in three languages for seniors and people with disabilities on Medicaid', *American Journal of Public Health*, 99: 2188–95.

Newton, S. and Appiah-Poku, J. (2007) 'The perspectives of researchers on obtaining informed consent in developing countries', *Developing World Bioethics*, 7: 19–24.

NHMRC (1991) *Guidelines on Ethical Matters in Aboriginal and Torres Strait Islander Health Research*, Canberra: National Health and Medical Research Council. Online. Available HTTP: <http://www.nhmrc.gov.au/_files_nhmrc/file/health_ethics/ahec/history/e11.pdf> (accessed 18 March 2013).

NHMRC (2007) *National Statement on Ethical Conduct in Human Research*, Canberra: National Health and Medical Research Council. Online. Available HTTP: <http://www.nhmrc.gov.au/_files_nhmrc/publications/attachments/e72.pdf> (accessed 18 March 2013).

NHS Management Executive (1992) *Local Voices: the views of local people in purchasing for health*, London: National Health Service Management Executive.

Nicolopoulou, A., Barbosa de Sá, A., Ilgz, H. and Brockmeyer, C. (2010) 'Using the transformative power of play to educate hearts and minds: from Vygotsky to Vivian Paley and beyond', *Mind, Culture, Activity*, 17: 42–58.

Nilsen, E.S., Myrhaug, H.T, Johansen, M., Oliver, S. and Oxman, A.D. (2010) 'Methods of consumer involvement in developing healthcare policy and research, clinical practice guidelines and patient information material', *Cochrane Database of Systematic Reviews*, 3. DOI: 10.1002/14651858.CD004563.pub2.

Nimegeer, A., Farmer, J., West, C. and Currie, M. (2011) 'Addressing the problem of rural community engagement in healthcare service design', *Health and Place*, 17: 1004–6.

Noar, S.M., Black, H.G. and Pierce, L.B. (2009) 'Efficacy of computer technology-based HIV prevention interventions: a meta-analysis' *AIDS*, 23: 107–15.

Nordentoft, H.M. and Kappel, N. (2011) 'Vulnerable participants in health research: methodological and ethical challenges', *Journal of Social Work Practice*, 25: 365–76.

North, N. and Werkö, S. (2002) 'Widening the debate? Consultation and participation in local health care planning in the English and Swedish health services', *International Journal of Health Services*, 32: 781–98.

NSW DoH (2001) *Partners in Health: sharing information and making decisions together. Report of the Consumer and Community Participation Implementation Reference Group*, Sydney: New South Wales Department of Health.

NT DoHCS, (2004) *Building Healthier Communities: a framework for health and community services 2004–2009*, Darwin: Northern Territory Department of Health and Community Services.

Nussbaum, M. (2003) 'Capabilities as fundamental entitlements: Sen and social justice', *Feminist Economics*, 9: 33–59.

Nyamu-Musembi, C. and Cornwall, A. (2004) *What is the 'rights-based approach' all about? Perspectives from international development agencies*, IDS Working Paper 234, Brighton: Institute of Development Studies.

O'Brien, J. (2008) 'Presenting the case for conscience', in *BPAS (British Pregnancy Advisory Service), Abortion, Ethics, Conscience and Choice*. Online. Available HTTP: <http://www.abortionreview.org/images/uploads/AR_SpecialEdition_1.pdf> (accessed 18 March 2013).

O'Brien, M. (1981) *The Politics of Reproduction*, London: Routledge and Kegan Paul.

O'Connor, C. and Stagnitti, K. (2011) 'Play, behaviour, language and social skills: the comparison of a play and a non-play intervention within a specialist school setting', *Research in Developmental Disabilities*, 32: 1205–11.

O'Dell, S. (2000) 'Psychotherapy with gay and lesbian families: opportunities for cultural inclusion and clinical challenges', *Clinical Social Work Journal*, 28: 171–82.

O'Leary, T., Burkett, I. and Braithwaite, K. (2011) *Appreciating Assets*, Dunfermline: International Association for Community Development/Carnegie UK Trust.

O'Neill, M., Woods, P.A. and Webster, M. (2005) 'New Arrivals: participatory action research, imagined communities, and "visions" of social justice', *Social Justice* 32 (1): 75–88.

O'Neill, M., Campbell, R., Hubbard, P., Pitcher, J. and Scoular, J. (2008) 'Living with the other: street work, contingent communities and degrees of tolerance', *Crime, Media, Culture*, 4: 73–93.

Oakley, A. (1981) 'Interviewing women: a contradiction in terms', in H. Roberts (ed.) *Doing Feminist Research*, London: Routlege and Kegan Paul.

OECD (2009) *Focus on Citizens: public engagement for better policy and services*, Paris: Organisation for Economic Co-operation and Development.

Ogilvie, K.K. (2012) in *Debates of the Senate (Hansard) 1st Session, 41st Parliament, Volume 148, Issue 92 Monday, June 18, 2012*. Online. Available HTTP: <http://www.parl.gc.ca/Content/Sen/Chamber/411/Debates/092db_2012-06-18-e.htm> (accessed 18 March 2013).

Okal, J., Luchters, S., Geibel, S., Chersich, M.F., Lango, D. and Temmerman, M. (2009) 'Social context, sexual risk perceptions and stigma: HIV vulnerability among male sex workers in Mombasa, Kenya', *Culture, Health and Sexuality*, 11: 811–26.

Okoli, C. and Pawlowski, S. (2004) 'The Delphi method as a research tool: an example, design considerations and applications', *Information and Management*, 42: 15–29.

Oldridge, N.B. (1996) 'Outcomes measurement: health-related quality of life', *Assistive Technology*, 8: 82–93.

Oleckno, W.A. (2002) *Essential Epidemiology. Principles and Applications*, Long Grove, IL: Waveland Press.

Oliver, M. (1990) *The Politics of Disablement*, London: MacMillan.

Ong, K., Kelaher, M., Anderson, I. and Carter, R. (2009) 'A cost-based equity weight for use in the economic evaluation of primary health care interventions: case study of the Australian indigenous population', *International Journal for Equity in Health*, 8: 34.

Osmani, S. (2008) 'Participatory governance: an overview of issues and evidence', in *Participatory Governance and the Millennium Development Goals*, New York: United Nations.

Ostrow, L. and Adams, N. (2012) 'Recovery in the USA: from politics to peer support', *International Review of Psychiatry*, 24: 70–8.

Owens, J. (2007) 'Liberating voices through narrative methods: the case for an interpretive research approach', *Disability and Society*, 22: 299–313.

Owuor, J. (2009) 'HIV prevention among black Africans in England: A complex challenge', *A Race Equality Foundation Briefing Paper*, London: Race Equality Foundation. Online. Available HTTP: <http://eprints.hud.ac.uk/7400> (accessed 18 March 2013).

Palmer, M., O'Kane, P. and Owens, M. (2009) 'Betwixt spaces: student accounts of turning point experiences in the first-year transition', *Studies in Higher Education*, 34: 37–54.

Panapasa, S., Jackson, J., Caldwell, C., Heeringa, S., McNally, J., Williams, D., Coral, D., Taumoepeau, L., Young, L., Young, S. and Fa'asisila, S. (2012) 'Community-based participatory research approach to evidence-based research: lessons from the Pacific Islander American Health Study', *Progress in Community Health Partnerships*, 6: 53–8.

Parker, R. (2002) 'The global HIV/AIDS pandemic, structural inequalities, and the politics of nternational health', *American Journal of Public Health*, 92: 343–6.

Parrott, L. (2009) 'Constructive marginality: conflicts and dilemmas in cultural competence and anti-oppressive practice', *Social Work Education*, 28: 617–30.

Pascarella, E.T. and Terenzini, P.T. (2005) *How College Affects Students: a third decade of research*, San Francisco, CA: Jossey-Bass.

Pate, A. and Horn, M. (2006) *Aids and Equipment for Victorians with Disabilities: entitlement or hand-out? A Position Paper: recommendations for an effective Victorian aids and equipment program for the 21st century*, Melbourne: Research and Social Policy Unit, Melbourne Citymission.

Paterson, T. (1996) 'Leaving well alone: a systemic perspective on the therapeutic relationship', in C. Flaskas and A. Perlesz (eds) *The Therapeutic Relationship in Systemic Therapy*, London: Karnac Books.

Patston, P. (2007) 'Constructive functional diversity: a new paradigm beyond disability and impairment', *Disability and Rehabilitation*, 29: 1625–33.

Patton, M. (2002) *Qualitative Research and Evaluation Methods*, 3rd edn, Thousand Oaks, CA: Sage Publications.

Pawar, M.S. (2009) *Community Development in Asia and the Pacific*, London: Routledge.

Pellegrino, E. D. and Thomasma, D.C. (2000) 'Dubious premises – evil conclusions: moral reasoning at the Nuremberg Trials', *Cambridge Quarterly of Healthcare Ethics*, 9: 261–74.

Pemberton G., Andía, J., Robles, R., Collins, C., Colón-Cartagena, Pérez del Pilar, O. and Vega, T.S. (2009) 'From research to community-based practice – working with Latino researchers to translate and diffuse a culturally relevant evidence-based intervention: The *Modelo de Intervención Psicomédica* (MIP) experience', *AIDS Education and Prevention*, 21: 171–85.

Pennington, J. and Knight, T. (2008) 'Staying Connected: the lived experiences of volunteers and older adults', *Ageing International*, 32: 298–311.

Peter, M. (2003) 'Drama, narrative and early learning', *British Journal of Special Education*, 30: 21–7.

Peterson, N.A. and Hughey, J. (2004) 'Social cohesion and intrapersonal empowerment: gender as moderator', *Health Education Research*, 19: 533–42.

Phillips, A. (2009) 'Health status differentials across rural and remote Australia', *The Australian Journal of Rural Health*, 17: 2–9.

Pholi, K., Black, D. and Richards, C. (2009) 'Is "Close the Gap" a useful approach to improving the health and wellbeing of Indigenous Australians?', *Australian Review of Public Affairs*, 9 (10): 1–13.

Picard, M. (2005) *Principles into Practice: learning from innovative rights-based programmes*, London: CARE International UK.

Pinkham, S. and Malinowska-Sempruch, K. (2008) 'Women, harm reduction and HIV', *Reproductive Health Matters*, 16: 168–81.

Pinquart, M. and Duberstein, P.R. (2010) 'Associations of social networks with cancer mortality: a meta-analysis', *Critical Reviews in Oncology/Hematology*, 75: 122–37.

Pittman, L.D. and Richmond, A. (2008) 'University belonging, friendship quality, and psychological adjustment during the transition to college', *The Journal of Experimental Education*, 76: 343–61.

Planning with Kids (2010) *Blanks Levels of Questioning – stimulating children's language development*. Online. Available HTTP: <http://planningwithkids.com/2010/03/18/blanks-levels-of-questioning-stimulating-children%E2%80%99s-language-development> (accessed 18 March 2013).

Plumridge, L. and Abel, G. (2001) 'A "segmented" sex industry in New Zealand: sexual and personal safety of female sex workers', *Australian and New Zealand Journal of Public Health*, 25: 78–83.

Pollock, V.L. and Sharp, J. (2012) 'Real participation or the tyranny of participatory practice? Public art and community involvement in the regeneration of the Raploch, Scotland', *Urban Studies*, 49 (14): 3063–79.

Popay, J., Escorel, S., Hernández, M., Johnston, H., Mathieson, J. and Rispel, L. (2008) *Understanding and Tackling Social Exclusion*, final report to the WHO Commission on Social Determinants of Health from the Social Exclusion Knowledge Network. Online. Available HTTP: <http://www.who.int/social_determinants/knowledge_networks/final_reports/sekn_final%20report_042008.pdf> (accessed 18 March 2013).

Pope, A. and Tarlou, A. (eds) (1991) *Disability in America: towards a national agenda for prevention*, Washington, DC: National Academy Press.

Pope, T. (2010) 'Legal briefing: conscience clauses and conscientious refusal', *Journal of Clinical Ethics*, 21: 163–76.

Postle, K., Wright, P. and Beresford, P. (2005) 'Older people's participation in political activity: making their voices heard: a potential support role for welfare professionals in countering ageism and social exclusion', *Practice*, 17: 173–89.

Power, L., Bell, M. and Freemantle, I. (2010) *A National Study of People over 50 with HIV*, York: Joseph Roundtree Foundation. Online. Available HTTP: <http://www.jrf.org.uk/publications/over-50-living-with-HIV> (accessed 18 March 2013).

Preston, R., Waugh, H., Larkins, S. and Taylor, J. (2010) 'Community participation in rural primary health care: intervention or approach?', *Australian Journal of Primary Health*, 16 (1): 4–16.

Price, C.A., Zavotka, S.L. and Teaford, M.H. (2004) 'Implementing a university–community–retail partnership model to facilitate community education on universal design', *Gerontologist*, 44: 697–702.

Prilleltensky, I. (2010) 'Child wellness and social inclusion: values for action', *American Journal of Community Psychology*, 46: 238–49.

Provis, C. (2007) 'Ethics and issues in public policy', *Politics and Society*, 26 (3): 21–33.

Przeworski, A. (2008) 'Democracy, social inclusion and development', in *Participatory Governance and the Millennium Development Goals*, New York: United Nations.

Punch, M. (1998) 'Politics and ethics in qualitative research', in N. Denzin and Y. Lincoln (eds) *The Landscape of Qualitative Research*, London: Sage.

Pungello, E. P., Iruka, I.U., Dotterer, A.M., Mills-Koonce, R. and Reznick, J.S. (2009)

'The effects of socioeconomic status, race, and parenting on language development in early childhood', *Developmental Psychology*, 45: 544–57.

Pyett, P. and Vichealth Koori Research and Community Development Unit (2002) 'Towards reconciliation in Indigenous health research: the responsibilities of the non-Indigenous researcher', *Contemporary Nurse*, 14: 56–65.

Pyett, P. and Warr, D. (1999) 'Women at risk in sex work: strategies for survival', *Journal of Sociology*, 35: 183–97.

Pyett, P., Waples-Crowe, P. and van der Sterren, A. (2008) 'Challenging our own practices in Indigenous health promotion and research', *Health Promotion Journal of Australia*, 19: 179–83.

QH (2006) *Developing a Consumers Health Council for Queensland: engaging Queensland consumers in health care*, Brisbane: Queensland Health.

Quadara, A. (2008) 'Sex workers and sexual assault in Australia: prevalence, risk and safety', *Australian Institute of Family Studies*, 8: 1–40.

Radcliffe, T. (2012) *Take the Plunge: living baptism and confirmation*, London: Bloomsbury.

Ramcharan, P. and Grant, G. (1994) 'Setting one agenda for empowering persons with a disadvantage within the research process', in M.H. Rioux and M. Bach (eds) *Disability is Not Measles: new research paradigms in disability*, Ontario: L'Institut Roeher Institute.

Ramsay, S., Jones, E. and Barker, M. (2006) 'Relationship between adjustment and support types: young and mature-aged local and international first-year university students', *Higher Education*, 54: 247–65.

Ramsland, J. (1992) 'The London Foundling Hospital and its significance as a child saving institution', *Australian Social Work*, 45 (2): 23–36.

Rausch, J.L. and Hamilton, M.W. (2006) 'Goals and distractions: explanations of early attrition from traditional university freshmen', *The Qualitative Report*, 11: 317–34.

Rayle, A.D. and Chung, K. (2007) 'Revisiting first-year college students' mattering: social support, academic stress, and the mattering experience', *Journal of College Student Retention*, 9: 21–37.

Read, B., Archer, L. and Leathwood, C. (2003) 'Challenging cultures? student conceptions of "belonging" and "isolation" at a post-1992 university', *Studies in Higher Education*, 28: 261–77.

Read, S. and Maslin-Prothero, S. (2011) 'The involvement of users and carers in health and social research: the realities of inclusion and engagement', *Qualitative Health Research*, 21: 704–13.

Reason, P. (1994) 'Three approaches to participative inquiry', in N.K. Denzin and Y.S. Lincoln (eds) *Handbook of Qualitative Research*, Thousand Oaks, CA: Sage Publications.

Reay, D., Ball, S. and David, M. (2002) '"It's taking me a long time but I'll get there in the end": mature students on access courses and higher education choice', *British Educational Research Journal*, 28: 5–19.

Reay, D., David, M. and Ball, S. (2001) 'Making a difference? Institutional habitus and higher education choice', *Sociological Research Online*, 5 (4). Online. Available HTTP: <http://www.socresonline.org.uk/5/4/reay.html> (accessed 18 March 2013).

Reece, M. and Dodge, B. (2004) 'A study in sexual health applying the principles of community-based participatory research', *Archives of Sexual Behavior*, 33: 235–47.

Reissman, C. (2005) 'Exporting ethics: a narrative about narrative research in South India', *Health*, 9: 473–90.

Rekart, M. (2005) 'Sex work harm reduction', *The Lancet*, 366: 2123–34.

Renner, S., Prewitt, G., Watanabe, M. and Gascho, L. (2007) *Summary of the Virtual Round Table on Social Exclusion*. Online. Available HTTP: <http://hdr.undp.org/es/indh/redes/respuestas/161.pdf> (accessed 29 March 2013).

Renton, T. (2011) *Guidelines for people interested in organising a like-minded group in the community*, Unpublished Bachelor of Public Health and Health Promotion report, Burwood, Australia: School of Health and Social Development, Deakin University.

Repper, J. and Breeze, J. (2007) 'User and carer involvement in the training and education of health professionals: a review of the literature', *International Journal of Nursing Studies*, 44: 511–9.

Reynolds, E., Stagnitti, K. and Kidd, E. (2011) 'Play, language and social skills of children aged 4–6 years attending a play based curriculum school and a traditionally structured classroom curriculum school in low socio-economic areas', *Australian Journal of Early Childhood*, 36 (4): 120–30.

Rhodes, R. (2005) 'Response to commentators on "Rethinking research ethics"', *The American Journal of Bioethics*, 5 (1): W15–8.

Rhodes, S.D., DiClemente, R.J., Cecil, H., Hergenrather, K.C. and Yee, L.J. (2002) 'Risk among men who have sex with men in the United States: a comparison of an Internet sample and a conventional outreach sample', *AIDS Education and Prevention*, 14: 41–50.

Rhodes, S.D., Hergenrather, K.C., Yee, L.J. and Ramsey, B. (2008) 'Comparing MSM in the southeastern United States who participated in an HIV prevention chat room-based outreach intervention and those who did not: how different are the baseline HIV-risk profiles?', *Health Education and Research*, 23: 180–90.

Rhodes, S.D., Vissman, A.T., Stowers, J., Miller, C., McCoy, T.P., Hergenrather, K.C., Wilkin, A.M., Reece, M., Bachmann, L.H., Ore, A., Ross, M.W., Hendrix, E. and Eng, E. (2011) 'A CBPR partnership increases HIV testing among men who have sex with men (MSM): outcome findings from a pilot test of the CyBER/testing Internet intervention', *Health Education and Behavior*, 38: 311–20.

Rice, K., Tsianakas, V. and Quinn, K. (2007) *Women and Mental Health: gender impact assessment No. 2*, Melbourne: Women's Health Victoria.

Rickard, W. and Growney, T. (2001) 'Occupational health and safety amongst sex workers: a pilot peer education resource', *Health Education Research*, 16: 321–33.

Rioux, M. H. and Riddle, C. (2011) 'Values in disability policy and law: equality', in M. Rioux (ed.) *Critical Perspectives on Human Rights and Disability Law*, Leiden: Martinus Nijhoff.

Ritchie, J. (2010) 'Why we need success stories in reporting the health of Australian Aboriginal and Torres Strait Islander peoples: a personal perspective', *Global Health Promotion*, 17 (4): 61–4.

Robinson, K. (2009) *The Element: how finding your passion changes everything*, New York: Penguin/Viking.

Robinson, K. (2011) *Out of Our Minds: learning to be creative*, Westford: Capstone Publishing.

Robinson, K.J., Campbell, B. and Campbell, T. (2010) 'YOUR Blessed Health: a faith-based, community-based participatory research project to reduce the incidence of HIV/AIDS and sexually transmitted infections', in T.S. Kerson, J.L.M. McCoyd and Associates (eds) *Social Work in Health Settings: practice in context*, 3rd edn, New York: Routledge.

Rodrigues, M.L.C.F. and Da Costa, T.H.M. (2001) Association of the maternal experience and changes in adiposity measured by BMI, waist hip ratio and percentage body fat in urban Brazilian women, *British Journal of Nutrition*, 85: 107–14.

Room, G. (1999) 'Social exclusion, solidarity and the challenge of globalization', *International Journal of Social Welfare*, 8: 166–74.

Rorty, R. (1989) *Contingency, Irony and Solidarity*, Cambridge: Cambridge University Press.

Rose, N. (1989) *Governing the Soul: the shaping of the private self*, London: Routledge.

Rose, N. (1998) *Inventing our Selves: psychology, power and personhood*, Cambridge: Cambridge University Press.

Rose, N. (1999) 'Interrogating the psychotherapies: an interview with Nikolas Rose', *Psychotherapy in Australia*, 5: 40–6.

Roshelli, K.M. (2009) 'Religiously based discrimination: striking a balance between a health care provider's right to religious freedom and a woman's ability to access fertility treatment without facing discrimination', *St. John's Law Review*, 83: 977–1016.

Ross, M.W., Crisp, B.R., Månsson S.-A. and Hawkes, S. (2012) 'Occupational health and safety among commercial sex workers', *Scandinavian Journal of Work, Environment and Health*, 38: 105–19.

Rovner, J. (1997) 'US budget bill contains surprise on abortion', *The Lancet*, 350: 573.

Rowe, G. and Wright, G. (1999) 'The Delphi technique as a forecasting tool: issues and analysis', *International Journal of Forecasting*, 15: 353–75.

Rowe, J. (2003a) *Who's Using? The health information exchange (St Kilda) and the development of a primary care response for injecting drug users*. Report for The Salvation Army Crisis Service, Melbourne. Online. Available HTTP: <http://www.salvationarmy.org.au/Global/State%20pages/Victoria/St%20Kilda%20Crisis%20Centre/Articles%20Journals%20Pub/Publication_Who%27s_Using.pdf> (accessed 18 March 2013).

Rowe, J. (2003b) 'In limbo and in danger: street based sex workers and the issue of tolerance zones', *Just Policy*, 30: 24–31.

Rowe, J. (2006) *Street Walking Blues: sex work, St Kilda and the street*. Melbourne: Centre for Applied Social Research, RMIT University, Australia.

Rowse, T. (2009) 'Indigenous Australia: treaty talk', *Australian Policy Online*. Online. Available HTTP: <http://apo.org.au/commentary/indigenous-australia-treaty-talk> (accessed 18 March 2013).

Russ, S.W. (2003) 'Play and creativity: developmental issues', *Scandinavian Journal of Educational Research*, 47: 291–303.

Russell, J. (2005) 'What are friends for', *The Guardian*. Online. Available HTTP: <http://www.guardian.co.uk/theguardian/2005/jan/24/features11.g2> (accessed 18 March 2013).

Rydin, Y., Bleahu, A., Davies, M., Dávila, J.D., Friel, S., De Grandis, G., Groce, N., Hallal, P.C., Hamilton, I., Howden-Chapman, P., Lai, K.M., Lim, C.J., Martins, J., Osrin, D., Ridley, I., Scott, I., Taylor, M., Wilkinson, P. and Wilson, J. (2012) 'Shaping cities for health: complexity and the planning of urban environments in the 21st century', *The Lancet*, 379: 2079–108.

Sadler, K. (2010) 'Art as activism and education: creating venues for student involvement and social justice education utilizing Augusto Boal's Theater of the Oppressed', *Vermont Connection*, 31: 82–95.

Sainsbury Centre for Mental Health (2009) *The Chance of a Lifetime: preventing early conduct problems and reducing crime*. London: Sainsbury Centre for Mental Health. Online.

Available HTTP: <http://www.centreformentalhealth.org.uk/pdfs/chance_of_a_lifetime.pdf> (accessed 18 March 2013).

Salimi, Y., Shahandeh, K., Malekafzali, H., Loori, N., Kheiltash, A., Jamshidi, E., Frouzan, A.S. and Majdzadeh, R. (2012) 'Is community-based participatory research (CBPR) useful? A systematic review on papers in a decade', *International Journal of Preventive Medicine* 3: 386–93.

Sallman, J. (2011) 'Living with stigma: women's experiences of prostitution and sub-stance use', *Affilia*, 25: 146–59.

Saltzburg, S. (1996) 'Family therapy and the disclosure of adolescent homosexuality', *Journal of Family Psychotherapy*, 7 (4): 1–18.

Sandelowski, M. (2000) 'Whatever happened to qualitative description?', *Research in Nursing and Health*, 23: 334–40.

Sanders, T. (2004) 'A continuum of risk? The management of health, physical and emotional risks by female sex workers', *Sociology of Health and Illness*, 26: 557–74.

Saunders, P., Naidoo, Y. and Griffiths, M. (2007) *Towards New Indicators of Disadvantage: deprivation and social exclusion in Australia*, Sydney: Social Policy Research Centre.

Schalock, R.L., Bonham, G.S. and Verdugo, M. (2008) 'The conceptualization and measurement of quality of life: implications for program planning and evaluation in the field of intellectual disabilities', *Evaluation and Program Planning*, 31: 181–90.

Scherer, M. J. (2005) *Living in the State of Stuck: how assistive technology impacts on the lives of people with disabilities*, Cambridge, MA: Brookline Books.

Schriner, K. and Scotch, R.K. (2001) 'Disability and institutional change: a human variation perspective on overcoming oppression', *Journal of Disability Policy Studies*, 12: 100–6.

Schulz, A.J., Parker, E.A., Israel, B.A., Allen, A., Decarlo, M. and Lockett, M. (2002) 'Addressing social determinants of health through community-based participatory research: the East Side village Health Worker Partnership', *Health Education and Behavior*, 29: 326–41.

Scotch, R.K. (2000) 'Models of disability and the Americans with Disabilities Act', *Berkeley Journal of Employment and Labor Law*, 21: 213–22.

Scotch, R.K. and Schriner, K. (1997) 'Disability as human variation: implications for policy', *The Annals of the American Academy of Political and Social Science*, 549: 148–59.

Scotland Bill (2004) *National Health Service Reform (Scotland) Act 2004*. Online. Available HTTP: <www.opsi.gov.uk/legislation/scotland/en2004/2004en07.htm> (accessed 18 March 2013).

Scotland, J. (1972) 'The centenary of the Education (Scotland) Act of 1872', *British Journal of Educational Studies*, 20: 121–36.

Scott, J.G. (2005) *How Modern Governments Made Prostitution a Social Problem: creating a responsible prostitute population*, Lewiston, NY: Edward Mellen Press.

Scottish Executive (2001) *Patient Focus and Public Involvement*. Online. Available HTTP: <www.scotland.gov.uk/library3/health/pfpi-00.asp> (accessed 18 March 2013).

Scottish Executive (2004) *Patient Focus and Public Involvement*. Online. Available HTTP: <http://www.scotland.gov.uk/Resource/Doc/158744/0043087.pdf> (accessed 18 March 2013).

Scottish Health Council Workplan (2006) *Scottish Health Council Workplan 2006–2007*, Glasgow: Scottish Health Council.

Scourfield, P. (2010) 'A critical reflection on the involvement of "experts by experi-ence" in inspections', *British Journal of Social Work*, 40: 1890–907.

Seib, C., Debattista, J., Fischer, J., Dunne, M. and Najman, J.M. (2009a) 'Sexually transmissible infections among sex worker and their clients: variation in prevalence between sectors of the industry', *Sexual Health*, 6: 45–50.

Seib, C., Fischer, J. and Najman, J.M. (2009b) 'The health of female sex workers from three industry sectors in Queensland', *Social Science and Medicine*, 68: 473–8.

Seja, A.L. and Russ, S.W. (1999) 'Children's fantasy play and emotional understanding', *Journal of Clinical Child Psychology*, 28: 269–77.

Sen, A. (1999) *Development as Freedom*, Oxford: Oxford University Press.

Sen, A. (2000) *Social Exclusion: concept, application, and scrutiny*, Social Development Paper No. 1, Office of Environment and Social Development Asian Development Bank. Online. Available HTTP: <http://www.adb.org/publications/social-exclusion-concept-application-and-scrutiny> (accessed 18 March 2013).

Sen, A. (2009) *The Idea of Justice*, London: Allan Lane.

Senate Community Affairs Reference Committee (2004) *A Hand Up Not a Hand Out: renewing the fight against poverty – report on poverty and financial hardship*. Canberra: Senate Community Affairs References Committee Secretariat.

Shakespeare, T. (2008) 'Disability: suffering, social oppression, or complex predicament?', in M. Duwell, C. Rehmann-Sutter and D. Mieth (eds) *The Contingent Nature of Life: bioethics and limits of human existence*, Berlin: Springer.

Shalowitz, M.U., Isacco, A., Barquin, N., Clark-Kaufman, E., Delger, P., Nelson, D., Quinn, A. and Wagenaar, K.A. (2009) 'Community-based participatory research: a review of the literature with strategies for community engagement', *Journal of Developmental and Behavioral Pediatrics*, 30: 350–61.

Shammas, N. (1996) *The Questionable Socio-economic Future of Lebanon*, Boston, MA: Harvard University Club.

Shield, M., Graham, M. and Taket, A. (2011) 'Neighbourhood renewal: an effective way to address social inclusion', *Journal of Social Inclusion*, 2 (2): 4–18.

Silva, M-L. (2003) *The Human Rights Based Approach to Development Cooperation Towards a Common Understanding Among UN Agencies*, Geneva: Office of the High Commissioner for Human Rights.

Silver, H. and Miller, S.M. (2003) 'Social exclusion: the European approach to social disadvantage', *Indicators*, 2: 1–17.

Simpson, E.L. and House, A.O. (2002) 'Involving users in the delivery and valuation of mental health services: systematic review', *British Medical Journal*, 325: 1265–8.

Skyrme, G. (2007) 'Entering the university: the differentiated experience of two Chinese international students in a New Zealand University', *Studies in Higher Education*, 32: 357–72.

Sluss, D.J. (2005) *Supporting Play: birth to age eight*, New York: Delmar Thompson.

Small, R. (2001) 'Codes are not enough: what philosophy can contribute to the ethics of educational research', *Journal of Philosophy of Education*, 35: 387–406.

Smith, K. (2002) 'School to university: sunlit steps, or stumbling in the dark?', *Arts and Humanities in Higher Education*, 2: 90–8.

Smith, K. (2004) 'School to university: an investigation into the experience of first-year students of English at British universities', *Arts and Humanities in Higher Education*, 3: 81–93.

Smith, K. and Hopkins, C. (2005) 'Great expectations: sixth-formers perceptions of teaching and learning in degree-level English', *Arts and Humanities in Higher Education*, 4: 304–18.

Smyth, G., Harries, P. and Dorer, G. (2011) 'Exploring mental health service users' experiences of social inclusion in their community occupations', *The British Journal of Occupational Therapy*, 74: 323–31.

Social Protection Committee (2011) *The Social Dimension of the Europe 2020 Strategy*, Luxembourg: Publications Office of the European Union.

Sonfield A. (2005) 'Rights vs. responsibilities: professional standards and provider refusals', *Guttmacher Report on Public Policy*, 8 (3): 7–9.

Sonfield A. (2008a) 'Provider refusal and access to reproductive health services: approaching a new balance', *Guttmacher Policy Review*, 11 (2): 2–6.

Sonfield A. (2008b) 'Proposed "conscience" regulation opposed widely as threat to reproductive health and beyond', *Guttmacher Policy Review*, 11 (4): 17–9.

Sonfield A. (2009) 'Delineating the obligations that come with conscientious refusal: a question of balance', *Guttmacher Policy Review*, 12 (3): 6–10.

South, J., Kinsella, K. and Meah, A. (2012) 'Lay perspectives on lay health worker roles, boundaries and participation within three UK community-based health promotion projects', *Health Education Research*, 27: 656–70.

St. James' Parish School, (2011) 'Self report', Unpublished report, Ballarat, Victoria: St. James School.

St Kilda Gatehouse (2013) Home page. Online. Available HTTP: <http://www.stkildagatehouse.org.au> (accessed 18 March 2013).

Stagnitti, K. (1998) *The Learn to Play Approach: an approach to increase the imaginative play skills of children*, Melbourne: Co-ordinates Publishing.

Stagnitti, K. (2004) 'Occupational performance in pretend play; implications for practice', in M. Mollineux (ed.) *Occupation for Occupational Therapists*, Oxford: Blackwell Science.

Stagnitti, K. (2009) 'Children and pretend play', in K. Stagnitti and R. Cooper (eds) *Play as Therapy: assessment and therapeutic interventions*, London: Jessica Kingsley.

Stagnitti, K. and Cooper, R. (2009) *Play as Therapy: assessment and therapeutic intervention*, London: Jessica Kingsley.

Stagnitti, K. and Jellie, L. (2006) *Play to Learn: building literacy skills in the early years*, Melbourne: Curriculum Corporation.

Statistics New Zealand (2010) *Census Night Population count*. Online. Available HTTP: <http://www2.stats.govt.nz/domino/external/omni/omni.nsf/wwwglsry/Census+Night+Population+Count> (accessed 18 March 2013).

Steel, E.J. and de Witte, L.P. (2011) 'Advances in European Assistive Technology service delivery and recommendations for further improvement,' *Technology and Disability*, 23: 131–8.

Steinert, H. and Pilgram, A. (eds) (2007) *Welfare Policy from Below: struggles against social exclusion in Europe*, Aldershot: Ashgate.

Sternberg, P. and Garcia, A. (1989) *Sociodrama: who's in your shoes?*, New York: Praeger.

Stevens, N.L., Martina, C.M.S. and Westerhof, G.J. (2006) 'Meeting the need to belong: predicting effects of a friendship enrichment program for older women', *The Gerontologist*, 46: 495–502.

Stevenson, M. (2010) 'Flexible and responsive research: developing rights-based emancipatory disability research methodology in collaboration with young adults with Down Syndrome', *Australian Social Work*, 63: 35–50.

Stevenson, R. (2011) 'Welcoming people with mental health problems into mainstream market research', *International Journal of Market Research*, 53: 737–48.

Stoljar, N. (2011) 'Informed consent and relational concepts of autonomy', *Journal of Medicine and Philosophy*, 36: 375–84.

Stone, E. and Priestly, M. (1996) 'Parasites, pawns and partners: disability research and the role of non-disabled researchers', *The British Journal of Sociology*, 47: 699–716.

Stone, T. (2004) 'Making the decision about enrolment in a randomised control trial', in M. Smyth and W. Williamson (eds) *Researchers and their 'subjects': ethics, power, knowledge and consent*, Bristol: Policy Press.

Strega, S., Casey, L. and Rutman, D. (2009) 'Sex workers addressing treatment', *Women's Health and Urban Life*, 8 (1): 42–53.

Strier, R. and Binyamin, S. (2010) 'Developing anti-oppressive services for the poor: a theoretical and organisational rationale', *British Journal of Social Work*, 40: 1908–26.

Subreenduth, S. and Rhee, J.E. (2010) 'A porous, morphing, and circulatory mode of self-other: decolonizing identity politics by engaging transnational reflexivity', *International Journal of Qualitative Studies in Education*, 23: 331–46.

Sullivan, H. (2002) 'Modernization, neighbourhood management and social inclusion', *Public Management Review*, 4: 505–28.

Summers, M. (2010) *NAERA Foundation Document*, Melbourne: NAERA.

Sunderland, M. (2007) *What Every Parent Needs to Know*, London: DK Books.

Sung-Chan, P. and Yuen-Tsang, A. (2007) 'Bridging the theory–practice gap in social work education: a reflection on an action research in China', *Social Work Education*, 27: 51–69.

Swain, J., French, S., Barnes, C. and Thomas, C. (eds) (2004) *Disabling Barriers: enabling environments*, London: Sage Publications.

Swain, S. (1986) *A Refuge at Kildare: the history of the Geelong female refuge and Bethany Babies Home, North Geelong*, Victoria: Bethany Child and Family Support.

Taket, A. (2012) *Health Equity, Social Justice and Human Rights*, London: Routledge.

Taket, A., Crisp, B.R, Nevill, A., Lamaro, G., Graham, M. and Barter-Godfrey, S. (eds) (2009a) *Theorising Social Exclusion*, London: Routledge,

Taket, A.R. and Edmans, T. (2003) 'Community led regeneration: experiences from London', *International Journal of Healthcare Technology and Management*, 5: 81–95.

Taket, A., Foster, N. and Cook, K. (2009b) 'Understanding processes of social exclusion: silence, silencing and shame', in A. Taket, B.R. Crisp, A. Nevill, G. Lamaro, M. Graham and S. Barter-Godfrey (eds) *Theorising Social Exclusion*. London: Routledge.

Taket, A.R. and White, L.A. (2000) *Partnership and Participation: decision-making in the multiagency setting*, Chichester: Wiley.

Tamakoshi, A., Tamakoshi, K., Lin, Y., Mikami, H., Inaba, Y., Yagyu, K., Kikuchi, S. and JACC Study Group (2011) 'Number of children and all-cause mortality risk: results from the Japan Collaborative Cohort Study', *European Journal of Public Health*, 21: 732–7.

Tekola, F., Bull, S., Farsides, B., Newport, M., Adeyemo, A., Rotimi, C. and Davey, G. (2009a) 'Tailoring consent to context: designing an appropriate process for a biomedical study in a low income setting', *PLoS*, 3 (7): e482. Online. Available HTTP: <http://www.plosntds.org/article/info%3Adoi%2F10.1371%2Fjournal. pntd.0000482> (accessed 18 March 2013).

Tekola, F., Bull, S., Farsides, B., Newport, M., Adeyemo, A., Rotimi, C. and Davey, G. (2009b) 'Impact of social stigma on the process of obtaining informed consent for genetic research on podoconiosis: a qualitative study', *BMC Medical Ethics*, 10 (13). Online. Available HTTP: <http://www.biomedcentral.com/1472-6939/10/13/ abstract> (accessed 18 March 2013).

Teliska, H. (2005) 'Obstacles to access: how pharmacist refusal clauses undermine the basic health care needs of rural and low-income women', *Berkeley Journal of Gender, Law and Justice*, 20: 229–48.

Tempfer, C.B. and Nowak, P. (2011) 'Consumer participation and organizational development in health care: a systematic review', *Wiener Klinische Wochenschrift*, 123: 408–14.

Tenthani, L., Cataldo, F., Chan, A.K., Bedell, R., Martiniuk, A.L.C. and van Lettow, M. (2012) 'Involving expert patients in antiretroviral treatment provision in a tertiary referral hospital HIV clinic in Malawi', *BMC Health Services Research*, 12: 140.

Tett, L. (2004) 'Mature working-class students in an "elite" university: discourses of risk, choice and exclusion', *Studies in the Education of Adults*, 36: 252–64.

The Guardian (2011) *NUJ chief Michelle Stanistreet's statement to the Leveson inquiry*. Online. Available HTTP: <http://www.guardian.co.uk/media/2011/nov/16/michelle-stanistreet-leveson-inquiry> (accessed 18 March 2013).

Thomas, C. (2007) *Sociologies of Disability and Illness: contested ideas in disability studies and medical sociology*, Basingstoke: Palgrave Macmillan.

Thomas, L. (2002) 'Student retention in higher education: the role of institutional habitus', *Journal of Education Policy*, 17: 423–42.

Thompson, E., Neighbours, H., Munday, C. and Jackson, J. (1996) 'Recruitment and retention of African American patients for clinical research: an exploration of response rates in an urban psychiatric hospital', *Journal of Consulting and Clinical Psychology*, 64: 861–7.

Thomson, H., Thomas, S., Sellstrom, E. and Petticrew, M. (2009) 'The health impacts of housing improvement: a systematic review of intervention studies from 1887 to 2007', *American Journal of Public Health*, 99 (Suppl 3): S681–92.

Tinto, V. (1987) *Leaving College: rethinking the causes and cures of student attrition*, Chicago, IL: University of Chicago Press.

Tisdall, E.K.M., Davis, J.M. and Gallagher, M. (2008) 'Reflecting on children and young people's participation in the UK', *International Journal of Children's Rights*, 16: 343–54.

Tomes, N. (2006) 'The patient as a policy factor: a historical case study of the consumer/survivor movement in mental health', *Health Affairs*, 25: 720–29.

Tomm, K. (1988) 'Interventive questioning', *Family Process*, 27: 1–15.

Tones, M., Fraser, J., Elder, R. and White, K.H. (2009) 'Supporting mature-aged students from a low socioeconomic background', *Higher Education*, 58: 505–29.

Transparency International (2012) *Advocacy and Legal Advice Centres in Asia Pacific*. Online. Available HTTP: <http://archive.transparency.org/regional_pages/asia_pacific/current_projects/advocacy_and_legal_advice_centres_in_asia_pacific> (accessed 18 March 2013).

Treloar, C., Rance, J., Madden, A. and Liebelt, L. (2011) 'Evaluation of consumer participation demonstration projects in five Australian drug user treatment facilities: the impact of individual versus organizational stability in determining project progress', *Substance Use and Misuse*, 46: 969–79.

Tsey, K., Patterson, D., Whiteside, M., Baird, L., Baird, B. and Tsey, K. (2004) 'A microanalysis of a participatory action research process with a rural Aboriginal men's health group', *Australian Journal of Primary Health*, 10 (1): 64–71.

Tutelian, M., Khayyat, M. and Abdel Monem, A. (2007) *Lebanon Family Health Survey 2004*, Beirut: The Pan Arab Project for Family Health, Ministry of Social Affairs.

Ulrich, W. (1998) *Systems Thinking As If People Mattered: critical systems thinking for citizens and managers*, Working Paper No. 23, Lincoln School of Management, Humberside: University of Lincoln.

UN (1948) *The Universal Declaration of Human Rights*, United Nations. Online. Available HTTP: <http://www.un.org/Overview/rights.html> (accessed 18 March 2013).

UN (1966) *International Covenant on Civil and Political Rights*, United Nations Office of the High Commissioner for Human Rights. Online. Available HTTP: <http://www.un.org/millennium/law/iv-4.htm> (accessed 18 March 2013).

UN (1989) *Convention on the Rights of the Child*, United Nations. Online. Available HTTP: <http://cyberschoolbus.un.org/treaties/child.asp> (accessed 18 March 2013).

UN (2006) *Convention on the Rights of Persons with Disabilities and Optional Protocol*, Geneva: United Nations.

UN (2010) *Monitoring the Convention on the Rights of Persons with Disabilities Guidance for Human Rights Monitors. Professional training series*, New York and Geneva: United Nations, Office of the High Commissioner for Human Rights.

UN (2012) *Realizing the Future We Want for All: report to the Secretary General*, New York: United Nations.

UN (n.d.) Article 55 Reportory suppl I vol II, 1946 to 1955, UN Treaty collection. Online. Available HTTP: <http://untreaty.un.org/cod/repertory/art55/english/rep_supp1_vol2-art55_e.pdf> (accessed 18 March 2013).

UNAIDS (2011) *Global Report: UNAIDS report on the global AIDS epidemic 2010*, Geneva: Joint United Nations Programme on HIV/AIDS (UNAIDS) UNAIDS. Online. Available HTTP: <http://www.unaids.org/globalreport/Global_report.htm> (accessed 18 March 2013).

UNDP (2005) *Human Development Report 2005*, New York: United Nations Development Programme. Online. Available HTTP: <http://hdr.undp.org/en/reports/global/hdr2005> (accessed 18 March 2013).

UNESCO (1994) *The Salamanca Statement and Framework for Action on Special Needs Education*, Spain: United Nations Education Scientific and Cultural Organisation and Ministry of Education and Science Spain.

Uren, N. and Stagnitti, K. (2009) 'Pretend play, social competence and learning in preschool children', *Australian Occupational Therapy Journal*, 56: 33–40.

van Bortel, G. and Mullins, D. (2009) 'Critical perspectives on network governance in urban regeneration, community involvement and integration', *Journal of Housing and the Built Environment*, 24: 203–19.

Van Criekingen, M. and Decroly, J.-M. (2003) 'Revisiting the diversity of gentrification: neighbourhood renewal processes in Brussels and Montreal', *Urban Studies*, 40: 2451–68.

Van Lerberghe, W., Ammar, W., El Rashidi, R., Sales, A. and Mechbal, A. (1997) 'Reform follows failure I: unregulated private care in Lebanon' *Health Policy and Planning*, 12: 296–311.

Vanclay, F., Higgins, M. and Blackshaw, A. (2008) *Making Sense of Place: exploring concepts and expressions of place through different senses and lenses*, Canberra: National Museum of Australia Press.

Vanwesenbeeck, I. (2001) 'Another decade of social scientific work on sex work: a review of research 1990–2000', *Annual Review of Sex Research*, 12: 242–89.

Vanwesenbeeck, I. (2005) 'Burnout among female indoor sex workers', *Archives of Sexual Behavior*, 34: 627–39.

Veatch, R. (2007) 'Implied, presumed and waived consent: the relative moral wrongs of under and over-informing', *The American Journal of Bioethics*, 7 (12): 39–54.

Visher, C., LaVigne, N. and Travis, J. (2004) *Returning Home: understanding the challenges of prisoner re-entry. Maryland pilot study: findings from Baltimore*, Washington, DC: Urban Institute.

Vos, T., Barker, B., Begg, S., Stanley, L. and Lopez, A. (2009) 'Burden of disease and injury in Aboriginal and Torres Strait Islander peoples: the Indigenous health gap', *International Journal of Epidemiology*, 38: 470–7.

Vromen, A. and Collin, P. (2010) 'Everyday youth participation?: contrasting views from Australian policymakers and young people', *Young*, 18: 97–112.

Vygotsky, L.S. (1966) 'Play and its role in the mental development of the child', *Voprosy psikhologii*, 12: 62–76.

Vygotsky, L.S. (1997) *Thought and language* (A. Kozulin, trans.), Cambridge, MA: MIT Press.

Walker, K. (2007) *Play Matters. Engaging children in learning: the Australian Developmental Curriculum*, Melbourne: ACER Press.

Walker, S., Chang, M., Powell, C.A. and Grantham-McGregor, S. (2005) 'Effects of early childhood psychosocial stimulation and nutritional supplementation on cognition and education in growth-stunted Jamaican children: prospective cohort study', *The Lancet*, 366: 1804–7.

Wallach, M.A. and Kogan, N. (1965) *Modes of Thinking in Young Children: a study of the creativity–intelligence distinction*, New York: Holt, Rinehart and Winston.

Wallcraft, J., Schrank, B. and Amering, M. (eds) (2009) *Handbook of Service User Involvement in Mental Health Research*, Chichester: Wiley-Blackwell.

Wallcraft, J., Amering, M., Freidin, J., Davar, B., Froggatt, D., Jafri, H., Javed, A., Katontoka, S., Raja, S., Rataemane, S., Steffen, S., Tyano, S., Underhill, C., Wahlberg, H., Warner, R. and Herrman, H. (2011) 'Partnerships for better mental health worldwide: WPA recommendations on best practices in working with service users and family carers', *World Psychiatry*, 10: 229–36.

Wallerstein, N. and Duran, B. (2010) 'Community-based participatory research contributions to intervention research: the intersection of science and practice to improve health equity', *American Journal of Public Health* 100 (Suppl 1): S40–6.

Wallerstein, N., Oetzel, J., Duran, B., Tafoya, G., Belone, L. and Rae, R. (2008) 'What predicts outcomes in CBPR?', in M. Minkler and N. Wallerstein (eds) *Community-Based Participatory Research: from process to outcomes*, San Francisco, CA: Wiley.

Walls, P., Parahoo, K., Fleming, P., McCaughan, E. (2010) 'Issues and consideration when researching sensitive issues with men: examples from a study of men and sexual health', *Nurse Researcher*, 18 (1): 26–34.

Walmsley, J. (2001) 'Normalisation, emancipatory research and inclusive research in learning disability', *Disability and Society*, 16: 187–205.

Walmsley, J. and Johnson, K. (2003) *Inclusive Research with People with Learning Disabilities: past, present and future*, London: Jessica Kingsley Publishers.

Walshe, K. and Rundall, T. (2001) 'Evidence-based management: from theory to practice in health care', *Milbank Quarterly*, 79: 429–57.

Wang, B., Li, X., Stanton, B., Fang, X., Yang, H., Zhao, R. and Hong, Y. (2007) 'Sexual coercion, HIV-related risk, and mental health among female sex workers in China', *Health Care for Women International*, 28: 745–62.

Wang-Letzkus, M.F., Washington, G., Calvillo, E.R. and Anderson, N.L.R. (2012) 'Using culturally competent community-based participatory research with older diabetic Chinese Americans: lessons learned', *Journal of Transcultural Nursing*, 23: 255–61.

Wehmeyer, M.L. and Bolding, N. (2001) 'Enhanced self-determination of adults with intellectual disability as an outcome of moving to community-based work or living environments', *Journal of Intellectual Disability Research*, 45: 371–83.

Welsh Assembly Government (2010) *Working for Equality in Wales: inclusive policy making guidance*, 2nd edn. Online. Available HTTP: <http://wales.gov.uk/docs/dsjlg/publications/equality/100607ipmrev2en.pdf> (accessed 18 March 2013).

Wenger, E. (1999) *Communities of Practice: learning, meaning, and identity*, Cambridge: Cambridge University Press.

Wernow, J. and Grant, D. (2008) 'Dispensing with conscience: a legal and ethical assessment', *The Annals of Pharmacotherapy*, 42: 1669–78.

Wesche, S., Schuster, R.C., Tobin, P., Dickson, C., Matthiessen, D., Graupe, S., Williams, M. and Chan, H.M. (2011) 'Community-based health research led by the Vuntut Gwitchin First Nation', *International Journal of Circumpolar Health*, 70: 396–406.

Wesley Mission Victoria (2009) *Social Inclusion and Belonging Policy*. Melbourne: Wesley Mission Victoria.

Westby, C. (1991) 'A scale for assessing children's pretend play', in C. Schaefer, K. Gitlin and A. Sandrund (eds) *Play Diagnosis and Assessment*, New York: John Wiley and Sons.

Westby, C. (2000) 'A scale for assessing development of children's play', in K. Gitlin-Weiner, A. Sandrund and C. Schaefer (eds) *Play Diagnosis and Assessment*, 2nd edn, New York: John Wiley and Sons.

Westra, H.A., Dozois, D. and Marcus, M. (2007) 'Expectancy, homework compliance, and initial change in cognitive–behavioral therapy for anxiety', *Journal of Consulting and Clinical Psychology*, 75: 363–73.

Wheeler, D. (2003) 'Methodological issues in conducting community-based health and social services research among urban Black and African American LGBT populations', *Journal of Gay and Lesbian Social Services*, 15 (1–2): 65–78.

White, M. (2007) *Maps of Narrative Practice*, New York: W.W. Norton.

Whiteford, H.A. and Buckingham, W.J. (2005) 'Ten years of mental health service reform in Australia: are we getting it right?', *Medical Journal of Australia*, 182: 396–400.

Whitington, V. and Floyd, I. (2009) 'Creating intersubjectivity during socio-dramatic play at an Australian kindergarten', *Early Child Development and Care*, 179: 143–56.

Whitlock, E.P., Orleans, C.T., Pender, N. and Allen, J. (2002) 'Evaluating primary care behavioral counseling interventions: an evidence-based approach', *American Journal of Preventative Medicine*, 22: 267–84.

WHO (2001) *International Classification of Functioning, Disability and Health*, Geneva: World Health Organization.

WHO (2002) *Active Ageing: a policy framework*, Geneva: World Health Organization.

WHO (2003) *The World Health Report 2003: shaping the future*, Geneva: World Health Organisation.

WHO (2005) *Promoting Mental Health: concepts, emerging evidence, practice*, Geneva: World Health Organization.

Wicclair, M. (2009) 'Negative and positive claims of conscience', *Cambridge Quarterly of Healthcare Ethics*, 18: 14–22.

Wiggins, N. (2011) 'Popular education for health promotion and community empowerment: a review of the literature', *Health Promotion International*, 27: 356–71.

Wilcox, P., Winn, S. and Fyvie-Gauld, M. (2005) 'It was nothing to do with the university, it was just the people: the role of social support in the first-year experience of higher education', *Studies in Higher Education*, 30: 707–22.

Wiles, J.L., Allen, R.E.S., Palmer, A.J., Hayman, K.J., Keeling, S. and Kerse, N. (2009) 'Older people and their social spaces: a study of well-being and attachment to place in Aotearoa New Zealand', *Social Science and Medicine*, 68: 664–71.

Wiles, R., Charles, V., Crow, G. and Heath, S. (2005) 'Researching researchers: lessons for research ethics', *Qualitative Research*, 6: 283–99.

Wilkinson, R. and Marmot, M. (eds) (2003) *Social Determinants of Health: the solid facts*, 2nd edn, Geneva: World Health Organization Regional Office for Europe.

Wilkinson, R. and Picket, K. (2009) *The Spirit Level: why more equal societies almost always do better*, London: Allen Lane.

Williams, M. (2010) 'Can you imagine a World AIDS Conference without the red umbrellas?', *HIV Australia*, 8 (3): 40–1.

Williams, V. and Simons, K. (2005) 'More researching together: the role of nondisabled researchers in working with People First members', *British Journal of Learning Disabilities*, 33: 6–14.

Wilson, A. and Beresford, P. (2000) '"Anti-oppressive practice": emancipation or appropriation?', *British Journal of Social Work*, 30: 553–73.

Wilson, E., Wong, J. and Goodridge, J. (2006) *Too Little Too Late: wait times and cost burden for people with a disability in seeking equipment funding in Victoria*, Melbourne: Scope (Vic).

Wilson, E., Pollock, K. and Aubeeluck, A. (2010) 'Gaining and maintaining consent when capacity can be an issue: a research study with people with Huntington's disease', *Clinical Ethics*, 5: 142–7.

Wilson, J. and Murdoch, K. (2006) *How to Succeed with Thinking,* Melbourne: Curriculum Corporation.

Winterson, J. and Russ, M. (2009) 'Understanding the transition from school to university in music and music technology', *Arts and Humanities in Higher Education*, 8: 339–54.

Withers, M., Dornig, K. and Morisky, D.E. (2007) 'Predictors of workplace sexual health policy at sex work establishments in the Philippines', *AIDS Care*, 19: 1020–5.

Włodarczyk, P. and Ziółkowski, A. (2009) 'Having children and physical activity level and other types of pro-health behaviour of women from the perspective of the Theory of Planned Behaviour', *Baltic Journal of Health and Physical Activity*, 1: 143–9.

Wolfberg, P.J. and Schuler, A.L. (1993) 'Integrated play groups: a model for promoting the social and cognitive dimensions of play in children with autism', *Journal of Autism and Developmental Disorders*, 23: 467–89.

Wolffers, I. and van Beelen, N. (2003) 'Public health and the human rights of sex workers', *The Lancet*, 361: 1981.

Women's Health in the North (2006) *Exploring community connectedness for women in Melbourne's North*, Melbourne: Women's Health in the North.

Wong, W.C., Holroyd, E and Bingham, A. (2010) 'Stigma and sex work from the perspective of female sex workers in Hong Kong', *Sociology of Health and Illness*, 33: 50–65.

Woodbridge, M.A. (1895) *Life and Labors of Mrs. Mary A. Woodbridge*, edited by A.M. Hills, Ravenna, OH. Republished 1995.

Woodill, G. (1994) 'The social semiotics of disability', in M.H. Rioux and M. Bach (eds) *Disability is Not Measles: new research paradigms in disability*, Ontario: L'Institut Roeher Institute.

World Bank (1994) *The World Bank and Participation* (fourth draft), Washington DC: World Bank.

World Medical Association (1964) *WMA Declaration of Helsinki - Ethical principles for medical research involving human subjects*. Online. Available HTTP: <http://www.wma.net/en/30publications/10policies/b3/index.html> (accessed 18 March 2013).

Wyver, S.R. and Spence, S. H. (1999) 'Play and divergent problem solving: evidence supporting a reciprocal relationship', *Early Education and Development*, 10: 419–44.

Yang H., Stanton, B., Fang, X., Zhao, R., Dong, B., Liu, W., Liang, S., Zhao, Y. and Hong, Y. (2005) 'Condom use among female sex workers in China: role of gate-keepers', *Sexually Transmitted Diseases*, 32: 572–80.

Yates, B.C., Dodendorf, D., Lane, J., LaFramboise, L., Pozehl, B., Duncan, K., Knodel, K. (2009) 'Testing an alternative informed consent process', *Nursing Research*, 58: 135–9.

Yorke, M. (2004) 'Retention, persistence and success in on-campus higher education, and their enhancement in open and distance learning', *Open Learning: The Journal of Open and Distance Learning*, 19: 19–32.

Youth in Mind (n.d.) Online. Available HTTP: <http://www.sdqinfo.org> (accesed 18 March 2013).

Zambrano, R. and Seward, R.K. (2012) *Mobile Technologies and Empowerment: enhancing human development through participation and innovation*, United Nations Development Programme. Online. Available HTTP: <http://www.undpegov.org/sites/undpegov.org/files/undp_mobile_technology_primer.pdf> (accessed 18 March 2013).

Ziff, M.A., Harper, G.W., Chutuape, K.S., Deeds, B.G., Futterman, D., Francisco, V.T., Muenz, L.R., Ellen, J.M. and the Adolescent Medicine Trails Network for HIV/AIDS Intervention (2006) 'Laying the foundation for Connect to Protect®: a multi-site community mobilization intervention to reduce HIV/AIDS incidence and prevalence among urban youth', *Journal of Urban Health*, 83: 506–22.

Index

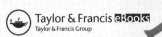